EVALUATION
and
DECISION MAKING
for
HEALTH SERVICES

SECOND EDITION

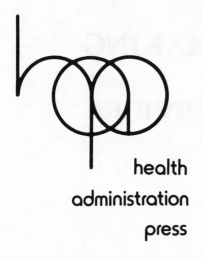

health
administration
press

EVALUATION
and
DECISION MAKING
for
HEALTH SERVICES
SECOND EDITION

James E. Veney
Arnold D. Kaluzny

 Health Administration Press
Ann Arbor, Michigan   1991

95   94   93   92   91   5   4   3   2   1

Library of Congress Cataloging-in-Publication Data

Veney, James E.
  Evaluation and decision making for health services / James E. Veney and Arnold D. Kaluzny. — 2nd ed.
    p.   cm.
  Rev. ed. of: Evaluation and decision making for health services programs. c1984.
  Includes bibliographical references and index.
  ISBN 0-910701-72-5 (hardbound : alk. paper)
  1. Health services administration—Evaluation.   2. Health services administration—Decision making.   3. Health services administration—United States—Evaluation.   4. Health services administration—United States—Decision making.   I. Kaluzny, Arnold D.   II. Veney, James E. Evaluation and decision for health services programs.   III. Title.
  [DNLM: 1. Decision Making.   2. Evaluation Studies.   3. Health Services Research—methods.   W 84.3 V457e]
  RA394.V45   1991   362.1'068—dc20
  DNLM/DLC for Library of Congress   91-7110 CIP

Health Administration Press
A division of the Foundation of the
  American College of Healthcare Executives
1021 East Huron Street
Ann Arbor, Michigan 48104-9990
(313) 764-1380

To Leslie Ford and Edward Sondik
of the National Cancer Institute
who presented many of the challenges and
opportunities for what follows.

Contents

Foreword

The U.S. health care system faces growing demands for both clinical and fiscal accountability. This is evidenced by the increased attention given to studies of medical effectiveness and patient outcomes and the near religious fervor with which many health care organizations have adopted continuous quality improvement/total quality management approaches to delivering care. Yet there can be no accountability without evaluation. Thus, this second edition of *Evaluation and Decision Making for Health Services* by Jim Veney and Arnold Kaluzny is particularly timely.

Grounded in a cybernetic approach emphasizing feedback for purposes of clinical and managerial decision making, the book provides a comprehensive, systematic discussion of major evaluation approaches and methods. The advantages and disadvantages of monitoring, case studies, surveys, trend analysis, and experimental and quasiexperimental designs are each discussed. They are richly illustrated by many "real world" examples ranging from family planning programs in developing countries to community clinical oncology programs to public television educational efforts. The chapters are well organized: the strategy behind each evaluation approach is discussed, followed by a chapter on techniques and interpretation. In this fashion, specific methods and techniques are considered along with program goals, the evaluation approach being used, and the organizational and political context within which the evaluation is being conducted. Further, the book does an outstanding job of describing how the overall approaches to evaluation are interrelated and how most evaluations require the use of several approaches to produce meaningful results for decision makers.

Perhaps the book's most striking feature is the clarity with which the material is presented. The authors deserve special recognition for making accessible to a wide variety of evaluation "doers" and "users" material which is often presented in a dense and arcane manner. Students and practitioners of evaluation will clearly benefit from using this book. But, perhaps even more important, so will clinicians and executives caught up in the everyday world of learning by doing. Veney and Kaluzny have written a book that will help all involved to better "capture the learning" and transfer the results into a more cost-effective service delivery.

Stephen M. Shortell
A. C. Buehler Distinguished Professor
of Health Services Management
Professor of Organization Behavior
J. L. Kellogg Graduate School of Management
Northwestern University

Preface

This second edition continues to emphasize that evaluation is considered an integral part of the decision-making process. Evaluation is not simply an academic effort but is a critical component of the managerial process. Additional knowledge for the sake of knowledge itself may be laudable, but it is not evaluation.

Building on the experience of the first edition, the text has attempted to incorporate a number of new features:

- clear designation of a cybernetic model as the overall paradigm of the book
- application of quantitative decision making to a variety of practice issues faced by managers
- inclusion of quality improvement concepts and techniques as an integral part of the larger evaluation scheme
- use of contemporary illustrations reflecting issues facing health service managers
- consideration of evaluation within the context of strategic management

The book continues to use an overall framework that combines three major dimensions of evaluation: levels, strategies, and techniques. From the standpoint of what we call "level," evaluation may address the substantive issues of program relevance, program process, effectiveness, efficiency, or impact. We consider five major evaluation strategies—monitoring, case studies, surveys, trend analysis, and experimental design—and present various techniques appropriate to each strategy. Finally, we present material on measurement, sampling, operations research techniques, and cost-benefit and cost-effectiveness analysis—techniques appropriate to all evaluation approaches. Since these are basic to all other chapters, readers not familiar with this material are requested to review Chapters 14, 15, 16, and 17 before beginning the study of specific evaluation strategies.

Acknowledgments

We have been fortunate in having had the opportunity to work with a large number of capable people over the course of our careers thus far, and this book, in both its first and second editions, has benefited significantly from the intellectual stimulation, insight, and knowledge afforded by that opportunity. In the preparation of this second edition, we have also been fortunate to have had the assistance of students and co-workers who deserve mention. These include Jay McCloud, Hong Li, Donna Cooper, Susan Lauffer, and Jean Allen. We thank them for their assistance.

We also wish to thank our colleagues in the field who, through their use of the first edition and their continued interest, encouragement, and occasional harassment, supported our development of the second edition.

List of Acronyms

ABNA	Achievable benefits not achieved
AHCPR	Agency for Health Care Policy and Research
APACHE	Acute Physiological and Chronic Health Evaluation
ARIMA	Autoregressive integrated moving average
CCOP	Community clinical oncology program
CIS	Cancer Information Service
CPM	Critical Path Method
DCPC	Division of Cancer Prevention and Control
DRG	Diagnostic-related group
EOQ	Economic ordering quantity
FTE	Full-time equivalent
GAO	Government Accounting Office
GNP	Gross national product
HCFA	Health Care Financing Administration
IRR	Internal rate of return
JCAHO	Joint Commission on Accreditation of Healthcare Organizations
LIFE	Labor and Industry Focus on Education
MBO	Management by objectives
NCI	National Cancer Institute
NIH	National Institutes of Health
NPV	Net present value
OSHA	Occupational Safety and Health Administration
PBS	Program budgeting system
PDQ	Physician data query
PERT	Program evaluation and review technique
PPS	Prospective payment system
RFP	Request for proposal
SAS	Statistical analysis system

SIPP   Survey of Income and Program Participation
SMSA   Standard Metropolitan Statistical Area
SPSS   Statistical Package for the Social Sciences
TQM   Total quality management
UNICEF   United Nations Children's Fund
URW   United Rubber, Cork, Linoleum, and Plastic Workers of
          America
USAID   United States Agency for International Development
WHO   World Health Organization
WIC   Special Supplemental Program for Women, Infants, and
          Children

Part I

Introduction

1

The Evaluation Framework

Health care organizations and programs are increasingly challenged to provide a rationale for their existence, document their operations, and present a strategic plan for their future activities. Hospitals and physicians are being judged by their clinical outcomes, existing programs are subject to termination unless there is clear evidence that they have met objectives, and managers are increasingly queried about a variety of evaluation-type studies that require their attention, if not understanding. All this leads to the conclusion that program evaluation continues to be serious business.

Despite the importance of program evaluation, it is often characterized as a unidimensional activity or as an activity that is isolated from the decisions of management or both. Evaluation is neither unidimensional nor is it an activity isolated from management. Program evaluation encompasses a number of different functions and a wide range of formal and informal research and management activities, including experimental design, survey research, cost-benefit/effectiveness analysis, aspects of operations research, as well as less formalized procedures, such as good management practice and even good guesses. Moreover, program evaluation is not an activity that can be relegated to the arcane world of academic scholarship. It has always been an integral part of the managerial process and provides important information for strategic and program planning, implementation, and control activities. In short, program evaluation is not a benign social science activity but a political decision-making tool. As described by Rossi and Freeman (1989):

> Perhaps the most challenging aspect of applying social research procedures to the study programs and the most distinctive feature of evaluation research is the inherent requirement that the evaluator do his or her work in a continually changing decision making milieu. (p. 38)

3

The objective of this chapter is to define *evaluation,* describe its role in the managerial process, and provide a framework for considering the various functions and different types of evaluation and their relationships to methodological strategies and methods.

What Is Evaluation?

Evaluation incorporates a broad range of activities with different objectives, procedures, and expectations. Because of the multiplicity of these activities, there is often a tendency to make evaluation more complex and mysterious than it need be. Although evaluation uses various methodological strategies and procedures borrowed from the social and management sciences, its basic thrust is central to the managerial process, and its application is often intuitive in nature. For our purposes, we shall define evaluation as the collection and analysis of information by various methodological strategies to determine the *relevance, progress, efficiency, effectiveness,* and *impact* of program activities.

The following discussion considers various functions of evaluation (WHO 1981) and provides examples to illustrate the kinds of issues involved in each type. The various methodological strategies and their relationship to the functions of evaluation, along with their role in managerial decision making, are discussed later in the chapter.

Relevance refers to whether the program or service is needed. This issue determines the basic rationale for having a program or set of activities to meet the health needs or service demands of a community. The development of relevance as a legitimate evaluation topic in health services is a recent phenomenon. Historically, health services were considered relevant a priori and critical questions concerned the delivery of services. But in more recent years delivery and extent of use have been supplemented by concern for the underlying rationale for a specific activity. The very basis of a program in terms of objectives, scope, depth, and coverage becomes the problematic issue. Questions central to this type of evaluation include the following:

- What problem does the program address?
- Does that problem need attention?
- How accurate is the information about the problem?
- How adequate is the definition of the problem?
- How adequate is the definition of the program?
- Is the program appropriate to the defined problem?

- How does the program fit with the overall strategy of the organization?

Progress refers to the tracking of program activities. Progress deals with analysis efforts made to assess the degree to which program implementation complies with the plan for it. This type of evaluation has long been considered an integral part of the management process. Illustrative questions concerning progress include

- Are appropriate personnel, equipment, and financial resources available in the right quantity, in the right place, and at the right time to meet program needs?
- Are expected products of the program actually being produced? Are these products of expected quality and quantity? Are these outputs produced at the expected time?

Efficiency refers to whether program results could be obtained less expensively. Questions of efficiency concern the relationship between the results obtained from a specific program and the resources expended to maintain the program. Efficiency as an evaluation focus is gaining increasing attention. The recognition that resources are limited and that programs must compete for them will increase the role that evaluations of efficiency have in determining whether new programs are funded or not funded, continued or terminated, expanded or contracted. Questions that evaluations of efficiency raise include the following:

- Are program benefits sufficient for the cost incurred?
- Are program benefits more or less expensive per unit of outcome than benefits derived from other programs designed to achieve the same goal?

Effectiveness refers to whether program results meet predetermined objectives. Emphasis is on program outputs or the immediate results of program efforts and whether these outputs are as expected. Evaluations of effectiveness are aimed at improving program formulation and thus have a relatively short-term perspective. The questions central to this type of evaluation include the following:

- Did the program meet its stated objectives?
- Were program providers satisfied with the effects of program activities?
- Were program beneficiaries satisfied with the effects of program activities?

- Are things better as a result of the program's having existed?

Impact refers to the long-term outcomes of the program. The issue of impact is concerned with changes observed over time in characteristics that the program is ultimately designed to influence. While evaluation of effectiveness focuses on program outputs, impact evaluation considers whether these outputs have had the desired effects on the ultimate problems that the program is designed to solve. It is possible that a program may prove both efficient and effective in producing short-run outputs and yet have minimal long-term impact. Illustrative questions for this type of evaluation include the following:

- Did a particular program produce the observed effect?
- Could the observed effects occur in the absence of the program or in the presence of some alternative program or set of activities?

Why Program Evaluation?

Why is program evaluation important? It seeks to find out more about the program, to ensure that it works, to keep track of program activity, and to be able to report on it if necessary are the reasons for evaluation. All seem like reasonable ends. But the view of the purpose of evaluation as taken by this book can be stated much more simply. There is basically one purpose for program evaluation: to make better decisions about program activities. The key point is decision making. Evaluation is not an activity to be undertaken for the fun of it. It is fine, for example, to find out more about a given program, but that additional knowledge must be directed toward some decision about the program. If there are no decisions to be made or the decisions are not ones that can be improved with the addition of information, then evaluation is meaningless.

Many programs are implemented for political rather than technical reasons. Programs often operate according to political rather than technical criteria. Under such circumstances evaluation is likely to be of little use. Of course, there is the possibility that in a highly political arena certain issues remain primarily technical and a legitimate subject for evaluation, or that in a basically technical arena certain issues remain political and not subject to evaluation. If so, fine, but it is incumbent upon the evaluator to know which issues can be evaluated and which cannot. Otherwise the effort may produce little of value.

Frequently evaluations are undertaken without a clear understanding or definition of what the decision points are. This is simply bad management. No evaluation activity should be initiated without a clear statement of which decisions will result from the information obtained. The decision might be as seemingly simple as determining whether a program works and thus needs no modification, or that the state of the program requires that some action be taken. In either case the decision area must be known a priori. Evaluation is undertaken to provide information for some decision process. If no clear decision-making process is served by the results, the effort may be an excellent piece of academic work, the design well thought out, the data collection thorough, and the analysis inspired, but it is not evaluation.

Even in the best of all possible worlds, of course, many well-planned and well-executed evaluations that were clearly aimed at decision making will remain unused. But if a conscious effort is made at the outset to define the decisions to be made, it is likely that information generated by evaluations will be used. A major purpose of this book is to increase the likelihood that such evaluations will be part of the decision-making process.

Evaluation and the Managerial Process

All managers are forced daily to make judgments and plan actions on the basis of what are essentially evaluations. These evaluations may deal with such apparently mundane affairs as determining whether program resources and personnel are in the right places at the right time (progress), or with more glamorous issues, such as whether a program has "made any difference" (impact). But any activity aimed at making decisions about whether or how a program should be implemented, how the program should be carried out, whether program activities are being pursued in a timely manner, if the program is producing expected outcomes, whether the outcomes are as desirable as anticipated at the initiation of the program, or how the program can be improved is essentially evaluation. Evaluation may range from highly structured, planned, and formalized activities to highly informal activities, many of which may verge on the intuitive. Whether structured or intuitive, evaluation is an integral part of the management cycle. Figure 1-1 shows a nonlinear model of planning, implementation, and control as three interconnected activities. Using this perspective, evaluation occurs during all phases of the management cycle. Program evaluation, for example, may accompany the planning

Figure 1-1   Nonlinear Model of Program
Planning, Implementation, and
Evaluation

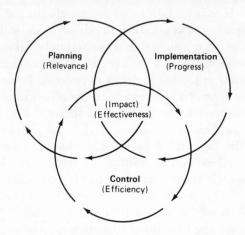

and design stage of a program and be directed at such issues as the current state of the system to be affected by the program, the specific nature of problems that the program is to address, and alternative approaches to solving these problems. Such evaluation basically deals with whether a program of some type is needed, how it should be structured, and what kind of problems it should solve. This evaluation concerns the question of program relevance, although relevance cannot entirely be decided a priori because a major aspect of relevance is evaluation of program impact. The clear decisions to be made at the level of planning and design include whether to implement a program and, if so, what type to implement.

Also integral to planning and design is whether a particular problem should be solved. To a certain extent, this question is one that can be addressed by evaluation. The basic issue is whether the problem involved is one that by virtue of its widespread impact or importance requires a solution. Surveys of selected populations can provide information about the prevalence or incidence of disease and associated morbidity and mortality that can, on a comparative basis, help to identify problems that may merit solutions or efforts at solutions. In a situation of limited resources, not all health problems merit the same attention.

Once a program has been designed and implemented, a number of other evaluation issues arise, many of which involve monitoring and improvements. One general question is whether the program is, in fact, implemented and whether the process works as expected. Do resources—whether funds, doses of vaccine, students to be trained, medical supplies, or other types of inputs—arrive at the proper place, on time, and in sufficient quantity? Are activities undertaken in a timely manner and in proper order? Do various components of the program interrelate properly? Do various personnel in the program coordinate appropriately? Is it possible to improve the process over time? These and many other questions are part of program monitoring. The point of such monitoring is to detect breakdowns in the process and the operation of the program and to take the decisions appropriate for corrective action.

Once the program has been implemented, is it effective and efficient? Are the costs of the program reasonable? Do results expected from the program appear in the projected time frame? Are there other cheaper or more timely ways of producing the same results? Are the results of the program meeting predetermined objectives? These questions are often studied by more formal evaluation, such as cost-benefit analysis, as well as fairly elaborate operations research and comparative studies. Particularly during the start-up phase of a program, it may be feasible to try several alternative program structures in order to compare costs, timeliness of results, and even effectiveness.

Finally, are the desired results achieved? Has the problem that the program was designed to solve been solved or is it being solved on a continuing basis? Would the problem have been solved in the absence of the program? Could any other program have solved the problem? This is the appropriate area of summative evaluation. If the problem has not been solved, other questions arise. Is the structure of the program adequate for solving the problem? Are the inputs adequate? Is the definition of the problem itself adequate?

Effectiveness and impact are the ultimate tests of a program. If a program has no effect or impact, decisions about the importance of the problem or relevance of the program for the problem, monitoring of program processes, and judgments about reasonableness of cost are all basically irrelevant. Yet effectiveness and impact of a program are often the most difficult aspects of the program to assess. The basic question involved is, Has the program caused the expected result to occur? Very often, however, there are no good objective criteria to measure the expected result.

Who Does Evaluation?

All managers do evaluation, and many social scientists have the skill necessary to conduct evaluations. The extent of involvement of both groups depends on the degree to which formal evaluation/research techniques are involved and the extent to which the manager collaborates with individuals skilled in evaluation techniques.

Figure 1-2 presents a continuum showing the various levels of involvement by managers and evaluation-type personnel. At one end of the continuum the manager has the most influence. Here emphasis is on evaluation focusing on relevance and program progress. At the other end of the continuum researchers have the most influence, and emphasis is on assessing impact. These evaluations involve the most sophisticated methodological approaches and technique.

In reality, evaluation must involve collaboration between program personnel and personnel trained in research/evaluation methodologies. This collaboration requires substantive changes in the way that both researchers and managers function. For managers, collaboration requires a recognition that they do not know whether program X will be effective or whether it is even relevant to the many problems faced by their organization. Instead of advocating a particular solution, the manager needs a better understanding of the basic functioning of the organization and the economic, political, social,

Figure 1-2   Manager-Evaluator Collaboration

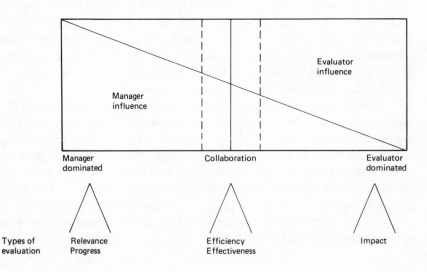

and financial context (Mintzberg 1989) and needs to present solutions as a series of options and develop ways to assess them as they affect the community as well as the organization. As described by Campbell (1969) over twenty years ago, this approach requires a

> . . . shift from the advocacy of a specific reform to the advocacy of the seriousness of the problem, and hence to the advocacy of persistence in alternative reform efforts should the first one fail. The political stance would become: "This is a serious problem. We propose to initiate policy A on an experimental basis. If after five years there has been no significant improvement, we would shift to Policy B." By making explicit that a given problem solution was only one of several that the administrator or party could in good conscience advocate, and by having ready a plausible alternative, the administrator could afford honest evaluation of outcomes. Negative results, a failure of the first program, would not jeopardize his job, for his job would be to keep after the problem until something was found that worked. (p. 410)

Within the world of health services, this approach is very difficult, yet possible. The Department of Medicine at Cleveland Metropolitan General Hospital has introduced a program that permits the experimental changes in the delivery of health services to be carried out on an ongoing basis (trials) and to be evaluated over time (Cohen and Neuhauser 1985). The department is organized into four similar teams of physicians associated with similar 28-bed inpatient units and similar outpatient clinics termed *firms*. Patients, as well as house officers, are randomly assigned, approximating a laboratory for ongoing clinical and health services research. A variety of evaluation issues have been addressed concerning physicians' behavior. For example, one project evaluated a program intended to improve physician compliance with the delivery of preventive interventions. In this trial, the health services and two independently, randomly selected firms were offered educational seminars and given checklists with medical records for their patients and encouraged to use pneumovax, influenza vaccines, and mammography. House officers in the control firm were not given checklists, although they were invited to seminars. The use of the preventive interventions increased significantly (5–45%) among eligible patients in the experimental group while remaining unchanged among controls (Cohen et al. 1982).

Moreover, the very essence of management, control, is bound up in the activity of performing evaluations of operations and outcomes. As described by Mick (1989):

> If comparison of behavior with norms or standards (i.e., evaluation) does not occur, or is flawed, or is not timely, management has breached the "control cycle." In a fundamental sense it is operating an organiza-

tion that is "out of control" because it lacks data on itself and the very organization it claims to run. (pp. 511–512)

For social scientists, an equally important shift must occur. The challenge to the social scientist is not just to disseminate information to the managerial community in order to enhance program operations but to work collaboratively with managers to achieve a clear understanding of the problem and its implications. This must be accomplished with a sense of timing vis-à-vis the managerial decision process and without the use of jargon or excessive theoretical conceptualization. This is not to say that the social scientist must abandon "rigor" or "theory," but only that it must be placed within the context of operations and be presented as underlying, often-implicit principles.

Recurring Issues in Evaluation

Every evaluation effort confronts a set of recurring generic issues, presented here to provide a context for considering various evaluation strategies.

Summative versus formative evaluation

A now classic distinction has been made between summative and formative evaluation (Scriven 1967). *Formative evaluation* refers to the activities associated with the ongoing operations of a program. Emphasis here is on data gathering and analysis designed to improve the program and its management. *Summative evaluation,* on the other hand, refers to activities associated with the more long-term effects of a program—whether the program, in fact, has any impact on given indicators of performance.

The requirement that evaluation must provide information for the decision-making process places a substantial burden on the evaluator, on the managers who seek the evaluator's expertise, and on the evaluation strategy itself. Unfortunately, the most powerful methodological techniques available for program evaluation are most appropriately directed at summative-type evaluations.

Because the methodological techniques available for formative-type evaluation are much less well defined and well specified, evaluators tend to concentrate on the summative aspects of evaluation. They are likely to place little importance on the value of formative evaluations, besides being less competent to undertake such evaluations. Only rarely can the evaluation of ultimate outcomes actually be useful in future decision making. By the time that outcomes have been evaluated, if they can, in fact, be evaluated, the program is already well under way or may have ended. Only in instances where similar programs are anticipated in the future will such summative evaluation clearly affect the decision-making process. It is incumbent on those charged with evaluation efforts to try to improve their techniques for formative evaluation.

Evaluability assessment

Although all programs can be evaluated, there is often merit in delaying any substantive evaluation and engaging preliminary assessment of the program's basic design. Specifically, evaluability assessment determines whether (Wholey 1983)

- program objectives are well defined. Have the individuals in charge of the program defined the objectives in terms of quantifiable measures of performance and are data on these measures obtainable at a reasonable cost?
- program assumptions/objectives are plausible. Is there evidence that program activities have some likelihood of meeting the objectives?
- intended uses of evaluation information are well defined. Have those in charge of the program defined any intended uses of the information generated by the evaluation?

Answers to these questions provide a basis for determining which programs are most likely to benefit from a more substantive evaluation activity. Evaluation resources, like program resources, are limited and should be allocated to those program activities likely to benefit from the evaluation.

Evaluation and evaluation research

Although the distinction between *evaluation* and *evaluation research* is not always precisely drawn, it usually refers to the difference between results based on the evaluator's judgments and those based on the scientific method (Shortell and Richardson 1978). Using this point of view, evaluation research becomes a more rigorous and serious effort than simple evaluation. It is often considered the sole property of social scientists who have entered the evaluation realm.

There are two major problems in viewing evaluation research in this light and as distinct from evaluation per se. The first is that the desire to use the scientific method is often translated into the idea that evaluation research can only be done by scientists applying specific types of experimental designs. From this perspective any lesser effort does not merit attention. Many useful and even necessary evaluations can be carried out by program personnel, using a variety of techniques that are not as powerful for answering specific cause-and-effect relationships as experiments but that are still important for improving decision making and for improving the overall process of providing service.

A second problem of defining evaluation research as distinct from evaluation is that it does, in effect, become the property of social scientists. But social scientists are often likely to be attracted to the program (and to its evaluation) from outside. They are brought in specifically for their assumed evaluation expertise and in that role are marginal to the program. They are rarely in the mainstream of decision making, and their evaluations are rarely central to program decision making despite the rigor of the method or the quality of the results.

In this book we hope to avoid the distinction between evaluation and evaluation research. Instead we prefer to view evaluation as an integral part of the management control cycle and, in effect, the very essence of organizations (Mick 1989). As described by Dornbusch and Scott (1975):

> Organizations are power structures in which some participants are given differential access to organizational rewards and penalties in order to control other participants. Evaluation is required if power is to be employed to control behavior. If A has power over B and wishes to use this power to control B's behavior, A must indicate to B what he or she wants to do, determine what criteria to employ in judging B's success or failure, and make some attempt to ascertain the extent to which B's behavior conforms to these criteria. A may then sanction B, rewarding conformity or success, or punishing non-conformity or failure. Evaluation is one of the most commonplace of human acts. (p. 6)

Plan for the Book

Figure 1-3 presents the basic structure of this book. The intent is not to make the reader an expert in either methodology or various types of evaluation but to give health professionals a better understanding of, and a set of basic tools to deal with, the evaluation problems frequently confronted in the provision of health services. This chapter has already defined the various types of evaluation and its relationship to the managerial process. Chapter 2 presents a cybernetic

Figure 1-3 Plan of the Book

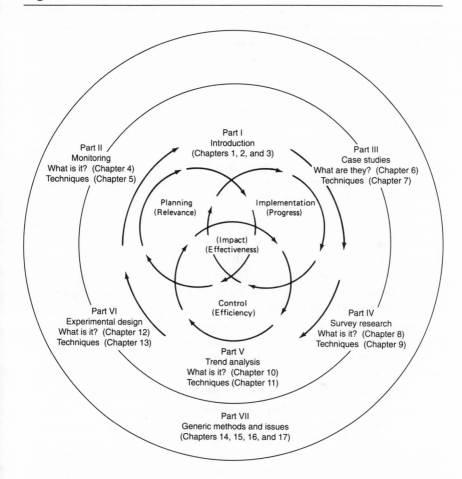

model of evaluation and illustrates its application to continuously improve program and organizational decision making. Chapter 3 continues this general introduction and focuses on the uses and non-uses of evaluation as a decision tool as well as the political context affecting evaluation activities.

The next 10 chapters outline various strategies appropriate to different types of evaluation and are divided into five major sections: monitoring, case studies, survey research, trend analysis, and experimental design. The last four chapters of the book represent methods—measurement, sampling, operations research, and cost-benefit analysis—that are useful in several of the evaluation strategies. The first chapter in each section defines the strategy, its limitation and the type of data required for its use, and the application of the approach to the various functions of evaluation. The second chapter outlines various techniques appropriate to that strategy and illustrates their use in different health services situations.

The presentation of respective strategies does not imply that any one strategy is to be used to the exclusion of others. In fact, any well-designed evaluation requires multiple strategies, as Denzin (1978) describes:

> No single method ever adequately solve the problem of rival causal factors—because each method reveals different aspects of empirical reality, multiple methods of observation must be employed. This is termed triangulation. (p. 28)

In reality, the use of multiple methods is somewhat idealistic given limited funds, short time frames, and the political constraints affecting most evaluative activities. Thus the evaluator is forced to select one particular strategy and supplement it with others, time and resources permitting. Let us consider briefly each of the strategies presented in Parts II through VII.

Part II deals with *monitoring* and begins with Chapter 4, which is concerned with monitoring program progress and improvement, whether necessary inputs are being provided, and if the program is operating as projected. In many settings monitoring is an overlooked and underrated aspect of the evaluation process; it is, however, often the total evaluation. The chapter deals with the appropriate setting in which monitoring should be conducted and outlines the types of data most appropriate for the monitoring task. Chapter 5 presents the analytical techniques that may be used with data collected for monitoring. The chapter deals with a variety of program-planning techniques, such as PERT (Program Evaluation and Review Technique), Gantt charts, and critical path method, as well as a variety of quality improvement techniques, such as control charts and run diagrams.

Part III presents the *case study* approach to evaluation. Chapter 6 discusses the appropriate setting for case studies, types of data that can be used, and various applications of case study results to program evaluation. Chapter 7 describes a series of analytical techniques helpful in using case studies as an evaluation strategy. The chapter offers various illustrations and emphasizes how the interpretation of case studies may facilitate or impede program decision making.

Part IV focuses on *survey research* as an evaluation approach, with particular emphasis on its use in addressing questions of efficiency, effectiveness, and program impact. Chapter 8 defines survey research and discusses the appropriate settings in which it can be applied to evaluation, plus the type of data that can be used in this approach. Chapter 9 discusses various data analysis techniques appropriate to survey research, including the use of contingency tables, regression, and structural equations. The chapter concludes with an interpretation of survey data and the application of survey results to program decision making.

Part V deals with *trend analysis*. This approach combines characteristics of monitoring, case studies, and survey research and can be particularly useful in the absence of an experimental design in providing information about program effectiveness and impact. Chapter 10 defines trend analysis and outlines the appropriate settings for it and the types of data required for its successful application. Chapter 11 focuses on the analytical techniques that can be employed in trend analysis and builds on techniques initially outlined in Chapter 9. Emphasis will be given to regression techniques and methods.

Part VI deals with *experimental design* as an evaluation format. Experimental design is the most powerful evaluation strategy, particularly when directed to evaluation issues of impact. Chapter 12 defines various experimental designs applicable to different health service settings. It considers the appropriate conditions for experimental design as well as types of data required for useful results. Special attention goes to various evaluation projects that have used experimental design to illustrate problems of interpretation and their overall impact on decision making. Chapter 13 discusses various analysis techniques appropriate to experimental designs, with emphasis on analysis of variance and the general interpretation of results and their use in decision making.

Finally, Part VII focuses on some *generic methodological techniques* basic to all evaluation approaches. Chapter 14 deals with measurement issues often encountered in evaluation projects. It defines measurement and describes the process by which measurement rules are developed and applied and the types of scales and techniques used in scale construction. Chapter 15 discusses various sampling techniques. It outlines basic issues and concepts of sampling and problems of sampling in different evaluation strategies; specific recommendations for sample selection appropriate to monitoring, case studies, surveys, trend analysis, and experiments are presented. Chapter 16 presents various operations research techniques and their application in decision making. Attention is given to model building, simulation, mathematical programming and queuing, and particularly their relevance to health services. Chapter 17 deals with cost benefit and cost effectiveness. Techniques involved in cost benefit and cost effectiveness and their applications to various health service settings are described. Readers not familiar with these basic issues are asked to acquaint themselves with this material before reading material on the various evaluation strategies, beginning with Part II and ending in Part VI.

Discussion Questions

1. Select a health service program with which you are familiar and define the types of issues resolved by the various types of evaluations: relevance, progress, efficiency, effectiveness, and impact.
2. Distinguish research from evaluation. What features are common to both activities? What features are unique to each activity?
3. Under what conditions is it advisable to undertake an evaluability assessment? Is it equally applicable to all types of evaluation? Why or why not?
4. What are some of the problems that evaluators experience when they work with program managers? Why do managers experience some of these problems when they work with evaluators? Consider mechanisms to use in overcoming these problems.

2

Evaluation and the Decision-Making Process

The purpose of this chapter is to set the stage upon which evaluation-based decision making takes place. While decisions are made continually during the implementation and operation of any program, this book is particularly concerned with decisions that are made within what will be referred to as the *cybernetic decision model*. The primary feature of this model is that decisions are based on two types of information:

1. information about the nature of the problem being addressed by the program
2. information about the effect of the program on the nature of the problem being addressed by the program

The evaluation process uses continuous feedback of information about the problem and about the effect of the program on the problem to make necessary modifications and changes in the program. The purpose of the evaluation at all points in time is to continuously improve program decision operations.

This chapter is presented in four sections, each dealing with an aspect of decision issues. The first section discusses what is meant by the cybernetic decision model and how this model relates to other decision models that may be employed to make program (or other types of) decisions. It is our underlying premise that the cybernetic decision model, the model based on feedback, is the appropriate context within which to discuss evaluation, in general, and by extension, evaluation of health services.

The last three sections of the chapter present a conceptual statement about three aspects of program evaluation that are generally associated with the temporal line of program implementation and that may all be seen as component aspects of the cybernetic decision model: needs assessment, program implementation, and assessing results. As seen in Figure 2-1, each of these phases of program operation is generally associated with particular types of questions in program evaluation and with related evaluation techniques. Needs assessment, for example, is most closely related to the issue of relevance and adopts survey-related techniques such as random sample surveys, Delphi studies and solicitation of expert opinion, and use of available data. Program implementation is most closely related to the issue of progress and adopts techniques like monitoring and related operations research techniques. Assessing results is related to issues of efficiency, effectiveness, and impact and adopts, again, survey techniques, cost-benefit and cost-effectiveness analysis, time series analysis, and experimentation. The detailed discussion of these methodological techniques is the major focus of the subsequent sections of the book.

The Cybernetic Decision Model

Since its introduction more than forty years ago (Weiner 1948), the word "cybernetics" has become popular as a way of defining a methodological approach to a wide variety of scientific and management

Figure 2-1 Schematic View of Components of Evaluation

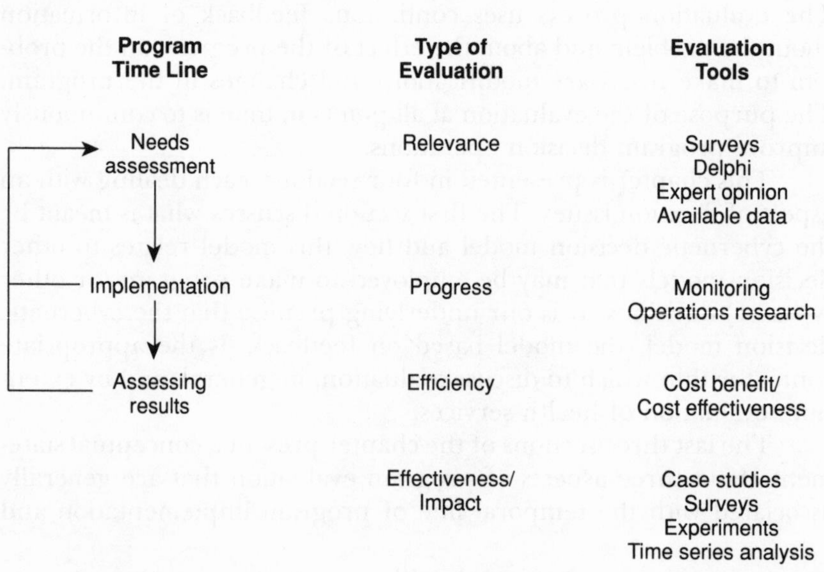

Program Time Line	Type of Evaluation	Evaluation Tools
Needs assessment	Relevance	Surveys Delphi Expert opinion Available data
Implementation	Progress	Monitoring Operations research
Assessing results	Efficiency	Cost benefit/ Cost effectiveness
	Effectiveness/ Impact	Case studies Surveys Experiments Time series analysis

endeavors. The idea of cybernetics has been closely linked with general systems theory, and its applications in the social, organizational, and management sciences has been extensively detailed by March and Simon (1958), Blau and Scott (1962), Katz and Kahn (1978), and Deming (1986).

Hage (1974), for example, has particularly discussed the application of a cybernetic model to health and welfare organizations and has identified two major components of the model:

1. There exists a system of interrelated variables that represent some production process (in the broadest sense, a process for accomplishing some end). These variables include inputs, throughputs, and outputs.

2. Some of the variables in the input-throughput-output system are being regulated and controlled by decisions made on the basis of the feedback of information about the state of the system.

The essence of the systems model of cybernetics may be seen in Figure 2-2. This figure is a schematic of the input-throughput-output model showing the feedback of information that leads to control. Also inherent in this view of cybernetics is the idea that the systems under observation tend to be large-scale and highly complex systems such as formal organizations, or even national political systems (Bryen 1971; Aulin 1982).

But Weiner (1948) did not necessarily assume large-scale or complex systems when he coined the term *cybernetics*. He defined cybernetics simply as the science of effective communication and control. The control is based on communication of information in any system, whether complex or simple. This view of cybernetics is the one that is taken by this book, that is, that cybernetics is concerned with communication and control. In the cybernetic decision model as we will use the concept, the concern is with the access and communication of information about the progress of a program

Figure 2-2   The Cybernetic Model

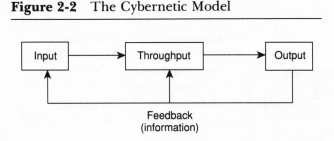

Feedback
(information)

from the evaluator to the decision maker (these may not be different persons).

The conceptual basis of the cybernetic decision model is relatively simple: Any process for accomplishing some end (input, throughput, output) may, in many cases, not produce the expected end (output) immediately, or there may be legitimate question as to whether the process can produce the expected end at all. In essence, the process is untested and unsystematized. The process is not "accepted" as the appropriate way to produce the desired outcome. The cybernetic approach to decision making in the conduct of the program assumes that there are verifiable ends (outcomes) that are expected to result from the process. The extent to which the process has been successful in producing these verifiable ends can be evaluated at various points during the life of the program and at its completion. The information about the gap between the expected outcomes and the actual outcomes is then used to modify either inputs or process, during program operation or before a similar program is launched in the future, to attempt to reduce the gap between the verifiable expected outputs and the actual outputs.

Alternate decision-making models

The cybernetic model is but one of the four models available to decision makers and must be viewed in the context of the other three alternatives, random walk decision making, traditional decision making, and mechanistic decision making.

In Figure 2-3, the four types of decision making are defined by the four cells of a two-by-two means/ends table. This table is defined on the horizontal axis as a verifiable versus a nonverifiable end (that is, it is possible to know when a process has been successful) and on the vertical axis by whether the means to obtain the end is accepted or not accepted. By accepted or not accepted, we mean that in a given

Figure 2-3   Means/Ends Decision Table

		Ends	
		Not verifiable	Verifiable
Means	Not accepted	Random walk	Cybernetic
	Accepted	Traditional	Mechanistic

setting a particular decision process (and hence, course of action) would generally be expected to produce the desired outcomes in a direct, linear manner, with no error along the way. An accepted means is essentially a recipe for moving directly to the desired output with no mistakes.

It should be understood that these decision-making modes are ideal types. By that, we mean that in virtually no real decision-making situation will the ideal type that we described be the only method that is likely to be brought to bear. Further, we do not claim that the ideal-type decision models we are going to suggest are totally exhaustive of all decision models. Nevertheless, it is useful to suggest these types as a point of departure.

To understand this typology, consider the category "accepted means and verifiable end." This is the *mechanistic model* of decision making (Deutsch 1968). Mechanistic decision making occurs when the ends are verifiable (that is, it is possible to know when the ends have been achieved) and the appropriate decision process, the means, is known and accepted. This is the realm, for example, of linear programming. If a hospital wishes to maximize its dollar profits from some course of action (a verifiable end) and subject to some set of constraints, the decision process (and hence, course of action) can be determined by a widely understood (and accepted) mathematical algorithm. The means is accepted, and at some point it can be verified that the result of the set of decisions is the optimum result. Yet it is generally not necessary to try other alternative decisions in this context because it is known (and accepted) that the linear programming model will produce the optimum result.

When there is a nonverifiable end or set of nonverifiable ends that are desired, and no accepted (known) means of reaching these ends, the decision process is in the realm of the *random walk*. Since it cannot be known if the goals or ends have been reached (they are not verifiable) and the appropriate decision process (and hence, course of action) for reaching the nonverifiable goals are not accepted or specified, any decisions will be as good or as bad as any others. In essence, a random decision process is adequate. The random process may ultimately arrive at a desired result, but it will not be verifiable, in any case.

But decision makers are, appropriately, uncomfortable with random decision making. What very often happens in this situation of discomfort is that a particular means is institutionalized—accepted—even in the absence of verifiable ends or in the absence of confirmation that the accepted means will produce a verified desired end. This is the mode of *traditional decision making*. In this mode of decision making it is possible to continue making decisions for long periods of time without ever subjecting these decisions to any further scrutiny than that they adhere to a particular institutionalized and accepted decision-making process. In effect, the process becomes the product.

If program goals or ends can be stated in ways that achievement of the ends can be verified, but there are no accepted means to obtain the ends, the decision-making process may be in the realm of *cybernetic decision making*. In cybernetic decision making, information about the extent to which a particular decision or set of decisions brings the program closer to the verifiable ends can be used to modify the decisions next taken. By doing this, an effort can be made to assure that the result comes ever closer to the desired ends.

The appropriate realm of evaluation as a decision-making tool, which is the appropriate use of evaluation, is the cybernetic decision-making mode. When ends are not verifiable or the necessary effort to verify them is not likely to be made (the realm of random walks or traditional decision making), evaluation cannot proceed because evaluation refers specifically to the assessment of the extent to which ends are reached. Further, there is no reason to conduct evaluation. In the absence of verifiable ends there will be no information produced that can be used for making better decisions than the ones already being made. Incidentally, the term "traditional decision making" does not necessarily refer to decisions that are made on the basis of long-standing tradition. The decision process may be in the traditional mode as soon as a particular set of decisions become the "right" set in the absence of any evidence that they produce a desired verifiable result.

Decision mode drift

Despite the efforts and good intentions of both decision makers and evaluators, much of program decision making follows closely either the random walk model or the traditional model. Moreover, much of what goes by the name of evaluation is actually a process of examining decisions that are made either on the basis of random walks or of tradition. To the extent that this is true, much that goes by the name of program evaluation is wasted effort since in both situations the ends are not verifiable.

There are a number of reasons why decision making tends to drift toward the random walk mode, and particularly toward the traditional mode. The ability to verify that an end has been achieved is, of course, a problem. What may begin as a clear effort to operate within the cybernetic decision realm (that is, clearly defined and verifiable ends available to assess results of decisions and courses of action through feedback) may quickly drift to either the random walk mode or to the traditional mode of decision making since verifiable ends are not easily accessible.

Decision mode drift may happen for several reasons. Program managers may decide that the cost of verifying program ends is greater than expected or greater than the value of verification. This perception is usually accompanied by a stated or unstated rationale that is something like "I know that this is the right course of action, so it is not reasonable to spend 25 percent of my program delivery budget on evaluation that will only confirm what I already know." In fact, this is probably often true.

Originally specified (and verifiable) goals may not express the full range of results expected from a program. It is unfortunate that verifiable goals may often be relatively trivial in the context of a program—the goal of a training program may be to impart the ability to deliver a complex skilled service, but the only verifiable (measurable) goal for the training program may be that a certain number of persons have been subjected to training. As goals become more complex, the decision-making process drifts toward the traditional or random walk modes.

Results that program managers see from a program may not be as attractive as they had hoped. In this situation, there is a tendency to kill the messenger by dismantling what might be a fairly serious cybernetic decision effort and falling back into the random walk or traditional modes, in which the lack of attempts to verify achievement of ends will not be a threat to program personnel or continuation of the program itself.

Mechanistic decision making, which is an appropriate realm of evaluation only to the extent that continued verification of the efficacy of a particular decision process is desired, may also drift toward traditional modes of decision making as ends become more complex. What may be a straightforward mechanistic decision process in the presence of a relatively simple set of goals (for example, a linear programming model to maximize hospital profits) may revert to traditional decision making as the goals become more difficult to measure (for example, improved community health status). The ideal situation would be that the mechanistic decision process would retrench at cybernetic decision making, but this will happen only if the necessary steps are taken to specify in measurable terms and to verify the more complex ends.

Cybernetic versus mechanistic decision making

Why is the cybernetic model, which implies feedback of information about the extent to which a given decision results in achievement of a given goal, the proper realm of evaluation, while evaluation is likely to be redundant in a setting in which mechanistic decision making, implying both a verifiable end and an accepted way to reach the end, is used? As a simple example, consider the problem of finding the square root of a number. The square root of a number is defined, of course, as that number, which when multiplied by itself will give the original number. Today, with the widespread availability of battery-powered calculators that provide square roots to ten decimal places at the push of a button, hardly anyone thinks of finding square roots as a decision problem of any kind, except possibly in the most trivial sense of "to find the square root of a number, enter the number into the hand calculator and push the square root button."

But there was a time, not too long ago, when the finding of a square root for a large number was far from a trivial matter. There were tables of square roots published in mathematics texts, but they always required some approximation. Some people learned to use logarithms to find square roots, but they usually required approximations also. Anyone going to school before the 1960s probably learned a tedious method for extracting square roots, which most have long forgotten. But this was a mechanistic method in the sense that if one learned the necessary steps, then followed them faithfully (without making any mistakes in arithmetic), one could produce the square root of any number to any number of decimal places desired without ever checking to see if the process was producing the right result. The result was assured by the decision-making process. Most books in mathematics or arithmetic no longer give this method, but it can be found, for example, in Swain and Nichols (1965, pp. 224–228).

But the square root of a number can also be found by a purely cybernetic (that is, feedback method) decision process that many of us hit upon independently when we first had access to electrically powered mechanical calculators that would multiply relatively quickly, but that would not take square roots directly. With this method there was no need to memorize an accepted decision process as was true for the mechanistic process. All that was required was to make a first guess at the square root of the number, then multiply the guess by itself. The result, however bad it may have been, was compared to the original number for which the square root was desired. If the result was bigger than the original number, then the original guess at the square root was too large and had to be adjusted down. If the result was smaller than the original number, then the original guess at the square root was too small and had to be adjusted up. The size of the adjustment in either direction depended on how bad the first guess was. On the basis of this adjustment, a new number to approximate the square root was selected, and the process repeated. This could be done as many times as necessary to obtain the accuracy required by the application.

In effect, this method used feedback of information (evaluation) about the difference between what was produced and what was desired to make a decision about what to do next. This was a cybernetic decision process, and the appropriate realm of evaluation. It is not necessary to determine which method was best in this situation. Either method produced a usable result. But there are many situations in which no mechanistic method of decision making is available. In such settings, only cybernetic decision making and evaluation are likely to produce the results desired.

Needs Assessment

Needs assessment is the first stage in program implementation. Needs assessment is a phrase to describe the process of determining the nature and extent of the problems that a program is designed to address. In World Health Organization (WHO) terms, it is the assessment of the relevance of the program. From the view of cybernetic decision making, needs assessment could very easily be seen as referring to the entire temporal range of program implementation, being concerned with providing information about a program as it begins, as it is being carried out, and when it has been concluded. In general, however, and as used in this book, needs assessment will be seen as referring primarily to the initial statement of the problem that the program is to address.

Though needs assessment refers to the initial statement of the problem to be addressed by the program, it can and should be carried out within the cybernetic decision-making mode as discussed above. In particular, this means that information about the problem—a gap between the desired state of some verifiable end and the actual state of that verifiable end—is used as the basis on which to structure and direct a program. This information may include the nature of the problem, its extent, who or what it affects, where and when it occurs, its frequency, and any other salient information. But it is information about the problem on which the nature of the program is based, and not, particularly, on guesses about the problem (random walk decision making) or the assumption in the absence of data that the problem fits into a previously defined mold (traditional decision making). It is possible that a needs assessment might indicate that the problem is amenable to solution by one or another systematic decision-making technique, such as linear programming. But this decision, in itself, should be made within the context of information about the actual nature of the problem.

There are at least two reasons that the cybernetic mode of decision making may fail to be used in determining the problem that the program is to address and how it will be addressed. The first of these is the problem of institutionalized (previously accepted) means, and the second is expert bias. Institutionalized objectives limit effective needs assessment particularly as they restrict the range of issues that a program may be permitted to address. Expert bias refers to the basic misconception that many experts may have about what the actual problem may be.

The issue of institutionalized objectives is one in which the problem is stated in such a way that only one or a limited number of program solutions can be adopted. For example, use of family planning services in a country may be a function of the quality and extent of training of service providers. But it will also be a function of the political situation, the degree to which people desire family planning, the availability of supplies and equipment and of attractive clinics in which to provide services, and a host of other factors. If the institutionalized means of training is the driving force behind the needs assessment, it is likely that it will result in finding that more training of service providers is needed, even if other interventions might have a greater effect on contraceptive use. Institutionalized objectives are often determined by agencies that fund programs in the first place, and no matter how good the needs assessment effort may be in a technical sense, it may not, by the very nature of institutionalized objectives, be useful in improving the situation relative to some selected verifiable ends.

Expert bias is the problem that those who are expected to carry out the needs assessment, the "experts," may have predetermined notions about what the needs assessment should show. Physicians assessing emergency medical care in a community may well determine that what is needed is expanded and improved medical services in emergency rooms. A representative of a law enforcement agency might conclude that the problem was the need for better control of highway accidents. The ambulance service might conclude that what is needed is a better distribution of emergency vehicles. A social scientist might conclude that the problem is the need to control domestic violence. This is different from the problem of institutionalized means since in the case of institutionalized means there may be a serious and detailed effort to examine the problem, but only from the standpoint of a single or limited number of programmatic aspects. In the case of expert bias, the problem may never actually be examined at all, but simply assumed to exist by an expert doing the assessment, who by virtue of expertise itself may not recognize the need to verify the assumed problem empirically.

Approaches to needs assessment

There are a number of strategies that can be used in the conduct of a needs assessment, the determination of the relevance of a program intervention. These include survey research, use of available data, Delphi and nominal group techniques, and expert judgments. Survey research techniques are discussed in detail in Chapters 8 and 9. The use of available data, Delphi and nominal group techniques, and expert judgments are discussed in Chapter 7. The challenge, however, is the sequence in which they are applied. Several steps are involved:

1. Develop a general statement of what the program is expected to accomplish.
2. Determine the degree and nature of the problem that the program is expected to address, and determine the level of accomplishment that might actually be realized.
3. Determine the strategies that should be employed by the program to attack the identified problem.
4. Specify criteria that are to be used to assess successful realization of the objectives.
5. Construct a conceptual causal chain that describes the process by which the program intervention is expected to influence the desired outcome.

Following is an illustration and discussion of each of these steps.

1. Developing program expectations: The case of a family planning program in a developing country

The first step in the needs assessment is to develop a general statement about what the family planning program is expected to accomplish. Is it expected to reduce overall birth rates? Is it expected to reduce the increase of the population? Is it expected to reduce the number of unwanted pregnancies? Is it expected to reduce the incidence of maternal and neonatal mortality and morbidity through child spacing? Or is the program expected to increase the number of first-time acceptors of family planning methods? Is it expected to increase the prevalence of family planning use? Is it expected to increase the number of women who have favorable attitudes toward the use of family planning services?

In fact, the program organizers are likely to say that the program is expected to do all of the things indicated in the paragraph above, and more. But herein lies the first stumbling block for cybernetic decision making. Program organizers are likely not to be willing to expend the resources necessary to define adequately, and then to measure routinely, each of the possible ends indicated above. A few of the ends may be measured and the rest are left to faith, and hence, to the traditional—or perhaps worse, random walk—decision mode. But agreement on the ends is only the first step in the needs assessment.

2. Determining the nature and degree of the problem: The case of a family planning program in a developing country (continued)

To determine what the level of the ends to be affected by the program actually are is likely to require a combination of techniques. Determination of the overall birth rate or rate of population increase may be made, if at all, by reference to fertility surveys, such as those conducted by Westinghouse as the International Fertility Surveys, or possibly to documents published by the government of the country in question. It is unlikely, however, that a program to improve family planning will have the resources to initiate its own data-gathering efforts to determine birth rates or rates of population increase.

The number of unwanted pregnancies in the society might be determined by direct questioning of women through household surveys about whether they had had an unwanted or unplanned pregnancy. But the interview would have to be carefully conducted and take into account the cultural milieu if it was to be expected to produce valid results. Determination of some general level of unwanted pregnancies might also be done through attempts to assess the extent of events that would be expected to be associated with unwanted pregnancies, such as abortions. But the valid measurement of abortions in a society might prove to be even more difficult than the valid measure of unwanted pregnancies.

The incidence of maternal and neonatal mortality and morbidity may be quite difficult to determine in a developing country. It is likely that the only available data will be based on results of births in hospitals or possibly in health centers and clinics. In this case, the use of available data would provide some information. But these data will generally exclude the large proportion of women who deliver at home or in the home of a relative. Very few such births are ever recorded at the time of birth. Hospital and health center data may also exclude stillbirths and spontaneous abortions, simply because they are not considered a birth. Moreover, the only information that is likely to be recorded accurately, at all, is mortality information. Morbidity data will almost certainly not be available in a valid form in either hospital or heath center records.

But it is also unlikely that any useful information could be obtained on maternal or infant mortality and morbidity either from household surveys or from surveys of health facilities. Because surveys occur at a point in time, they tend to pick up only what is happening at the point in time when they are conducted. This is likely to produce a highly skewed view of the extent of mortality or morbidity.

If the program is expected to increase the number of first-time acceptors of family planning methods, the present number of family planning acceptors might be available from the existing family planning facilities in the country. But it is likely that the information these facilities will have will not give specific information on numbers of new acceptors, but rather on total service users over some period of time. It will generally not be easy to separate the new users in a given time period from people who are coming back to the facility for a second or third or subsequent time.

The prevalence of family planning use is a measure of the number of users at any point in time. This could be an absolute prevalence measure, or it could be a measure of prevalence relative to the total eligible population. Absolute prevalence could be determined from available data in family planning service sites if the records were well kept. But there could be a great deal of difficulty in separating out the number of users if recording periods are relatively long, or getting a real count if recording periods are short. Population surveys based on a random selection of eligible users would give as good a measure of prevalence as might be obtained, if the program could support such an effort. Data might be available from contraceptive prevalence surveys, such as those conducted by Westinghouse, for the country in question, and this is probably the best source of prevalence information. But these surveys are not always up-to-date and do not exist for all countries. If prevalence rates are desired, it will require a valid estimate of the eligible population. Many developing countries cannot produce such estimates, particularly for small areas.

The number of women who have favorable attitudes toward the use of family planning services can only be determined directly from household surveys of potential users. Such surveys would have to be based on a probability selection of households to assure valid data. The number of women with favorable attitudes might be inferred from other data, such as the number of women who request family planning services from health clinics that do not provide such services or provide them only in limited quantities. But data of this type are likely to be anecdotal, at best.

There are two reasons that the determination of the level of the problem to be considered is important to establish during the needs assessment. First, it provides the baseline of verifiable information against which the program is to be assessed and which serves as the initial statement of the level of the verifiable end that the program is expected to change, about which the evaluation strategies employed will provide information for program modification over time to assure that the program achieves the projected ends. Second, it provides a critical assessment of whether the assumed problems that the program is expected to address are, in fact, real problems. For example, it may be found in a well-conducted needs assessment that contraceptive use is low, but the attitude of women toward family planning is highly favorable. In this context it will be of little value to devise a program for improving women's attitudes toward contraception. It might also be found, for example, that child spacing— especially in a highly traditional society—might not be a real problem, in the sense that children may already be well spaced by traditional methods, such as separation of parents for extended periods after the birth of a child. If this is the case, then the family planning program may not need to address child spacing, per se, as an issue.

3. Determining strategies

A third step in needs assessment is to determine what strategies should be employed by the program to attack the problems specified. A first part of this is the specification of what the problems actually are. A program to improve the attitude of women toward family planning techniques might be different and have different components from a program to make services more readily available, which might have different components from a program aimed specifically toward spacing children two years apart.

It is likely that the most common approach to determination of strategies for program implementation is expert judgment. Expert judgment is probably the most important source of information about how a program should be structured. But this expert judgment may be developed in a number of different ways. It may be that program directors will simply decide how a program will be structured on the basis of their own judgment. But it is also possible to use the Delphi technique, or the nominal group technique, or focus groups, as examples, to generate data both from program directors and from other experts, about how a program should be structured to address the problems indicated, and even about what the problems actually are. The use of these techniques is discussed in Chapter 7.

Expert judgment may be particularly useful in determining what may feasibly be done. But what should be done may be determined by asking the people whom the program will be expected to affect.

Illustration: King-Drew Medical Center (Kosecoff and Fink 1982). As part of the activities associated with the establishment of a primary health care service, respondents from about 700 households (consumers) were asked to rate, on a response scale of five levels of importance, a list of 38 possible objectives that might be met by a primary health services center. Objectives were scored on the five-point scale from one to five according to the average value given by all respondents. Nineteen objectives received average scores of four or more.

Consumers, along with a sample of 224 physicians and 74 administrators (providers), were asked to rate these same objectives on a three-point scale of availability (or the degree to which the objective was already being met in the community). It was determined from this rating that 12 of the 19 objectives received scores of two or more on availability, indicating that the objectives were already being met. This left 7 candidates from the original list of possible objectives of a primary health care service on which there was consensus on the part of consumers that the objectives were important, and consensus on the part of both consumers and providers that the objectives were not being met. The 7 objectives were

1. to set up health services that are close to the people in the community

2. to identify and assist with family problems that are threats to health

3. to adequately treat common or frequent health problems in the same clinic

4. to make better use of community resources

5. to reduce the cost of health care

6. to reduce the time a patient has to wait for health services

7. to make home visits when indicated

The involvement of consumers (or more particularly, the people who will be affected by the program) in the determination of objectives for a new program (or in the determination of how the program will be delivered, what it will consist of, etc.) is likely to lead to a program that is closer to the perceived needs of the people it is designed to serve, and a program that is more likely to be accepted by those people. In the case of the King-Drew needs assessment, however, the types of needs identified by the community survey had already been circumscribed by the types of objectives presented to the consumers as the original list of 38. This is a common characteristic of needs assessments. The results are often, at least in part, predetermined by the types of questions that are asked.

An additional step was taken in the King-Drew needs assessment: determining the extent to which the seven objectives with high priority and low availability were actually feasible for a primary health care service. Feasibility of all objectives was assessed on a three-point scale by providers; Kosecoff and Fink report that consumers had difficulty rating feasibility and were not asked to do so in the final survey (p. 31). The consensus of the providers was that the first four objectives in the list above had high feasibility scores (two or more) while the last three objectives were assessed as having low feasibility (scores less than two). Through this needs assessment, the first four objectives in the list above became the priority items for the primary health care service.

A well-designed needs assessment carried out in anticipation of the initiation of, or expansion of, family planning services in a developing country would include both an assessment of what should be provided from the view of experts (directors of health services, service providers, managers of services, external consultants and an assessment of what the expected recipients of services, the clients, thought of as their needs and the kinds of services they would like to receive. Both pieces of information are critical to a complete needs assessment. Providers, or experts, for example, may feel that the most important aspect of a family planning service is the availability of a wide range of methods to meet the varying individual needs of clients. Clients may be happy to have access to a wide range of methods but may feel that the most important aspect of a service is its convenience, or its confidentiality, or that the clinic is a pleasant and friendly place to visit. Without having both views, program success will be jeopardized.

4. Specifying criteria

Once objectives of the program have been identified in a general way, as was done in the King-Drew example given above, a next and critical step in a needs assessment is to specify the criteria that are to be used to assess successful realization of the objectives. This addresses, specifically, the question of verifiable ends. Consider, for example, the first of the King-Drew objectives (one that was assessed as feasible): "to set up health services that are close to the people in the community." This objective is certainly desirable, but it is not particularly assessable as stated. There are two points in this objective that require further clarification and specification before it can be assumed that verifiable ends exist. These are the phrases "health services" and "close to the people." The issue, of course, is what do these mean for purposes of assessment, and how can the realization of these goals be empirically verified?

So as not to become bogged down in the example, consider only the phrase "health services." Specifically, to what health services is reference made? It is likely that emergency x-ray services are included, but probably not CAT scans. It is likely that suturing of wounds is included, but not thoracic surgery. So one component of this step in needs assessment is to draw up a list of the specific services to be provided. This list does not have to be exhaustive, but should specify the services that must exist for the objective to have been realized. For example, it may be that a health service center will provide for dispensing of over-the-counter drugs as a convenience to patients, but this might not be specified as one of the services that *must* be provided to assure the overall objective will be met.

Having drawn up a list of services to be provided, it might also be important to indicate, for assessment of the overall objective, whether all the services will be available at all times, or some at only some times; the hours of operation of the centers; and the numbers and certifications of persons who are to staff the center. There are also other possible criteria that might be specified. In order to realize the first objective as stated, some specification on most of these points is necessary. Perhaps more importantly, in order to remain in the cybernetic decision mode, to be able to use information about the extent to which the medical services *are* close to the people, in order to continue to assure the objective is being realized, it is necessary to have verifiable ends: in simple terms, a list of specific medical services that will be provided. Without such a list, it is anybody's guess as to how well the program is doing, and decisions made to assure success will be either random walk decisions or traditional decisions.

This does not mean that it is not possible to be concerned about ultimate good that may come from the program. The objective of having medical services close to the people is an end in the sense that it is the objective as stated and it will be likely to make the people more comfortable. But the penultimate purpose of this objective is to improve people's medical care services; and the ultimate purpose, to improve their health and happiness. It may be argued that confining the assessment of this objective to a sterile list of services to be provided robs the objective of its depth, its importance, or its meaning. Granted that we are all interested in ultimate purposes, it still cannot hurt to be sure that you have accomplished the specified task. It is pretty certain that if a specified set of essential services is not provided in close proximity to the people who need them, the objective itself will not be met, and the penultimate and ultimate purposes are likely to suffer.

5. Constructing a general causal chain

The final step in a needs assessment is the construction of a conceptual causal chain that describes the process by which the program intervention is expected to influence the outcome desired, the verifiable end to which the program is addressed. This is an important last step to assure that there is a logical pathway by which the expected effect of the program can come about, and also as a means of assuring program implementors that program inputs will be substantial enough to produce program results desired.

Illustration: Family planning in Nigeria. To consider how a conceptual model can be applied in a needs assessment, take as an example a program intervention that is now being carried out in Nigeria as a way to improve continuity of contraceptive use. As a bit of background, it was found in a review of clinic activities in one of the Nigerian states, that although women coming to the clinic often expressed a desire to use oral contraceptives or depo-provera for periods of time up to two or three years, less than 25 percent of women who initially visited the clinics for contraceptives came back more than one time. From a review of record-keeping systems in the clinics, it was found that none of the providers were aware at any particular time whether any of their clients were expected to return for resupply of contraceptives; that is, there was no "tickler file" to assure that providers knew which women had exhausted their supply of contraceptives and thus should return to the clinic.

A simple program intervention was devised consisting of a filing system, designed and constructed with local materials, that allowed the providers to file client records by the month in which they were expected to return to the clinic. This system was put into place in 12 experimental clinics in hopes of improving continuity of service use by women coming to the clinics. The causal model underlying this intervention is shown in Figure 2-4.

The model assumes that the revised filing system will provide better information to the provider, specifically information about which women should be returning to the clinic any month. This information will, in turn, allow the provider to recognize a gap (when women do not return) between expectations about how the system should operate, and what is actually happening (following the logic of the concept of visibility of consequences). Recognition of the gap in service provision will then lead to efforts on the part of the provider to bring the women who have not returned back to the clinic (one component of the program is active recruitment on the part of community outreach workers under the direction of the service provider). Efforts to recruit women back to services are expected to lead to a significant proportion of the women returning to the clinic, which then leads to greater continuity of service use. The verifiable outcome of the project will be the number of months that a woman continues using contraceptives, which can be ascertained from her clinic record.

Figure 2-4   Schematic Presentation of the Links between a Change in a Family Planning Record System and Continuation of Use

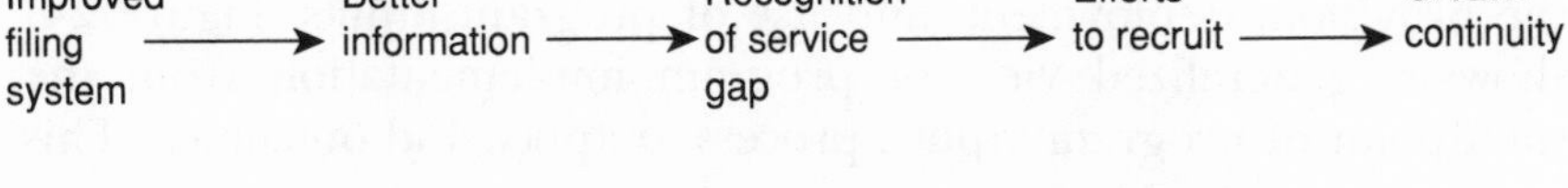

| Improved filing system | → | Better information | → | Recognition of service gap | → | Efforts to recruit | → | Greater continuity |

There are two clear benefits to producing a conceptual causal model such as the one shown in Figure 2-4 as a part of a needs assessment. The first is to be assured that there is a logical causal link between the program as implemented and the change in the verifiable end anticipated. If it is not possible to specify such a causal link, the intervention or the expected end should be rethought. The second benefit, which derives from the first, is a model for determining what activities (in addition to the program intervention) must be carried out, or assured, in order for the link between program and end to be established and maintained. For example, in the causal chain shown in Figure 2-4, it is clear that some way must be devised for contacting women who do not return for their next appointment. If this piece of the link is broken, the program is likely to fail. Monitoring of program activity—to be discussed in the next section—should include collection and maintenance, where possible, of information that demonstrates the continuity of these links.

Program Implementation

During the implementation stage of a program, the evaluation issue is primarily that of assuring that the program as designed is "in place and on track." This is the issue of progress. While managers and evaluators often assume the extent of implementation, implementation varies by site, over time, and even among program recipients as their characteristics interact with the attributes of the intervention (Scheirer 1989). For example, a review of 23 evaluation studies that included measures of implementation (Scheirer and Rezmovic 1983) revealed that less than one-third reported a high level of implementation; another third, mixed or moderate levels; and one-third, low levels of implementation.

Assessment of progress is generally considered to be an issue of monitoring. The program is expected to have progressed to a certain point by a certain time, for example. The point to which the program is expected to have progressed will be associated with the assurance of anticipated funding; with the delivery of program equipment; with the construction of a facility; with the hiring, or training, of personnel; and with the provision of services to some client population. To better visualize the province of monitoring as an evaluation activity, consider Figure 2-5.

In general, what is monitored in the assessment of progress is the provision, deployment, and use of program inputs. Figure 2-5 shows a generalized view of program implementation from the standpoint of program inputs, process, outputs, and outcomes. This might be considered as an expanded view of the implementation process presented in Chapter 1 and illustrated in Figure 1-1. Program monitoring, as an evaluation activity, is concerned particularly with program inputs and process. The questions raised in program monitoring will be particularly questions of whether such critical inputs as funding, equipment, facilities, and personnel have been made available in the quantities and at the times specified by the program plan. It will be concerned with whether the process of the program—which will include the way in which inputs are deployed and expended, and the timing of this use—conforms to the program plan. It will be concerned with determining whether the persons expected to be served by the program have actually been served in the quantity and with the level of quality expected and how the program can be improved.

In all of these monitoring activities, the cybernetic approach to decision making has a clear role. The verifiable ends are, in this case, the inputs and deployment of inputs (program process) specified by the program plan, or evolving on a real-time basis in the minds of the program managers. Evaluation in this context is concerned with determining whether the actual deployment of resources fits the existing or evolving plan. If it does not, it is the responsibility of the program managers to make those decisions necessary to assure that the deployment and use of resources does fit the plan. Statisticians speak of type one error, the finding of a program result when none actually exists, and of type two error, the finding of no program result when a result does exist. Program evaluators also speak of a type three error, the assumption that a program was implemented, when in fact it was not. Monitoring serves the purpose of allowing the manager to make the decisions necessary to assure that a program is implemented as expected and also serves the purpose of providing the basis for its continuous improvement. Monitoring fits into the cybernetic mode of decision making, with the verifiable ends being the program plans for provision and deployment of inputs. Chapters 4 and 5 provide further discussion of the relevant strategies and approaches.

Figure 2-5 A Schematic of Program Inputs, Process, Outputs, and Outcomes

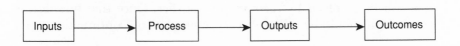

Assessing Results

The assessment of program results includes the three categories of evaluation: efficiency, effectiveness, and impact. By the WHO formulation of efficiency and effectiveness, these are program characteristics that may be assessed, in large part, while the program is ongoing. But as formulated by WHO, impact is concerned with the long-term effects of a program and, in particular, program influence on such difficult-to-measure concepts as quality of life. In the case of each of these categories of evaluation, however, the cybernetic approach to decision making should be served by the evaluation approach.

The difference between the use of the cybernetic process in the case of program results as compared to program implementation is that often with program implementation, evaluation information (results of program-monitoring efforts) will be available and may produce changes in a program, on a real-time and continuing basis, while in the case of program results, evaluation information (assessments of efficiency, effectiveness, and impact) may come too late in the life of a program to inform decisions for significant changes in the program itself, but rather may be most valuable in decisions about how a similar program should be structured next time around.

Effectiveness

Effectiveness is concerned with the question of whether the expected program outputs are produced. In Chapter 1, one of the questions raised as being of the type that might be addressed in an assessment of effectiveness was: Did the program meet its stated objectives? This is an example, perhaps the central feature of an evaluation of effectiveness. From the standpoint of the cybernetic decision-making model, a critical feature of this question is whether the objectives of the program are stated in such a way as to allow the evaluator to assess whether the objectives have been met—in short, to verify the achievement of program ends. If, for example, a family planning program has been upgraded for the expressed purpose of increasing the length of time that women continue to use contraceptives, the verifiable program end is an increase in the length of time that women who begin family planning actually continue use. There can be legitimate questions raised as to how much of an increase in length of time is actually an increase, but this is, in part, a technical question that can be resolved by recourse to statistics. Once that question is resolved, it should be relatively easy to get data on continuation from records that are almost certain to be available in family planning clinics.

On the other hand, if the stated objective of the program is to increase the quality of care provided in the clinics, it may be very difficult to devise a verifiable measure of quality of service provided. The quality of training of providers and their knowledge and skills at training might be assessed, but these are essentially program inputs and what is to be assessed are outputs. Quality of service, as provided, might be assessed through the technique of observation or demonstration, but this is not only a costly activity, requiring a substantial amount of time in observation of the providers, but it also requires a specification of precisely what service provision actions are to be assessed, how they are to be assessed, and what measuring instruments are to be used. In the absence of such specification, not a trivial matter, any decisions that result from the evaluation effort will have drifted back into either the traditional or the random walk decision modes.

Although effectiveness is concerned with program outputs, this does not always mean that evaluation of effectiveness comes only at the end of the program. Efforts to determine whether the program inputs are associated with greater continuity of contraceptive use might reasonably occur during the course of the program life, and the determination that no increase in continuity of use was occurring might lead directly to a decision to modify the program in some way. There is, of course, a downside to this. Decisions to change a program in midcourse could have significant and unexpected results in terms of the determination that the program—as opposed to other factors, including the changes in the program—was actually the causal agent in the change in outputs. But in this regard, assessment of effectiveness can also be seen to occur on a real-time basis and to have an input to decisions made about program operation.

There are a number of ways in which effectiveness may be assessed, depending on the nature of the program itself and on the nature of the verifiable end under assessment. These include, with varying degrees of internal validity, case studies, trend analysis, surveys, experiments, and even simulation techniques. Each of these topics is discussed in detail later in the book.

Efficiency

The issue of efficiency is essentially one of whether the verifiable ends of the program are sufficient to justify the costs incurred. This may also be considered in the context of the question of whether the verifiable ends are realized through the program under assessment at a lower cost than they might be realized through some other program. Either of these issues implies that the ends have, in fact, been reached and that they can be verified. Assessment of the cost of increasing the length of time that family planning acceptors continue to use family planning can move forward relatively easily if a way is found to determine the costs of the program. But efforts to assess the cost of increases in quality in the same program depend not only on the ability to determine costs, but also on the other problematic issue of how to determine that quality has increased. In either case, however, it would make little sense to speak of the efficiency of a program that had failed to meet the verifiable ends specified. Moreover, it follows from this that if program outputs cannot be stated as verifiable ends, assessment of efficiency is simply not possible.

On the strength of the (possibly optimistic) assumption that program ends can be stated in ways that allow them to be verified, the assessment of efficiency, like the assessment of effectiveness, has the potential of providing input to decisions made about the program at two times: (1) while the program is under way, comparing costs to expected costs or to costs realized under some other scheme, and (2) at the end of the program, with the same types of comparisons. Decisions taken as a result of the evaluation effort may influence the nature of the program as it is ongoing or may be used to determine how a future program to produce similar results should be structured. In either case, the assessment of efficiency is usually subsumed under the topics of cost-benefit or cost-effectiveness analysis. Chapter 17 is devoted to these topics.

Impact

The evaluation of impact stands in a somewhat different position relative to the cybernetic decision model than do the other four aspects of evaluation. Impact refers to the long-term results of the program—in particular, improvements in health and quality of life. The word "impact" itself—though a term used in most evaluation literature and frequently invoked by funding agencies, planners, and program managers—seems much too dramatic to describe the results—even long-term—to be expected from most programs. An earthquake has an impact. A program to increase the use of family planning services has a result or an effect, or even a long-term outcome, but it is hard to think of it as having an impact. Semantics aside, however, there are several aspects of the concept of impact that make it a questionable issue for program evaluation (although funding agencies, planners, program managers, and even evaluators are going to continue to talk of evaluation of impact).

Long-term effect

Impact must be thought of as the long-term effects, the outcomes, of program activities. This definition itself makes an interest in an assessment of impact problematic for the program manager. In general, managers are and should be concerned with decisions (and hence, evaluations) that bear on the decisions they will make about the continued progress of the program to assure that the results of the program are as expected, or at the very least, to assure that they can demonstrate where the program failed to meet its short-term (outcome) objectives. It is not the job of managers to assure that two or five or ten years after the program ends there will be salubrious changes in health or education or quality of life. In any case, program funders are not going to include the necessary resources to do such an assessment as part of the program. So on the basis of long-term results, the assessment of impact seems clearly problematic.

Verifiable ends

It has been argued that the cybernetic decision mode, the appropriate realm of evaluation, depends on the specification of verifiable ends against which the results of the program can be assessed. But it is in the nature of such long-term outcomes of a program as improved health, welfare, or quality of life, that it is both difficult to reach consensus on what the components of these things are (what goes into a measure of quality of life?) and that the components, even if agreed upon, are difficult or impossible to measure (verify). Take, for example, the concept of health as expressed by WHO. The WHO constitution defines health as a "state of complete physical, mental and social wellbeing . . ." (WHO 1981). How many different aspects of complete physical, mental, and social well-being would we have to specify to assure that we had all the important ones? And once we had them, how would we measure them? The likely recourse would be to fall back on specific indicators like infant mortality rates as a measure of well-being. But then why not just admit that the purpose of the program is to reduce infant mortality rate, which is a verifiable end.

Causal links

The final problem with assessing impact (long-term effects on quality of life) is the difficulty of assuring, demonstrating, or proving the causal link between the program inputs and process and the long-term outcomes expected.

Illustration. Figure 2-6 shows a causal model of the links between the quality of family planning services and contraceptive prevalence and fertility (Jain 1989). Also shown in Figure 2-6 are two posited relationships that were not included in the original model: an arrow from training of providers to provider competence and from fertility to quality of life. If we wish to consider the impact of a training program for contraceptive service providers, this model provides useful insights.

As Figure 2-6 shows, Jain posits a direct and known causal chain from demand for services, through acceptance and continuation, to contraceptive prevalence and fertility. He also indicates hypothesized but unproven links from quality of service to acceptance and continuation. But the quality-of-life "impact" measures are on the right side of the figure, with only a hypothesized, unproven link from fertility, while the program input, training of providers to improve provider competence, is on the extreme left side of the model, albeit with a (posited) real effect on provider competence. In this long chain of causation, the effect of training on quality of life may be so small as to be unmeasurable. Even the effect of training on fertility may be so small (even if real) that the error in measurement of changes in fertility may be greater than the (real) effect of training on fertility. This suggests the difficulty of showing, in any concrete way, that a program input may produce an impact, in the sense of long-term changes in health, welfare, quality of life.

This may seem to be an invented example with little real import. But recently the United States Agency for International Development (USAID) issued a request for proposal (RFP) for a program in a developing country in which they sought to influence several measures of maternal and child health through program interventions. One of the measures they wished to affect was maternal mortality associated with childbirth, which they wanted to show as being reduced by 15 percent. The rate of maternal mortality as stated in the RFP was 3 per thousand. In order to show a 15 percent reduction in that rate with a reasonable degree of statistical confidence, data on about 60,000 completed births would have to be collected. This could be a monumental data collection task in a country in which most births are never registered. The result is that even though we can define the end that the program (in this case) is to achieve (a reduction in maternal deaths of a given amount), the likely error of measurement (assuming we may be able to get, for example, information on even 10,000 births) will be larger than the expected program effect.

Figure 2-6   Chain of Causation for Family Planning Services between a Training Program and Health Impact

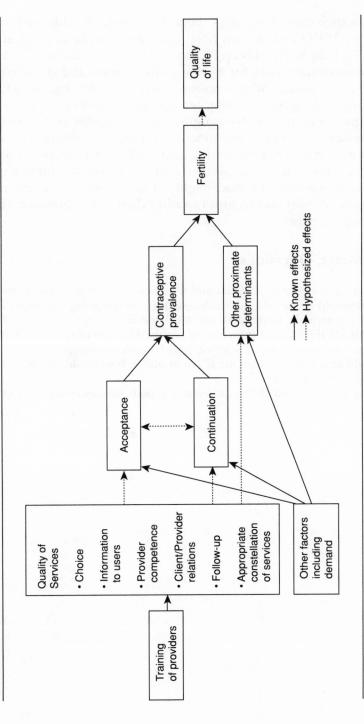

Source: Reprinted with permission from Anrudh K. Jain, "Fertility Reproduction and the Quality of Family Planning Services," *Studies in Family Planning* 20, no. 1 (1989): 3.

Despite these misgivings about the assessment of impact as defined by WHO and as used here, evaluation can be applied in this area. Techniques for this application include, essentially, those same techniques appropriate for assessing effectiveness and are discussed in the same context. Where resources exist for assessing impact, it is certainly in the interest of long-term program development (even if, perhaps, not relevant to the program decision maker as the program progresses) to carry out assessments of impact. A program that has no long-term effect on improving quality of life may be questionable, no matter how much of a specified output it produces. But to a great extent, assessments of impact might better be conceived as the province of academics and of history rather than as the province of the program manager.

Discussion Questions

1. Select a health care program and illustrate the type of decision making that would be carried out under each decision-making model: random walk, cybernetic, traditional, and mechanistic.
2. Illustrate the types of information required in each of the five steps of a needs assessment for a selected health services program. How readily available is this information? If not available, how would you propose to obtain the information?
3. Why is implementation a problem for both managers and evaluators?

3

Political and Organizational Context of Evaluation

$\mathbf{E}$valuation is an integral part of the managerial process and provides useful information for decision making. As part of that process, evaluation is influenced by the organizational and political context within which it is conducted. The objective of this chapter is to assess some of the uses and nonuses of evaluation data and to consider the context within which evaluation is likely to occur.

Uses and Nonuses of Evaluation as a Decision Tool

If we view evaluation as part of the managerial process, then information for decision making and the ability to continually improve the process itself are the clear products of the evaluation effort. Information derived from evaluation efforts can be used to affect decisions at all stages of the managerial process: planning, implementation, and control.

As described in Chapters 1 and 2, information derived from evaluation efforts should influence decisions at any one of several stages of the decision-making process: planning, implementation, or control.

While there is some indication that, at least among congressional committees, there is a growing reliance on evaluation information to inform decisions (Weiss 1989), many remain pessimistic about the use of evaluation results by decision makers (Rossi and Freeman 1989). The extent to which evaluation is incorporated into the decision-making process of managers continues to be a function of their ideology, their interests, and information (Weiss 1983).

Ideology

Evaluations are inevitably carried out with specifically defined goals or objectives and often overlook important outcomes or results from program efforts that are guided by a series of philosophies, principles, values, and political orientations. For example, in 1980 the Robert Wood Johnson Foundation initiated a national demonstration program to encourage community hospitals and their medical staffs to provide care in underserved areas. As described in the brochure mailed to potential applicants (National Planning Association 1974):

> . . . To strengthen the role of community hospitals and ambulatory care by developing affiliated (not necessarily hospital-based) group practices. It is the Foundation's hope that these groups may serve as a single, identifiable source of continuing care for the whole family with around the clock, front line coverage in an integrated and coordinated referral system. (p. 5)

The program, as implemented by a number of hospitals, took on a variety of objectives quite independent of those intended by the foundation (Shortell, Wickizer, and Wheeler 1984). For example, in one case, the hospital thought the primary objective of the program was to provide a setting to attract a more evenly balanced financial mix of patients and capture referral markets in outlying communities. In another community, the primary objective was to provide a setting to upgrade the quality of its medical staff and deliberately attract good, young primary care physicians, who in turn would help hospitals attract needed specialists. Clearly, any evaluation of the program must, in fact, be broad enough to adequately cover the multiple objectives, which were not intended in the original solicitation.

In trying to broaden the basis of evaluation and ensure that evaluation results are not so narrowly defined that major and important unintended consequences of programs are overlooked—or, further, to try to consider results of programs that are intended but difficult to assess—the evaluator is in an extremely difficult situation. Evaluation must be relevant to the issues with which decision makers are concerned. At the same time, evaluation must not be so narrow as to miss important aspects of programs that may be either unforeseen and unintended or that cannot be measured on an objective or quantitative basis.

One approach is to actively develop a theoretical model to assure that the evaluation identifies the full range of potential impacts (Browne and Wildavsky 1987) and, based on this range, narrows the focus on those that are most likely to have important managerial implications. While the theoretical and managerial may be of "different worlds," they are not mutually exclusive. As described by Lawler (1985):

> Theory and practice are not competing mistresses. Indeed, research [evaluation] that is useful to either the theoretician or to the practitioner is suspect. If it is useful to the practitioner but not the theoretician then one must wonder whether it is a valid finding and whether it has addressed the correct issue. If it is useful to the theoretician but not to the practitioner, then one must wonder whether the research is capturing a critical issue. Indeed, it can be argued that we should always ask two questions about research [evaluation]: Is it useful for practice and does it contribute to the body of scientific knowledge that is relevant to theory? If it fails either of these tests, then serious questions should be raised. It is a rare research [evaluation] study that can inform practice but not theory or vice versa. (p. 4)

Interests

Practicing administrators often do not see the work of researchers or evaluators as relevant to their decision-making needs (Boyle 1989; Petasnick 1989). This situation is illustrated by the contrast between formative and summative evaluations. Summative evaluations seek, in general, a single decision that the program is good and should go on or that it is bad and should be terminated. Unfortunately, these decisions are almost invariably reached after the fact and are irrelevant to the decision-making process of program managers. Evaluation must shed light on questions of interest to program administrators as they go through the decision-making processes necessary to directing the program. Information presented six months after the termination of a program is of little practical consequence. On the other hand, evaluation data suggesting to the manager that program activities have not been up to expected standards for the past two weeks or that the program is not using resources at the level expected will be much more valuable for program management and decision making. Administrators clearly need continual information feedback about how a program is progressing. It may, in certain circumstances, lead to less than optimum results over the long term, but the information derived will be relevant to the decisions that program administrators must make. Moreover, given the dynamics of the field, interests—and the conditions that determine interest—change, providing evaluation activities with a relatively narrow window of opportunity.

An example of an extremely costly evaluation that may not be worth the effort in the long run is the RAND Corporation experiment to assess the effect of various types of health insurance coverage on use of services (RAND 1988). Begun in 1972, this project, although a well-designed, experimental study, probably will have little influence on policymaking with regard to any national health insurance scheme. While the issue of national health insurance will undoubtedly be addressed, a study conducted in the 1970s may well be considered too dated to be of value.

One conclusion from this example is clear: for evaluation to be useful to managers, it must provide information when they require it and relevant to their current interests. This does not necessarily mean that evaluation cannot be scientific, systematic, or formal. It does mean, however, that the evaluator must recognize the needs and interests of administrators for information that they can use as the program develops. Evaluators must be willing to abandon the notion that they can deal only with summative evaluation of the overall contribution of a program and be willing to make observations and judgments about the quality of a program as it progresses.

Information

Information based on some form of evaluation is not the only source of knowledge about program activities and their effectiveness. As described by Mintzberg (1989): "Organizational effectiveness does not lie in [the] narrow minded concept called 'rationality'; it lies in a blend of clear-headed logic and powerful intuition." Similarly, as Lindblom and Cohen (1979) point out:

> Information and analysis constitute only one route among several to social problem solving. And [evaluation] is one method among several of providing information and analysis to the extent that they are required. Information and analysis provide only one route because . . . a great deal of the world's problem solving is and ought to be accomplished through various forms of social interaction that substitute action for thought, understanding or analysis. Information and analysis are not a universal or categorical prescription for social problem solving. (p. 10)

Lindblom and Cohen go on to indicate that a significant portion of decision making depends on ordinary knowledge, social learning, and interaction. *Ordinary knowledge* refers to knowledge that does not owe its origin, testing, degree of verification, truth status, or currency to distinctive professional social inquiry techniques but rather to common sense, causal empiricism, or thoughtful speculation and analysis. Decision making regarding any health and social welfare program will always depend heavily on ordinary knowledge.

Social learning refers to the actual participation in ongoing social phenomena through which individuals learn new behavior. In many situations, information generated from evaluation is likely to be of little use until required learning occurs. It may, however, be useful to supplement social learning by answering questions that arise after or as a result of such learning.

Interactive problem solving refers to the resolution of problems by actions rather than by thought. Through this method, solutions are introduced to resolve a problem or improve a situation without any understanding of it or systematic assessment of remedies or preferred outcomes; instead the problem is resolved by various forms of interaction among people, in which what they do rather than what they or anyone else thinks (or understands or analyzes) about the problem moves toward the solution or preferred situation.

Evaluation efforts must take intuition and these other sources of information and methods of resolving problems into account. Intuition, ordinary knowledge, social learning, and interactive problem solving are real approaches. Yet each can be supplemented by information generated by systematic evaluations when the evaluations are designed with the decision maker in mind.

Climate of Evaluation

In the best of all possible worlds, evaluation is a rational process that provides valuable information for program decision making. No conscientious program manager could oppose evaluation; there is a growing belief that no program or process should be without evaluation, that it should be designed into the process at the outset to ensure that the program will reach its established goals. Certainly political considerations should not enter into the technical issues that evaluation efforts address. Decisions using information provided by evaluation activities should not be subject to the whims of politics.

The real-life situation is quite different. Politics are an important issue in evaluation, and the political climate surrounding the evaluation process must be understood if the evaluator is to have any serious impact on program activities. At least four aspects of the political climate of evaluation should be understood by anyone who expects to become involved in evaluations. Understanding or being aware of these political aspects may not ensure the evaluator's success but will greatly improve its likelihood, and in those instances where success is not forthcoming, the evaluator will at least have some perspective on one of the possible reasons that evaluation efforts may fail.

Unrealistic program objectives

The evaluator must realize that programs develop as part of a political process and are likely to survive or fail on the basis of political, as opposed to technical rationality. Programs that are the focus of evaluation have emerged from the rough and tumble of political support, opposition, and bargaining (Weiss 1975, 1989). Attached to them are the reputations of legislative sponsors, the careers of administrators, the jobs of program staff, and the expectations of the clients. In this environment it is naive to assume that the criterion by which program decisions are made is technical rationality based on some clear and rigorous evaluation process.

The politics involved in the establishment of a program are such that it is necessary for the program to appear as a solution to all problems for all people. The passage of some type of national health insurance, for instance, is pictured variously as providing not only funds to finance hospital services for the American public but also a means for improving physicians' decision making, improving the quality of care, reducing the cost of hospital stays, and generally improving the nation's health. Although it is highly unrealistic to expect any program, particularly an insurance scheme, to do all this, nevertheless, it will probably be necessary to use such arguments to gain the passage of any national health insurance scheme.

Similarly, the World Health Organization is promoting primary health care as a means of ensuring "health for all by the year 2000." The very idea of a reference to "health for all" suggests that WHO is involved in a political process. The notion of an absolute level of health that can be achieved, according to some objective criteria, can only be accepted as a political statement. Still, the successful promotion of primary health care by the World Health Organization will depend in large part on the hyperbole and rhetoric involved in statements about health for all by the year 2000. The evaluator who undertakes an evaluation of a program of this type will immediately be on the defensive. Moreover, programs that require political support and compromise for their initiation will probably be influenced more by the political decisions in their progress than by technical, nonpolitical decisions.

Explicit versus implicit objectives

The second climate problem confronting evaluation is the issue of explicit versus implicit program objectives. Regardless of the high-sounding, altruistic, or rational statements made for the existence of a program, the basis of any program may be hidden goals that are acknowledged only rarely and very seldom in public or, in fact, may not even be recognized at all. As Kierkegaard observed, "Life is to be lived forward but understood backward." Mintzberg (1987) has applied that perspective to much of what happens within the managerial process and has suggested that managers may have to live strategy (programs) in the future, but they must understand it, then, through the past. Even when goals are understood, they are likely to be viewed differently by a variety of important constituent or stakeholder groups and, in fact, may have multiple and potentially conflicting sets of activities. Organizations are composed of coalitions or stakeholders, each of which have a claim on a particular problematic activity. For example, program X may be viewed by one constituency or set of stakeholders as enhancing the overall quality of the service provided, yet viewed by another as an opportunity to gather a larger market share within the community. Similarly, programs may have a series of goal achievements that are not easily combined. For example, in clinical research a program may aspire to diffuse state-of-the-art therapy and affect national mortality and morbidity levels. Similarly, within such programs there may be a need to emphasize both prevention and treatment strategies, thus raising the potential for conflict as they compete for limited resources and attention.

Secondly, any evaluation effort needs to recognize that program objectives are not a priori developed in a totally rational and deliberate process but can also be viewed as an emergent process evolving from the very dynamics of the organization over time. As described by Mintzberg (1987), strategies (program objectives) can form as well as be formulated. In other words, they need not be planned, but can emerge in response to an evolving situation.

Finally, consideration must be given to situations in which program staff might be characterized as "true believers." True believers are committed not only to a goal or set of goals but, in general, are also committed to a specific process for achieving those goals. Improving the health of the U.S. population may be a desirable goal, but most physicians in private practice are likely to believe that it should not and, in fact, cannot be done by providing medical services through public financing. Certainly they are apt to agree that it cannot be done by providing medical services under public control. The physician is a true believer in the efficacy of the private pursuit of and payment for medical care services.

The belief that providing more medical services will, in itself, improve health status is another aspect of the true believer phenomenon. There is little objective evidence of a relationship between health status as broadly defined and use of or access to medical care services. But, in the case of medical services, not only are program providers—physicians, hospitals, and clinics—populated by true believers, but the served population itself also tends to be a population of true believers.

Evaluation is almost impossible in programs in which true believers are in control. Because they believe a priori in the efficacy of a particular process, they are unwilling to allow that process to be subjected to evaluation. Moreover, they are likely to be unaware of the fact that the views they hold about the efficacy of a particular process are even subject to the possibility of evaluation. In such circumstances, the evaluator is likely to have substantial difficulty in affecting program activities.

Externally imposed evaluation

An external agent or agency may represent a higher-echelon decision-making level to which a program director reports; it may be some outside resource important in terms of funding or an expert in evaluation working within the program itself. In any of these cases, however, the politics of the situation are such that the evaluator will be in the position of power and authority with regard to the program. Few people, including managers, are so ingenuous as to welcome a free scrutiny of their affairs no matter how benign, uncritical, or even helpful that scrutiny is meant to be. If the data-gathering phase of the evaluation is successful, the evaluator is in possession of a great deal of information about a program that may have serious ramifications for its continuation and for the positions of the people in it.

If the evaluation is imposed from the top, program personnel are immediately on the defensive. They are likely to view the evaluation as an effort of the superordinate agency either to control program operations or to find reasons and excuses to modify or terminate the program. In this case, the evaluator is already at a clear disadvantage.

Even if the evaluation is not imposed from the top down or from the outside in, even in that highly desirable circumstance where the manager personally requests the evaluation or where evaluation has been built into the program at the outset, a problem that is basically political and that affects the use of evaluation results still exists. Evaluators are apt to be people who consider themselves professionals in the realm of evaluation. As professionals, they must demonstrate their expertise, which means that the evaluation must be both methodologically elegant and conceptually comprehensive. The evaluator is probably trained in one of the social sciences, partly because social science training usually includes a large measure of work in research methodology and statistics. Although this training is highly appropriate to evaluation efforts, it may be quite different from training that would lead logically to the ability to view the program from a manager's perspective. One problem of social science training, for example, is the fact that simplifying a research effort so that it confronts issues specifically of interest to and relevant for decision making is extremely difficult. Social scientists have a long tradition of launching large-scale research efforts without much thought about specific information requirements or the ability or desire to limit the amount of information gathered. As a result, many evaluation efforts become overblown, and miss an opportunity to contribute to important management questions.

Large-scale studies launched without much thought about how the information will be used or with little effort to limit the activity to essentials may be acceptable for academic endeavors but are highly inappropriate for evaluation. Not only are the audiences to whom the evaluation is addressed likely to question the relevance and value of this specific evaluation, and hence the relevance and value of every such effort, but managers will probably also be quite unhappy about being required to cooperate with and perhaps participate in an activity they do not understand. The politics of evaluation are often such that there is conflict between the evaluator and manager. Successful evaluation requires the evaluator to begin with the agenda of the manager.

Evaluation as a political process

Those involved in evaluation often prefer to deny the reality of politics vis-à-vis their evaluation activity, yet the fact that evaluation is an integral part of the management process places it squarely in a political context. Weiss (1989) discusses three ways in which politics and evaluation are related:

1. The programs being evaluated are political: they have legislative sponsors and supporters, administrative careers attached to them, and the support of program staff, clients, and interest groups.
2. Evaluation reports are fed into a political arena and become part of the political decision process.
3. Evaluation reports themselves unavoidably take a political position even if they claim to be objective.

Clearly, programs that are evaluated are the result of a long and complicated political process in which there are winners and losers and various important constituents. Moreover, each of these groups has their own perceptions of what the program is trying to accomplish, independent of its explicit goals. Evaluation results must fit into this ongoing process and must take into account the shifting in alliances and expectations that occur between the onset of the evaluation and its report of findings.

Finally, the evaluation itself implicitly assumes a political position. Presenting results, no matter how well designed and executed, has political overtones. For example, what is selected or not selected for study has important consequences since the unexamined program or program aspect has not become the focus of political debate centered on the allocation of scarce resources (Palumbo 1987). Moreover, programs may be in trouble even before evaluation occurs. Gurel (1975) points out that it is precisely when programs are in trouble—particularly when the trouble is a threat to funding—that evaluators are invited to assess the program. He goes on to point out that it takes little imagination to visualize the chilly reception that evaluation and the evaluator are then likely to receive from program managers. Documentation for this view comes partly through his description of the Veterans Administration Psychiatric Evaluation Project. This project underwent nine major evaluation studies. Seven originated from pressures and queries conveyed with congressional or budget bureau threats of financial reprisal. Evaluation efforts are often used as a tool to placate the agencies that may have power over program funding or other aspects of program control.

The political environment of evaluation leads even the most optimistic evaluator to doubt the probability of having a useful impact on program decisions and operations. Certainly if evaluators are to be effective, they must have a fundamental understanding of the political climate surrounding the evaluation effort in which they participate. Evaluators will probably be more effective if they recognize the characteristics of decisions that may result from evaluation efforts. An understanding of these categories can be useful to the evaluators in trying to make the work meaningful to program managers.

Using Decision-Making Models

Chapter 2 presented four different models that are available to decision makers: cybernetic, mechanistic, traditional, and random walk. Given the complexity within which evaluation occurs, what criteria are appropriate in the use of each model? Thompson (1967) suggested that there are three tests that managers can apply in a variety of situations: instrumental, efficiency, and social tests (pp. 84–87). The appropriateness is a function of (1) the degree of clear formulation or ambiguity of standards of desirability and (2) the completeness or incompleteness of cause-and-effect relationships, and corresponds to the means of analysis presented in Chapter 2. Table 3-1 presents the relationship of these tests to our four decision-making models.

Instrumental tests

As seen in Table 3-1, instrumental tests are primarily appropriate for decision making within the cybernetic model. Here the standards of desirability are reasonably clear, and the cause-and-effect relationships are uncertain. For example, will national health insurance produce greater access to health services for all people? Will managed care programs contain costs of providing services to various segments of the population, and does consensus conferences as a means of technology assessment change physician practice patterns? These are essentially technical questions in which the major criterion is to ascertain only whether the desired ends were achieved, without considering the exact means by which this was accomplished and/or without consideration of resource utilization.

It is in this area that the evaluator can make the most important contributions to program decision making. The tools available to the evaluator—measurement techniques, sampling, survey designs, experimentation—are all techniques that conform to the instrumental approach to information. As long as an issue is basically technical, the evaluator is in the most effective realm, although the evaluator is always at risk of challenge if the results do not conform to the expectations of important constituent groups. For example, in a randomized clinical trial of coronary care units, an initial report showing a greater death rate for those treated in hospitals than those treated at home was mistakenly reversed. When these data were presented to

Table 3-1 Decision Models and Criteria

| | Decision Models | | | |
Criteria	Cybernetic	Mechanistic	Traditional	Random Walk
Instrumental	X			
Efficiency		X		
Social			X	X

a group of cardiologists, they demanded that the trials be declared unethical and the study be stopped immediately since the results did not conform to their expectations. When the mistake was identified and the data presented correctly, the same group could not be persuaded to declare the trials unethical but found all sorts of problems with the study sampling and measurement procedures (Cochrane 1972).

Not all questions can be answered on the basis of instrumental tests, of course. Many questions of belief and values are simply not subject to technical verification or refutation. Even in those areas where technical criteria—empirical verification—can apply, measurement may be so difficult or complex that it is impossible to arrive at even a technical answer. Furthermore, the myriad of desirable ends that a particular program is to accomplish and the difficulty of objectively measuring all these ends usually make it impossible to hope that technical rationality alone can resolve all decision-making problems for program operation.

Efficiency tests

Where instrumental criteria in the broad sense raise the question of whether it is possible to demonstrate empirically that the means employed produces the ends desired, efficiency criteria tackles the question of whether the specific means employed is the most efficient means for producing the ends desired. This is critical to the mechanistic model, in which cause-and-effect relationships are well understood. The assumption, of course, is that there are alternative means by which a particular end may be reached or, at the very least, that the program has the option of producing a certain amount of a desired end and that the means will be exercised only to the extent that the cost of producing the amount of the end desired is acceptable.

Again, if evaluation is limited to the aspect of technical rationality that may be seen as economic rationality, evaluators are generally on firm ground. Cost-benefit analysis, cost-effectiveness analysis, and optimization techniques available from operations research are all capable of producing useful information about the most efficient means of realizing desired ends.

Social tests

As seen in Table 3-1, social tests are appropriate to random walk and traditional decision-making models, where standards of desirability are ambiguous regardless of cause-and-effect relationships. Under these conditions, criteria are validated by authority or consensus.

Abortion, for example, is technically an effective means of birth control. Yet in many countries both its legal and social acceptability remain in contention, if not doubt. Many genetic defects and genetically transmitted diseases could be effectively controlled from a technical standpoint through programs to control procreation. Again, in most societies these programs would be neither legally nor socially rational. Substantial questions could be raised as to whether the notion of primary health care as currently promoted by the World Health Organization and the United Nations Children's Fund (UNICEF) is technically the most rational way to approach the goal of "health for all by the year 2000." There is no question, however, that this modality, which relies heavily on local self-help and to a great extent on lay practitioners, has a substantial degree of social rationality for many of the developing nations in which it is to be implemented. On the other hand, because of the continuing restrictions on what nonphysicians may legally do in many of these societies, the legal rationality of the primary care programs may still be subject to question.

Similarly, a given program may be more a means of controlling resources, maintaining a particular elite in power, or providing a hope to special interest groups or disgruntled portions of the population than a way of actually eliminating or reducing the problem to which the program is manifestly addressed. Every large-scale program, despite its true relationships to desired ends from the technical standpoint, is likely to have a substantial component of political rationality in its formulation. The Medicaid program was passed at the same time as the Medicare program, largely for political reasons. Similarly, the passage and 1989 repeal of the Medicare Catastrophic Coverage Act of 1988 (P.L. 100-360) was a clear demonstration of political activity.

When the prevailing criteria of program planners and program managers are primarily social, the evaluator may have little effect on decision making. In fact, the evaluator's findings will probably be largely irrelevant to decision making because decisions are being made on the basis of criteria that are not essentially technical and that cannot be verified empirically. In this case, the evaluator may provide useful insights to decision makers about the technical characteristics of the program and perhaps clarify political trade-offs but cannot expect the work to have significant decision impact. It would be well for the evaluator to be aware of the appropriate tests within each decision model. Failure to apply the appropriate tests within each model will limit the ability of the evaluation to influence the decision-making process—as well as elucidate one's own role in that process.

Discussion Questions

1. Why are health service managers reluctant to use information generated by evaluation activities?
2. Why is it difficult to conduct evaluations on most health service programs? What might health service managers do to encourage program evaluation? What might evaluators do to overcome problems of nonuse by health service managers?
3. Differentiate between instrumental, efficiency, and social tests. What are the implications of each for evaluating health service programs?

Part II

Monitoring

4

Monitoring as an Evaluation Strategy

Program monitoring as an evaluation strategy may be one of the least discussed but most important aspects of program evaluation. Although often considered mundane or nonscientific, monitoring is, in fact, a critical component of evaluation. Monitoring is particularly important to formative evaluation and critical to the evaluation of progress and continuous improvement. The objective of this chapter is to describe monitoring as an evaluation tool. Consideration is given to the type of data on which monitoring is based, its application in various health settings, and its relationship to the various types of evaluation.

What is Monitoring?

Monitoring is the comparison between the program and expectations and involves the continuous endeavor to learn about all aspects of a process and to use that knowledge to improve the quality of the program. When the plan and expectations do not coincide, there are three courses of action: either the plan can be modified, the process can be modified, or steps can be taken to change expectations. In each case, data generated by the evaluation are critical to the decision.

A useful way to perceive monitoring is to view it in the context of general program activity. Figure 4-1 shows in a cybernetic schematic the five stages of program activity that are the primary subjects of monitoring as an evaluation activity. These stages are problem identification, program planning, program implementation, program output, and feedback.

Figure 4-1   Stages of Program Activity Subject to Monitoring

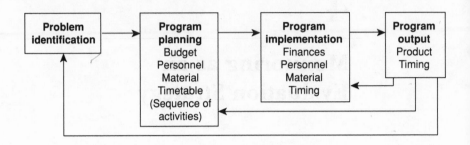

Problem identification and program planning

Monitoring has little to do with problem identification. But once a problem is identified and a program plan initiated, the issue of monitoring becomes critical. Any program plan is likely to address the six issues of *what, where, how, why, who,* and *when.* What is the program? Where will the program be implemented? How is it to be implemented? Why is it necessary? Who is to carry out the program? When is it going to be done? And how can it be improved? Monitoring is particularly concerned with the issues of *how, who,* and *when.*

The monitoring issues associated with these questions center on the specific sequence of activities that make up the program. A program to train new health auxiliaries, for example, may begin with the identification or establishment of institutions to provide the appropriate training, the definition and establishment of specific course content, and the identification of faculty to teach the courses. These activities may be followed by the admission of students to the curriculum, the actual training period itself, and the students' subsequent graduation. A continuing training program may then repeat the steps of student admission, training, and graduation any number of times. This is a very simple, but fairly clear, sequence of activities that must occur if a training program for health auxiliaries is to be carried out effectively. Obviously admission of students to a program that does not yet exist or graduation before training would be nonsensical. So any program plan must specify *how* the program is to be carried out—and hopefully how can it be improved.

The monitoring issues associated with the question *who* center on available resources: What resources will be allocated to reach the goals of the program? Resources are generally defined in terms of a projected budget but will also include structures, material, and personnel. A program plan to train health auxiliaries, for instance, must specify who will do the training and the amount of budget allocated to purchase training materials and training space. Monitoring efforts provide an opportunity to track whether these resources were allocated as originally planned.

Finally, the monitoring issues associated with the question *when* center on the actual timing of program activities. Specific techniques for planning, monitoring the timing of activities, and improving activities are the Gantt chart, PERT or CPM, and various statistical monitoring techniques discussed in detail in the next chapter.

Program implementation and impact

With the program plan constructed, including the budget, specification of personnel, specification of other resources, sequence of activities, and a timetable, the monitoring aspect of evaluation can be carried out. As the program is implemented, finances are acquired and expended in a specific manner, personnel are deployed, and material is used. All is done according to a specific sequence of activities and a specific timetable. Finally, through the implementation of the program, program output is generated. A specific product or products are produced, again according to an anticipated time schedule.

Monitoring is simply the activity of determining whether the finances are available according to the budget, whether the personnel of the program meet the personnel needs of the plan, whether the material available as other resources meets the plan specifications, whether the timing of activities follows the timetable of the plan, and whether the program output is produced as the plan projects. Few monitoring efforts consider all aspects simultaneously.

Effective monitoring requires a distinction between macroimplementation and microimplementation (Berman 1978). In macroimplementation the focus is on the process by which some sponsoring agencies execute policy so as to influence local delivery agencies as they operate the program, for example, the extent to which the National Cancer Institute or the National Heart, Lung, and Blood Institute would implement a particular program initiative dealing with early detection and prevention in a variety of communities. Microimplementation focuses on the individuals within one or more of the affected organizations and examines the nature of behavior and organizational change involved in actually operating the program in the respective locations. In addition to the actual unit of analysis, implementation must further distinguish between implementation as a process and implementation as an end point (Scheirer 1989). As a process attention is given to a series of repeated activities through which and by which services and activities are fully delivered. The extent of implementation or end point is the actual delivery of program activities. Figure 4-2 summarizes these various dimensions of implementation.

At both the macro and micro level, monitoring is critical to the implementation process and extent of implementation. Extent of implementation can be measured by counting the number of times a program is used, by counting resources consumed by the program, direct observation, activity logs, written questionnaires for providers and recipients of service, interviews with providers and recipients, or some combination of these.

The implementation process is more complex and is dependent on the particular disciplinary perspective employed by the evaluator. Scheirer (1989) suggests that three general approaches are available: political, organizational process, and individual/cognitive. Each perspective focuses on different elements of the implementation process. The political perspective emphasizes the way decisions are reached within the organization and how these decisions are communicated to individuals. Data are collected by using case studies of events associated with the process. The organizational process highlights the structure and process that facilitate the implementation process, and data may be gathered by use of case studies, survey methodology, or both. The individual/cognitive perspective presents

Figure 4-2   Dimensions of Implementation that Require
             Monitoring

		Measurement focus	
		Extent of implementation	Implementation process
Theoretical perspective	Micro	• Accuracy of delivery • Number and types of participants	• Individual or organizational delivery actions
	Macro	• Scope of use among relevant organizations	• Organizational links • System change

a fairly micro view of the implementation process emphasizing pre-existing attitudes of individuals involved with the process as well as training needs by individuals actually involved with service provision.

Once the program is implemented it is equally important that monitoring occurs to assure the continual improvement of the overall process, that is, to continuously endeavor to learn about all aspects of a process and to use that knowledge to change the process and thus improve overall service. Here attention is given to the identification of specific processes involved in the overall program that represent opportunities for improvement. For example, within a hospital, monitoring activities may be directed toward continually improving the nurse response time on various nursing units or reducing the antibiotic intravenous waste in central services. In monitoring these processes it is important to distinguish between "special causes" and "common causes" of variation. Common causes result from variations within the system. These are random variations even if the process is operating in accordance with its fundamental design. Special causes are deviations from the intended process specifications that are due to controllable, attributable, and nonrandom events. The role of management in the monitoring process is to distinguish between special and common causes of variation and to redesign the system to reduce variation in common causes (Deming 1986; Berwick, Godfrey, and Roessner 1990).

Limitations

Although monitoring is an important aspect of evaluation, its application to health service programs is subject to several limitations. These limitations are in part generic to the monitoring process and in part a function of the unique characteristics of health services. As described by Freeman and Rossi (1981):

> In the health services area, it is not easy to monitor most programs. First, the practice of medical care is rooted in the idea that "professionals" are responsible people, and it is regarded as insulting to question the performance of such professionals. This sensitivity of health professionals, of course, not only affects monitoring efforts but also day-to-day efforts at cost containment, maintaining quality of care, and increasing provider productivity. We may have come a long way from the sanctimonious position the physician had earlier in this century regarding privacy and autonomy, but cries of "interference" still persist when the turf of the provider is invaded.
>
> A second aspect is that monitoring, at best, is inconvenient; at worst, it uses up time and resources that providers feel should be devoted to "practice." (p. 365)

These difficulties have a direct effect on the monitoring process applied to health service programs. First, much of what might be considered monitoring may be carried out in a highly informal manner. Frequently a program manager will be aware of the finances and personnel available to the program, materials needed, and the timetable for conducting various tasks. If program inputs, process, or outputs do not adhere to the plan, the manager will probably intuitively recognize any discrepancy and consider this good management rather than evaluation. In programs that are not exceedingly complex or that involve a limited number of actors, it is possible that no formal monitoring activity is ever undertaken or, for that matter, needed.

As programs become more complex, as they involve more resources, as their expected products become more extensive or diffuse, program monitoring becomes increasingly important. With a large, relatively complex program, it may be exceedingly difficult for a single program manager, or even several managers, informally to maintain the body of information needed to keep the program on track. Under such circumstances formal monitoring systems and networks need to be established to facilitate the task of program management and decision making.

A second problem of monitoring is that although more complex programs are likely to require sophisticated monitoring efforts, the resources, timetable, sequence of events, personnel, and finances involved in a large complex program are likely to be much more difficult to measure and thereby monitor. Unfortunately, the dilemma is often resolved by ignoring or giving only limited attention to monitoring activities. A more realistic approach would be to focus on those areas where monitoring is feasible. It is likely, for example, that the budget specified for program activities, personnel, and most resources will be critical to program outputs and thus should be of concern in program monitoring. It may be less clear that a specific sequence of activities or a specific timetable or even certain outputs are either necessary or sufficient to produce longer-range outputs and outcomes that are desired from the program.

Third, monitoring of activities may become a substitute for program performance. Program evaluators who are actively involved in program monitoring must be careful not to make monitoring a substitute for the actual products desired from the program. In the area of family planning, for instance, monitoring the number of condoms dispensed may be useless if they are never used. Monitoring the number of contraceptive pills distributed may also be useless in attempting to ensure the expected outcomes of a program if they are used for a few days or weeks and then abandoned or are used in a highly irregular fashion. Monitoring the number of community hand pumps installed might be useless for ensuring the success of a safe water program if the people expected to be served by a particular water source continue to use other unsafe water supplies.

There must be a clear relationship between what is monitored and what is desired as a program outcome. In many instances, the outcome must be assumed even though it is not demonstrated clearly. But every effort should be made to monitor those aspects of the program related to desired outcomes.

Finally, when monitoring occurs, there is always the propensity to gather too much information or information in too great detail. The evaluator should be conscious at all times of the need for economy. Monitoring should refer to those aspects of the program directly relevant to decision making and not be conceived of as a general data collection activity to cover all aspects of program operations. This aspect is particularly critical, for data collection is expensive and always time consuming.

Appropriate Data for Monitoring

Data required for monitoring can be conceived of as being related primarily to inputs, process, or outputs. Figure 4-3 is a restructuring of Figure 4-1 that focuses specifically on inputs, process, and outputs. *Inputs* are the resources and guidelines necessary to carry out the program. *Process* is the specific set of activities, their sequencing, and timing for the sequencing, which actually represents program operation. *Outputs* are the products of the program, which consist of direct outputs, intermediate effects, and long-run or ultimate effects or outcomes.

To specify data needed for monitoring is a difficult task. Our first inclination is to say that data should be available about all aspects

Figure 4-3   Monitoring Focused on Inputs,
Process, and Outputs

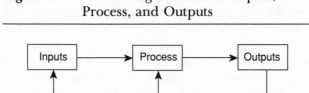

of program operation that bear on decision making. But such a statement requires clarification. On the one hand, the term *all* may not be descriptive enough to be useful in decisions about what specific items of information should be maintained. On the other hand, taking the term *all* literally may result in the collection and maintenance of data that will not be relevant to decision making either because such data simply do not bear on decisions required for the program or the collection of large amounts of data may overwhelm the evaluator's ability to process, analyze, and use it. Data needs for program monitoring within the areas of inputs, process, and outputs follow.

Data for monitoring inputs

All inputs to a program can be considered the resources by which the program is carried out. Resources, however, can be divided into a number of different categories.

1. *Finances*. It is useful to maintain records of the amount of money budgeted and subsequently of the amount actually allocated.

2. *Personnel*. Information to be maintained in regard to personnel might include the number of positions required to carry out the project and qualifications required for positions. Such a listing might involve specification of approved positions and the number under recruitment, characterized as either full-time and part-time positions or as full-time equivalents.

3. *Transportation and space (capital and rental)*. Transportation and space may best be characterized in terms of dollars available for transportation and for capital construction or rental. The category might also include specifics of expected trips— durations, costs, and times. Space requirements might be specified in terms of offices, laboratories, treatment rooms, or other categories germane to the project.

4. *Equipment and supplies*. The category of equipment and supplies will be quite program specific. The list of equipment and supplies as inputs to a primary care program will be quite different from the list for the establishment of an emergency medical services program or a managed care program. Nevertheless, certain categories are probably germane to any program-monitoring effort. In general, equipment will be considered relatively nondisposable; supplies, on the other

hand, are primarily disposable items. Categories for classifying equipment and supplies might include

- clerical equipment such as typewriters and dictating machines, disposable supplies such as paper, envelopes, and pencils
- laboratory equipment and supplies (for example, microscopes, slides, test tubes)
- service delivery equipment and supplies (for example, syringes, vaccines, bandages, well-drilling machines, insecticides, or whatever other equipment and supplies may be necessary to a specific program)

5. *Information guidelines.* Guidelines are standardized specifications for service (care) developed by a formal process that incorporates the best scientific evidence of effectiveness with expert opinion (Leape 1990).

Specific ways in which finances, personnel, transportation, space, equipment, supplies, and guidelines are broken down within categories and specific information kept within categories will be highly program specific. It will be an important task of the evaluator to work with program planners to determine (1) which categories of inputs are or will be useful for monitoring purposes, (2) which information should be maintained, (3) which categories will not be important in a monitoring effort, and (4) which information can be disregarded.

Data for monitoring process

The major pieces of information for monitoring program process will probably include specific activities to be carried out in completing the program, the sequence in which they are to be carried out, and their timing. The timing specification, for example, should also include the specification of use of resources, such as when specific expenditures will be made, when a certain number of inoculations should have been given, a certain number of fields sprayed, or a certain number of hospital expansion plans reviewed. Again in the category of process, the actual specific data elements to be maintained will be highly program specific. It will be important for the program evaluator to work closely with program planners and managers to ensure that important activities are specified, that their sequence is well specified, and that timing of this sequence is agreed on.

It is also important that every effort should be made to limit the amount of information to be collected and maintained to those pieces

Exhibit 4-1   Process Focus Worksheet for Food Delivery

In a hypothetical HCA hospital, the food delivery process works in the following manner. A patient completes a menu card which is sent by nursing personnel to the Dietary Department. Dietary workers check the menu card with the diet prescribed by the patient's physician and complete a food production sheet. The food production sheet is sent to the kitchen. The

What is a simple statement describing the process and its boundaries?

The food delivery process from the point the patient completes a menu card to the point a food tray is delivered to a patient's room.

Who is the owner of the process?

Dietary

Suppliers	Inputs	Actions	Outputs
Patient	Menu card	Send card to dietary	Food tray
MD	Diet order	Compare with diet order	
Food distributor	Food	Complete food production sheet	
		Prepare food	
		Assemble trays	
		Load cart	
		Deliver cart to floor	
		Deliver tray to room	

Source: Data used with the permission of HCA West Paces Ferry Hospital.

of information that are actually important in ensuring the operations of the program and its continual improvement. For example, in a hospital, the food delivery process is one component of the larger dietary program. In the process, a patient completes a menu card, which is sent by nursing personnel to the dietary department. Dietary workers check the menu card with diet prescribed by the patient's physician and complete a food production sheet. The food production sheet is sent to the kitchen. The food is then prepared by the kitchen staff, the patient tray is assembled, and the delivery cart is loaded. The cart is taken by dietary personnel to the patient's floor via the service elevator. The ward clerk checks the food on the tray against the order tray, and the tray is distributed by nursing person-

Exhibit 4-1 Continued

food is then prepared by the kitchen staff, the patient's tray is assembled, and the delivery cart is loaded. The cart is taken by dietary personnel to the patient's floor via the service elevator. The ward clerk checks the food on the tray against the order sheet, and the tray is distributed by nursing personnel to the patient.

Customers	Needs/Expectations	Key Quality Characteristics
Patient	Hot	Cold food complaints
	Correct	Disagreements with menu card
	Timely	Variance from schedule

nel to the patient. Exhibit 4-1 presents various designated inputs, actions, outputs, and indicators associated with the process.

Data for monitoring outputs

The outputs are the results of the program. Outputs can be classified in three types:

1. *Direct outputs*—such as specific services or goods provided by the program, for example, immunizations
2. *Intermediate effects* of direct outputs—impacts of the direct outputs, such as a person or population that is immunized
3. *Ultimate effects* of direct outputs—the purposes served by or

the usefulness of the impact, such as avoidance of economic
and other costs of the disease against which the persons have
been immunized (Schaefer 1973)

Direct outputs and the data necessary for monitoring them are
usually quite obvious. They are the actual items that the program is
to produce. In the case of an immunization program, it will be the
number of immunizations; in the case of a birth control program, it
may be the number of condoms dispensed or IUDs inserted; in a
cancer screening program, it will be the number of mammograms
provided.

Depending on the particular program, data to measure the intermediate effects or impacts of direct outputs may be relatively difficult to obtain in a form useful for monitoring purposes. If the intermediate effect of an immunization program is an immunized person
or population, for example, several factors may intervene between
the actual number of immunizations given (direct outputs) and the
existence of an immunized population (intermediate effects). In order for immunizations to be effective, a sequence of actual inoculations given at properly spaced intervals or to children of appropriate
ages is required. It may be very difficult to acquire and obtain the
data necessary to ensure that this sequence is carried out. Similarly,
there is likely to be a discrepancy between inoculations given and
immunized persons. An immunization program may inoculate a
number of children more than once. Consequently, other persons
may not receive immunizations. If 30,000 inoculations are given in a
population consisting of 30,000 children, it is still possible that only
90 percent of the children have actually been immunized. It should
be clear from this brief discussion that a serious effort to monitor
intermediate effects of even such a straightforward program as immunization requires a sophisticated record-keeping system.

Consider another type of program—for instance, one in family
planning and birth control efforts. The direct output might be numbers of condoms distributed or IUDs inserted or pills distributed.
The intermediate effect is the actual use of these birth control procedures or materials in an effective way. In one sense, a measure of
the extent to which these birth control measures were used effectively might be derived from a measure of the ultimate effect or
outcome for such a program: a change in the birth rate. It is possible,
however, to monitor effective usage by conducting an interview survey once or at several intervals on a sample of the population receiving birth control support. This interview could provide information

about the proper and continuous use of birth control methods as a way of monitoring intermediate effects of the program.

For hospital-sponsored primary care group practice, monitoring of intermediate and outcome effects presents a different type problem (Shortell, Wickizer, and Wheeler 1984). Here, intermediate outcomes are defined as provider productivity and provider turnover. Productivity as measured by the visits per full-time equivalent (FTE) provider is seen as critical to the development of a financially viable practice, to the meeting of the hospital's overall financial needs, and to its efforts to improve the organization of primary care services to the community. Physician turnover is likewise seen as influencing performance outcomes, particularly the ability to provide continuity of care.

The ultimate outcomes represent explicit criteria for measuring the effectiveness of the program. Generated from the major objectives of the program, ultimate outcomes represent the hospital's ongoing commitment to primary care, improvement in the organization of access to care, the degree to which group practice contributes to the overall financial health of the institution, and the degree to which the group practice itself is financially viable. For each of these, activities are monitored to provide evidence that these outcomes are, in fact, occurring. For example, to determine the hospital's ongoing commitment to primary care, the following activities are monitored over time:

1. increased number of primary care services provided by the group practice itself
2. increased number of primary care services provided by the hospital
3. development of spin-off programs such as satellite clinics over time
4. ongoing hospital sponsorship after the expiration of the grant that established the primary care group practices

Similarly, the ultimate measure of improved organization of access to care can be monitored by gathering data on such items as

1. net addition of primary care physicians to the community as a result of the group practice
2. development of after-hours service
3. transfer of emergency room patients to group practice
4. development of affiliations or relationships with family prac-

tice residency programs that would strengthen the hospital's ability to provide primary care

The ultimate effects or outcomes of a program represent its true justification. If the outcomes are not those desired, or are not beneficial at the very least, it is difficult to justify the program's existence. Monitoring, however, provides little information about the ultimate effects or outcomes of a program. For one thing, they are likely to appear well after a program is under way. Evaluation will probably have moved out of the process stage to which monitoring is appropriate and into the effectiveness and impact stages, which may be more effectively addressed by other strategies. Another reason that monitoring is seldom used to assess ultimate effects is that they may not be known or measurable at a time consistent with the program modifications with which monitoring is usually concerned. Finally, it is often impossible to measure the ultimate outcomes of a program with enough precision and clarity to make judgments about the program's impact per se on such effects. For example, mortality rates are irrelevant to evaluating ambulatory care, partly because death is such a rare occurrence, and partly because so many factors other than ambulatory care services influence mortality (Lohr 1988).

Despite these difficulties, it is still useful to discuss some of the data that might be involved in monitoring outcomes. These types of data usually focus on some aspect of health status. Health status is a difficult concept to define and even more difficult to measure. Nevertheless, we can talk about some specific proxy measures that provide approximate indicators of health status. The most readily accessible indicator, and the one often considered a proxy outcome measure, is mortality or mortality rate and its refinements, such as age-, sex-, and perhaps race-specific mortality rates. For example, this measure has been used by the Health Care Financing Administration (HCFA) in the release of hospital-specific mortality rates to identify outlier hospitals whose overall or diagnosis-specific death rates are higher than expected by chance after controlling for case-mix severity (*Federal Register* 1987).

A second general category of information useful for measuring health status is morbidity. In general, morbidity data will not be as readily available or as accurate as mortality data. Clearly it is difficult to maintain any type of accurate record on such items as venereal diseases or malnutrition conditions, items that may have a substantial impact on overall health and quality of life but that are almost impossible to measure effectively. On the other hand, it may be possible to maintain certain disease-specific morbidity data, particularly for diseases likely to be reported to public health or other authorities or diseases or conditions likely to be relatively clear at the onset. Diseases and conditions in this category might include various cancers, stroke, tuberculosis, and trauma. Other such indicators include disability and functional status (Lohr 1988). Disability indicators, including measures of premature retirement days of disability and work loss, are useful in tracking the impact of large-scale programs. Functional status indicators focus on overall health, attempting to assess physical and psychosocial dimensions of daily living.

If data on morbidity are maintained, it is desirable to have age-, sex-, and race-specific morbidity data for monitoring purposes. In addition, as disease data are maintained, it is useful to maintain them either as incidence or prevalence data. *Incidence* refers to the specific onset of a disease; *prevalence* refers to its actual existence in a population. Diseases of relatively short duration may have high incidence but low prevalence; diseases of long duration, on the other hand, may have low incidence and high prevalence.

In monitoring the outcomes of a program, it would be possible to maintain morbidity and mortality data over time and to examine continually the changes that occur in these data, if any. Although not a highly scientific test of the ultimate effect of a program, it provides at least some indication of whether the program does have an ultimate effect.

Data for Monitoring from Two Different Settings

To illustrate the type of data appropriate for monitoring, consider two different programs. Although differing in scope of activity and in purpose, each can benefit from various types of monitoring activity.

Illustration: Community clinical oncology program

The program is an organizational network initially designed to increase participation in National Cancer Institute (NCI) clinical trials composed of three major components: the individual community clinical oncology programs (CCOPs), the designated research bases, and the National Cancer Institute Division of Cancer Prevention and Control (DCPC).

The CCOP is the organizational unit for cancer control and treatment research at the community level. Specifically, a

CCOP is a working group of hospitals, physicians, and support staff, which can range from as few as one or two physicians and staff affiliated with a single hospital or office to as many as 50 physicians and staff affiliated with many hospitals and offices.

- Research bases can be NCI-funded cooperative groups, core grant cancer centers, or state health departments. Each CCOP may affiliate with up to five eligible research bases, only one of which may be a national multispecialty cooperative group.

- The Division of Cancer Prevention and Control is a constituent part of the National Cancer Institute, one of the National Institutes of Health. The division is responsible for overseeing the CCOP program through its associate director for centers and community oncology. The DCPC cooperates with the Division of Cancer Treatment in the protocol approval process and with other committees and units in NCI to oversee the quality and accountability of patient care for NCI-approved studies.

The CCOPs are led by a single clinician–principal investigator or coinvestigators who are responsible for the conduct of the CCOP activities. They are assisted by a data manager, usually a nurse specializing in oncology, who helps recruit patients and manages the flow of information and data between the research bases and the clinicians and the record-keeping sections of the component facilities. Additional nurse managers or coordinators are sometimes funded through the program, depending on the projected patient enrollment. One of the incentives built into the CCOP funding is support for travel expenses for the investigators, data managers, and other staff to attend the scientific and organizational meetings of the research bases. These meetings present opportunities for the staff to develop skills and provide scientific input to the development of specific protocols, and they reinforce CCOP commitment to the clinical trials network.

The goals of the program are fivefold:

1. Bring the advantages of treatment and other cancer control research to individuals in their own communities by having practicing physicians and their patients participate in clinical treatment and other cancer control research protocols.

2. Provide a basis for involving a wider segment of the community in cancer control research and investigate the impact

of cancer therapy and control advances in community medical practices.

3. Increase the involvement of primary health care providers and other specialists (for example, surgeons, urologists, gynecologists) with the CCOP investigators in treatment and other cancer control research approved by NCI.

4. Reduce cancer mortality by accelerating the transfer of newly developed cancer prevention, detection, treatment, and continuing care technology to widespread community application.

5. Facilitate wider community participation (including minority groups and underserved populations) in future treatment and other cancer control research approved by NCI.

The overall evaluation of the program focuses on three areas:

1. the implementation of the program in the selected areas

2. the impacts of the program within the communities

3. the characteristics of CCOPs, research bases, the NCI and their interaction that affect implementation and impact

The evaluation is a four-year longitudinal study examining environmental and organizational factors that affect the implementation of treatment and cancer control research in the CCOP network, and the impact of these activities on diffusion of state-of-the-art cancer care into community practice (Kaluzny et al. 1989). Implementation is measured by the ability of CCOPs to accrue patients to NCI-approved treatment and cancer control research protocols, the relative efficiency by which this is achieved, and the extent to which programs are institutionalized within their respective communities. Impact is measured by changes in practice patterns for selected disease sites (breast, colon, and rectum) and the readiness of primary care physicians to participate in cancer control research.

To assure that any changes documented in practice patterns or readiness of primary care physicians, or both, are in fact a function of the CCOP and not part of larger secular trends, CCOP community practice patterns are being compared to practice patterns in non-CCOP communities participating in the Surveillance, Epidemiology, and End Results Program of the NCI. Likewise, a national sample of primary care physicians is being surveyed and compared with primary care physicians located in the CCOP communities.

A range of organizational and environmental factors is being examined to characterize CCOPs, their designated research bases, and their interaction with NCI/DCPC to determine how these characteristics affect selected aspects of implementation and impact. Environmental factors include urban/rural setting, competition among local oncologists and hospitals, and basic demographic data about the community within which the CCOP is located; organizational factors focus on the structures and processes characterizing these organizations and their relationships.

This is obviously a complex program involving various approaches to evaluation. Monitoring is one part of the overall design. What are the pieces of information that might provide useful data for such monitoring vis-à-vis inputs, process, and program outputs?

Inputs

Initially listed in terms of finances, personnel, transportation, space, equipment and supplies, and information, inputs are not all equally relevant to a monitoring strategy. In terms of the community clinical oncology program, finances may be important only to the extent to which some programs are able to receive additional resources from other sources such as endowments at participating hospitals. Since this is an NCI-funded grant, all participating programs receive resources to fund a required set of personnel, provide for transportation, and pay for data processing costs. In this particular case, however, the critical input is the availability of protocols from research bases. While each CCOP is expected to accrue a certain number of patients to treatment and cancer control protocols, this accrual is contingent on the actual availability of such protocols to individual CCOPs. Thus, the principal investigator of a CCOP and the administrator of the overall program as part of a monitoring strategy would maintain a clear record as to the availability and timing of these protocols. Clear decision information from this particular monitoring effort would include the availability of the protocols, the lag times required for local clearance by respective institutional review boards, and whether they remain open for sufficient time for the individual CCOPs to accrue patients. For example, if few protocols are available and the individual CCOP has difficulty clearing these protocols within the local institutional review board process, corrective action might be required at both the research base and the local CCOP. Failure to take such action would result in protocols being closed before patients could be placed on protocols in local communities.

Process

The monitoring of process for this community clinical oncology program is somewhat more complicated. At one level, it is simply to monitor the extent to which patients are in fact being accrued to available protocols within the individual CCOP. At a more complex level, however, is the ability to accrue patients vis-à-vis the number of eligible patients for particular protocols; this requires a clear understanding of the number of eligible patients within the geographic area being served by the CCOP. Data, here, thus would include cancer incidence and demographic information for the CCOP communities.

Outputs

The primary output of the program is a change in physician practice patterns with respect to treatment of cancer patients within the local community. Three tracer conditions (5 breast, 1 colon, and 1 rectum) have been selected, and data are abstracted from the medical record within a subset of CCOPs. Specifically, data are collected for:

- women older than age 50 with localized breast cancer (Stage I–III), positive nodes, and ERA negative, and whether they are receiving chemotherapy
- women younger than age 50 with negative nodes and ERA positive, and whether they are receiving hormonal therapy
- women with localized breast cancer, and whether surgery is performed
- women younger than age 50 with negative nodes and ERA negative, and whether they are receiving chemotherapy
- women younger than age 50 with positive nodal status, and whether they are receiving chemotherapy
- men and women with operable Duke's B and C colon cancer, and whether they are receiving chemotherapy
- men and women with operable Duke's B and C rectal cancer, and whether they are receiving chemotherapy and/or radiation

Illustration: Primary health care program

Monitoring the implementation and operations of a primary health care program is a task of considerable magnitude and complexity. Successful primary health program efforts require serious planning effort, realistic allocation of resources, and continuing effective management practices. Monitoring as an evaluation tool can be extremely useful when applied to the development and implementation of a primary health care program. At the same time, monitoring a program of such magnitude is definitely not a simple or casual undertaking. Monitoring again should focus on program inputs, process, and outputs.

Inputs

Inputs to a primary health care program are basically the same categories described earlier—that is, finances, personnel, transportation, space, equipment and supplies, and information. Although a primary health care program is often viewed as a major program innovation by many health care organizations or many communities, it is not expected to need major budget allocation or budget shifts. Possible sources of expenditures or requirements for finances will include the recruitment and training of primary care personnel and the acquisition of initial supplies of limited pharmaceuticals, including materials for immunizations, contraceptive materials, and so forth.

A continuing assumption about a primary health care program is that a program, once initiated, will be financially self-supporting. This premise may or may not be realistic. In any case, an important source of data for monitoring inputs will be budget changes and modifications specifically for the purpose of implementing and operating the primary health care program and, as the program progresses, allocations of funds to specific budget categories. The decision point with regard to finances is the extent to which allocations reflect budget lines.

The basic personnel input for the primary health care program will be nursing and allied health personnel. The program will need to identify specific persons in the community to fill these roles and determine the extent to which they will require additional training to meet the objectives of the program. Data for monitoring personnel inputs should include information about the recruitment of individuals to staff various types of primary care activities, the extent of training required, and ultimately whether they are meeting expectations. Because primary care often involves teams of providers—physicians, nurses, and so on—monitoring should include information about the performance of the various teams. Such information will allow program decision makers to determine whether a given strategy for recruiting and training providers is working satisfactorily or if modifications must be made in recruitment, training, and placement policies.

Transportation is a major concern, particularly in rural programs. Public health personnel, for example, often indicate that a major portion of their time, perhaps as much as 80 percent, is used simply in getting from one point to another in the area that they are expected to cover. If part of the input to the primary health care program is some provision of transportation for primary health care personnel, data should be maintained on the number of personnel who have been provided transportation and, as the program progresses, on the number of vehicles in working order.

Similarly, the equipment and supplies category may be a continuing problem in primary health care programs. Many programs obtain initial supplies of drugs and other necessary items at no cost but are expected to replenish their stock at cost to the community, either by charging fees or by organizing collective community purchases. Whether or not such practice succeeds, an important component for monitoring inputs to the primary health care program will be the extent to which personnel have available a stock of required supplies. It is assumed, of course, that a standard set of supplies has been specified by a primary health care plan. If monitoring of available supplies shows that personnel are unable to replenish stocks under a particular strategy for doing so, such as purchases from local vendors with funds from fees charged to persons treated, then some strategy for modifying this approach can be developed.

A final input of concern to the primary health care program is information. A major type of important information will be a plan of implementation and operation. This plan will be critical in evaluating and monitoring the process of the primary health care program.

Process

At least three major areas of process deserve monitoring efforts:

1. the sequence of activities and time schedule for implementing primary health care services within a community
2. the protocol specifying which activities the primary health care personnel are expected and empowered to carry out
3. a continuing examination of the expenditure of funds and use of resources

The specification of a sequence for implementation and continuing operation of primary health care programs should be a major component of an overall plan for the implementation of primary health care in the community. Such a plan should specify major milestones, targets, or goals to be achieved at specific times: for example, when primary health care personnel will train, when primary health care programs will be staffed in a certain proportion of local centers, or when the program will be responsible for providing care to a given percentage of the population. The techniques of Gantt charting or PERT analysis, discussed in some detail in Chapter 5, are valuable for providing specification for the sequence of setup and operation. Data for monitoring process should include information about whether the various steps in the sequence have occurred; this information can then be compared to the plan and necessary modifications made if the sequence is not proceeding as desired.

A second major concern of the primary health care program should be the extent to which appropriate activities are being carried out. Many observers of the progress of primary health care are concerned because primary health care should cover all aspects of health, including education about sanitation, nutrition, housing, safe water supplies, family planning, treatment of disease, and provision of medical services. However, the majority of primary health care personnel are probably most heavily engaged in the diagnosis and treatment of disease and the dispensing of such drugs and pharmaceuticals as family planning materials. Observers note that this is both the major status-conferring activity for local primary health care personnel and the activity for which they are most likely to be reimbursed, either in money or in kind. Once recognized as a problem, it is probable that an important monitoring activity will be to maintain data on the types of activities carried out by primary health care personnel and the extent to which they spend their time in these various activities. One form of acquiring these data could be through direct reporting of activities by primary health care personnel. Doing so, however, may require a great deal of their time and may be viewed unfavorably. Nevertheless, a general reporting of activities on a weekly or monthly basis might be useful; if not too complex, a more detailed evaluation of what primary health care personnel actually do might require some type of survey approach. Characteristics of such an activity are discussed in more detail in Chapter 8.

An important aspect of the monitoring process will be the continuing expenditure of funds and use of resources. The budget, in conjunction with a protocol for expenditures, such as a Gantt or PERT chart, should specify in general terms times of budget expenditures, uses of resources at hand, and amounts to be used by these times. A reporting scheme must be devised to ensure that this information is kept on a routine basis. It could, of course, be the same reporting system used to keep track of inputs.

Outputs

Monitoring the outputs of a primary health care program can be discussed in terms of direct outputs, their intermediate effects, and their ultimate effects or outcomes. Monitoring per se, however, will be more concerned with direct outputs and, to a lesser extent, their intermediate effects than with ultimate effects.

The single most important direct output of a primary health care program will be contact between primary health care personnel and citizens of the community. These contacts will be the means through which common diseases and injuries are diagnosed and treated; appropriate and essential drugs and pharmaceuticals, including family planning materials, are dispensed; health education, including information about proper nutrition, basic sanitation, family planning, and maternal and child health, is provided; and immunizations are given. To monitor the extent of such contacts at the local level, to keep track in some consistent way of the nature of the contact—whether for diagnosis and treatment, dispensing of drugs and pharmaceuticals, health education, immunizations, and so on—and to determine whether the contact is appropriate, of high quality, and acceptable to community people will all be extremely difficult. Perhaps the most that can be done in this area is to ask the primary health care personnel to maintain a record of contacts and some record of their purpose. Despite the difficulty of obtaining accurate information, however, it would seem important to the success of the program in other communities to maintain records about the nature of contacts between primary health care personnel and community persons. This step would give an indication of the extent of local acceptance of the primary heath care program, the degree to which personnel are being used, and information on the range of services actually provided by the program.

Intermediate effects of direct outputs—that is, intermediate effects of contacts between the primary health care personnel and the community—are more difficult to measure and specify but may still at times be subject to monitoring as an evaluation approach. Records may be kept of certain improvements in such matters as water supplies and sanitation methods. Program personnel may keep records of the number of people immunized as a means of monitoring the immunized population. The use of basic family planning materials might be estimated for the community on the basis of supplies. Changes in diet that might lead to better nutrition could be followed. But generally it is probable that attempts to monitor intermediate effects of direct outputs would be both expensive and not overly effective. Possibly a more cost-effective approach to evaluation of intermediate effects might be some type of survey approach.

In general, it is also probable that any information about or evaluation of ultimate outcomes or effects of the primary health care program would best be approached either from a survey standpoint or on an experimental basis. An experiment, of course, would be extremely difficult, costly, and time consuming and would have little value for modifying day-to-day aspects of the primary health care programs; it will be discussed at some length in the chapter on experiments. For a more realistic evaluation of ultimate outcomes or effects on the community, surveys taken at two or more points in time may be more useful.

Application to Decision Making and Types of Evaluation

Monitoring as an approach to evaluation and its associated techniques are no more than good management. In fact, evaluation using monitoring techniques is a component of good management. Types of decisions that can be made and should be made as a result of a well-designed program-monitoring effort at the types of day-to-day management decisions that program managers are required to make during the course of a program to ensure its operations and continual improvement. These include that the program has available and uses all the resources necessary for its operations and improvement, and that the sequence of events is appropriate and appropriately ordered, and that anticipated short-term results are being generated. The relationship of monitoring to each of the five types of evaluation—relevance, progress, effectiveness, efficiency, and impact—is discussed next.

Relevance

In general, monitoring as an overall format and specific monitoring techniques have little impact on decisions about relevance. As discussed in Chapter 1, relevance is concerned primarily with the particular problem that a program should consider, how well defined the problem is, whether the appropriate agency is attacking the problem, and whether the planned program will actually have an impact on the problem. Monitoring is relatively weak in confronting any of these issues seriously. It can provide some limited output data that may serve to shed light on whether the program can produce a solution to the problem, but it is not capable of providing information about whether alternative programs would have produced better results unless the alternative programs are actually in place as well.

Progress

Monitoring can and does provide information for decision making about program progress. In fact, monitoring activity is primarily directed to program progress and efficiency. Monitoring provides systematic information about whether a program is going according to plan and is on schedule, the expected activities are being carried out in the manner they should be and at the appropriate time, and resources are being expended as they should be. Again, this may seem simply an aspect of good management. Although possibly true, it is also true that programs designed as part of more technically sophisticated evaluations involving applications of survey research or experimental design must be monitored to make certain that they are carried out as specified. The importance of this point can be seen from the following discussion.

Suppose that a relatively sophisticated experimental design has been devised to test the effectiveness and impact of one way of instituting and implementing primary health care as opposed to an alternative method. Such an experiment might involve undertaking the two alternative strategies in a sample of different communities or within selected areas in the same communities. A result that showed no difference between the two approaches (or perhaps more importantly, between the effort to establish a primary health care program and no activity at all) could have two quite different meanings. On the one hand, such a result could mean that, in fact, the programs are not different (or a program is no different from no program). Alternatively, it is possible that the primary health care program efforts were not carried out as designed. It is critical to a good evaluation study of the experimental type to provide for a monitoring of the program activities that will at least indicate the extent to which the programs have been carried out in the manner specified. Otherwise, negative results cannot be adequately understood.

Effectiveness and efficiency

Monitoring can provide important information for decision making about effectiveness. If effectiveness is considered the production of direct outputs, monitoring provides extensive information about whether expected outputs have been produced. As so well described by Freeman and Rossi (1981):

> In the human services field, when evaluation after evaluation indicated that programs more often failed to have any significant effects than to be successful in achieving their intended purposes, attention began to be given to an earlier question whether programs were being delivered as intended. After all, if a program is not being delivered, or is being delivered with changes that undermine its effectiveness, then it is no wonder that experimental or quasi-experimental evaluations arrive at the diagnosis of ineffectiveness. In human service after human service it was quickly found that program implementation was problematic; indeed, some programs were found not to exist at all after supposedly having been implemented; others were delivering treatments at such weak levels or in such transformed modes that the program could not be said to exist. (p. 364)

The monitoring format can also produce information regarding efficiency in the sense that it may be possible, if adequate records are kept, to determine average cost of a program for immunizations or the average cost of getting someone to schedule a clinic appointment under one form of communication or another. From the standpoint of efficiency, cost can be perceived as finances, or time, or some other resources.

Impact

The monitoring approach provides little or no information about program impact. In general, most programs are under way for a long period of time before any assessment of impact can be made. Moreover, an impact evaluation assumes the ability to compare program outcomes with outcomes of alternative programs or of no program at all. The monitoring approach does not take this factor into consideration.

In short, then, the importance of monitoring can be summarized primarily by saying that monitoring can be used (1) to detect when a program is not progressing or improving as designed, either in terms of inputs, process, or outputs; (2) to provide limited information about effectiveness and efficiency to the program; and in particular

(3) to ensure that the program is carried out in the manner in which it was designed. Two valuable results are that monitoring allows the evaluator's decision making to keep the program on track and permits a more adequate evaluation of effectiveness, efficiency, and impact via more sophisticated approaches of survey research or experimental design.

Discussion Questions

1. Why is monitoring often excluded as an approach to evaluation?
2. What are the strengths and limitations of monitoring as an evaluation strategy?
3. Select a health service program—for instance, an outreach program or well-baby clinic—and identify the critical input, process, and output indicators. How is this information helpful in the management of the program?

5

Monitoring Techniques and Interpretation

Monitoring may be done without using any formal data analysis methodology. Its primary analytical effort centers around a comparison of expectations to actual results. Although this area may seem intuitive and monitoring is possible on a relatively informal basis, a set of related techniques is useful mainly in monitoring and evaluating the sequence of events by which a program progresses and, to a lesser extent, in monitoring the costs involved in the sequencing of events. The objective of this chapter is to present these methodologies and illustrate their use in various health service programs.

Gantt Charts

A Gantt chart can be a significant aid in monitoring program activities in a way that will be useful and effective for decision making about that program. It provides a means of visually indicating the sequence of events or activities that make up a project as it proceeds through time.

Figure 5-1 shows an example of a Gantt chart. The chart illustrates the schedule of events through time that take place in the design and evaluation of a training manual for primary care physicians. The overall objective of the project was to facilitate the implementation and use of selected cancer detection regimes among rural primary care physicians (Kaluzny, Harris, and Strecher 1990). To meet this objective it was necessary to develop and produce education regimes for early detection of breast, cervical, colorectal, and skin cancer.

Figure 5-1   Sequence of Events for one Module through a Single
Testing and Evaluation

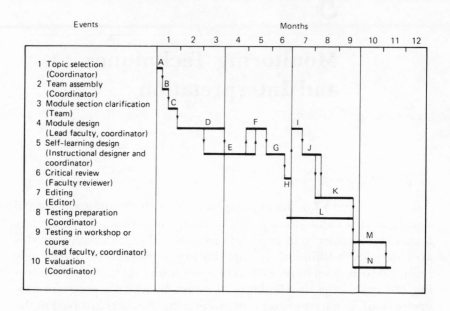

As the chart indicates, module development requires approximately 11 months. The wide horizontal lines represent the conduct of each specific activity to be carried out as part of module development. The thinner vertical-directed lines represent the flow of information. The first week of the 11-month development period is devoted to topic selection by the project coordinator. The second week is devoted to team assembly, and the final two weeks of the first month to clarification of the module with the team. The second month of the project begins with actual work in the design of the module, which continues intermittently through the seventh month. Concurrent with the design of the module but beginning in the third month of the project, the design of the self-learning materials will begin, and there will be a more or less free flow of information between the module design activities and the self-learning design activities. The last week of the sixth month will be devoted to a critical review of the learning module by a faculty reviewer, and preparation for testing the module will begin. Again, there will be input from critical reviews to module design, to self-learning design, and finally to editing. Testing begins in the final week of the ninth month and lasts approximately eight weeks. The last activity is an evaluation of the project.

Figure 5-1 is an idealized statement of how the process should be carried out. As such, it provides a useful monitoring tool. Knowing, for example, that the total development work for the module is to be completed in eleven months makes it clear that all development work must be completed by the ninth month if testing in an eight-week course is to be carried out. Other specific milestones of the project have similar relationships. A major value of the Gantt chart, then, is to allow the project decision maker to see easily the state of project progress at any point in time. To the extent that progress deviates from the projected schedule, modifications and adjustments can be made to meet that schedule.

A Gantt chart is relatively easy to formulate and can provide useful information in project or program evaluation. But its usefulness hinges on two factors. First, a Gantt chart is useful to the extent that it is realistic. Second, the usefulness of a Gantt chart depends, in large part, on the degree of control that can be maintained over the project.

If a Gantt chart is prepared primarily for the use of or to impress an external funding agency or as a requirement for the submission of a proposal, it will probably have little value in monitoring the project. If, on the other hand, it is prepared with serious attention to the problems of carrying out the aims of the program or project and a realistic schedule or timing of events, then it can be used for serious monitoring purposes. Such a chart does not require any special expertise for its construction, but it does need a fair understanding of the project, how it is to be carried out, and the realistic relationship of the various events.

A Gantt chart also assumes a substantial degree of control over project or program activities. Regardless of how realistic or well planned the activities and milestones may be, serious treatment of them for progress monitoring may be useless if the program coordinator is not actually in total control. In the module development example, the project coordinator needed to rely on faculty members —who have their own agendas and priorities—for module development, teaching, and evaluation. Consequently, a great deal of the actual conduct of the project is beyond the control of the project coordinator, and adherence to the specifics of the schedule for individual module development is difficult.

PERT and CPM

A natural extension of the Gantt chart is PERT (Program Evaluation and Review Technique) and CPM (Critical Path Method). PERT was originally developed by the U.S. Navy for the control of a Polaris missile project; Dupont developed CPM. Both PERT and CPM deal with exactly the same type of information as the Gantt chart. Although these two techniques have somewhat different origins, they are now quite similar in application and both deserve some discussion.

To employ PERT (or CPM) as an evaluation tool, the first step, just as with the construction of a Gantt chart, is to break the project down into a series of relatively self-contained activities. The breakdown of activities shown in Figure 5-1 is a reasonable classification to begin to develop a PERT network. Two activities, module design and self-learning design, however, are actually divided into three components each in the Gantt chart. In discussing the development of a PERT chart, it might make sense to see each of these three activities within module design and self-learning design as separate activities.

After the project is broken down into a set of relatively self-contained activities, the next step is to develop a precedence table for them. If we concentrate on the development of a teaching module as shown in the Gantt chart as the example, the precedence relationships for that project might be as shown in Table 5-1. The first activity (A) is topic selection, that is, what early detection regime is to be selected for module and self-learning design. No other activity precedes it. Activity B, team assembly, must be, according to this formulation, preceded by topic selection; presumably the structure of the team would depend on the topic selected. Then activity C, module section clarification, would necessarily follow team assembly, since the module section is clarified to the team. Activities D and E, module design and self-learning design, could presumably begin at the completion of module section clarification. Phase 2 of module design would follow phase 1, as phase 3 of self-learning design, and editing, would follow critical faculty review. Testing preparation need follow only team assembly, but testing in a workshop and course evaluation both must follow editing and testing preparation.

With such a precedence relationship established, a PERT network can be produced. A PERT network is constructed of circles that represent discrete events (such as the beginning of the project, the end of a specific activity, the completion of a report) and arrows that represent activities. Figure 5-2 shows an example of how events and activities are designated in PERT. The circled numbers 1, 2, 3, and 4 represent discrete events; for example, 1 might be the beginning of the project; 2, the specific point at which a first activity of the project is completed and other activities may begin; and 3 and 4, again points at which specific activities are completed. The activities themselves are represented by the arrows. Activity A requires two weeks; activity

Table 5-1   Precedence Relationships in Module Development

Activity	Description	Required Preceding Activities
A	Topic selection (Coordinator)	None
B	Team assembly (Coordinator)	A
C	Module section clarification (Team)	B
D	Module design (phase 1) (Lead faculty, coordinator)	C
E	Self-learning design (phase 1) (Instructional designer and coordinator)	C
F	Module design (phase 2) (Lead faculty, coordinator)	D
G	Self-learning design (phase 2) (Instructional designer and coordinator)	E,F
H	Critical review (Faculty reviewer)	G
I	Module design (phase 3) (Lead faculty, coordinator)	H
J	Self-learning design (phase 3) (Instructional designer and coordinator)	H
K	Editing (Editor)	H
L	Testing preparation (Coordinator)	B
M	Testing in a workshop or a course (Lead faculty, coordinator)	L,K
N	Evaluation (Coordinator)	L,K

B, five weeks; and activity C, one week. Activities B and C cannot begin until activity A is completed. This is the basic framework of the PERT network. Notice that the length of the arrow is not related to the time that the activity will require, as is the length of the horizontal line in a Gantt chart, but is arbitrary and selected simply for the construction of the network.

Using the PERT network conventions for events and activities

Figure 5-2 Example of PERT Events and
Activities

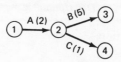

and relying on the precedence relationship shown in Table 5-1, it is possible to construct a PERT network for developing, testing, and evaluating a teaching module. Such a PERT network might be as shown in Figure 5-3. According to the precedence relationships from Table 5-1, activity A must precede B, as the network in Figure 5-3 shows. Activity C and activity L can begin after activity B is complete. Activities D and E can begin after activity C has been completed. Activity G may begin after activities E and F have been completed, and so on. The length of time required for each activity is shown in parentheses. The broken lines from event 9 to 10, from event 10 to 11, and from event 12 to 13 are known as "dummy" activities. They require zero time and zero resources. Their function is only to designate a precedence relationship. Dummy activities are always shown by broken lines.

The major value of a PERT network is the ability to determine what is known as a *critical path*. The critical path represents the sequence of activities and events that defines or determines the longest time from the start of the project to its end. The critical path for developing, testing, and evaluating a teaching module is shown in the PERT network in Figure 5-3 by the heavy directed line. The critical path for the development of the teaching module is 34 weeks.

Figure 5-3 PERT Network for Developing, Testing, and
Evaluating a Teaching Module

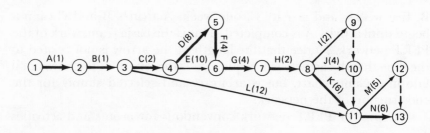

There are two advantages to knowing the critical path. First, given knowledge of the critical path, it is possible to recognize the critical path activities that must be completed on time if the project is to be completed totally within the 34-week period. Furthermore, it should be clear that if one of the critical path activities extends past its projected deadline by 2 weeks, other things being equal, the project will require 36 weeks.

A second value of identifying the critical path is that it allows the project coordinator to recognize activities not on the critical path. Activities not on the critical path, such as activities E, I, J, L, or M, are activities that provide a certain amount of slack to the project in terms of time and other resources. The critical path from event 3 to event 11, for example, is 26 weeks. Activity L, which must follow event 3 and precede event 11, requires only 12 weeks. This means that activity 11 can theoretically be stretched over a 26-week period if it is possible to carry out the activity on a part-time basis or if it can take place within any 12-week segment of the 26 available weeks. Either strategy might release personnel, financial, or other resources, which can then be made available to ensure that the critical path activities are completed on schedule.

Use of the module development project to introduce the PERT/CPM methodology is reasonable because it is simple enough for the relationships and sequence of events to be easily perceived. In real-life situations, PERT would probably be employed only in settings where the number of activities was so great and their precedence relationships so complex that the critical path activities and the set of noncritical path activities could not be determined by casual observation. Then it would be quite helpful to use computer programs designed to analyze PERT-type data.

Several modifications to PERT (or CPM) provide additional information to the planner and the evaluator. One approach to PERT, for example, uses a most pessimistic time period for completion of a task, a most optimistic time period, and the probable time period, thus providing a range for the project and for the value of the critical path. In many ways, this is a more realistic approach than a straight single-time estimate. CPM goes further and estimates the cost of completing specific activities within the estimated time period or the cost of "crashing" the activity by putting excess resources into the project and completing it in a shorter time period.

Regardless of the specific additions made to the basic PERT or CPM approach, it has much the same value for evaluation as the Gantt chart approach—that is, as a framework against which project directors, monitors, or decision makers can determine whether the project is moving forward in a timely fashion. To the extent that activities are not completed on time, the evaluator–decision maker has the option of redistributing resources to ensure the completion of various activities, particularly critical path activities, or of redefining the project.

Disadvantages of Gantt, PERT, and CPM

Gantt charts, PERT networks, and CPM appear, on the surface, to be useful tools for program monitoring and are requested by many funding agencies and apparently are widely used in various types of project development, but they do have some fairly clear shortcomings. First, in order to produce a realistic Gantt chart or PERT or CPM network successfully, program planners or managers must have a clear-cut idea of how to go from the point of beginning the program or the project to the point of completing it. Despite all the planning tools and the best intentions, it is often true that the activities that make up a project are so poorly understood or poorly specified that any Gantt chart or PERT network constructed on the basis of that understanding will be highly inaccurate. In this case, the manager must eventually try to reconcile the true state of affairs with the original plan. If unaware of the inaccuracy or naivete of the plan, he or she might be tempted to try to make adjustments in the project in order to adhere to a totally unrealistic plan.

A second problem of Gantt charts or PERT networks is that they are often constructed not for the purpose of program planning and subsequent monitoring but to impress a funding agency or higher-level management. Under such circumstances it is highly unlikely that they will have real value as a monitoring tool.

Input/Effort Analysis

Data from certain kinds of monitoring efforts might best be analyzed in terms of percentage of activity. Using these simple calculations, budget allocation by category can be compared to actual appropriations by category, which can be compared to expenditures by category. Again, such a comparison, particularly at the point of expenditures, would be most valuable if some type of timing for expenditure of funds could be built into the budget or allocation. Major divergences between allocations and budgeted amounts or between expended amounts and allocated amounts could be readily detected and corrective action initiated. This situation can be achieved by (1) establishing the cost of all resources mobilized for those services, (2) determining the work hours available of key professionals, (3) reflecting these costs or hours as a capacity to serve some number of clients per period of time, or (4) some combination of the above.

Illustration

An outpatient clinic has just been established in a hospital with an approved budget. Some staff members were transferred to the clinic and some were hired, equipment was purchased, and services were offered. At the end of the first six months the monthly cost of operation can be determined by accounting for all salaries, fringe benefits, medical and office supplies, utilities, travel, educational materials, maintenance, and so forth. The expenditures may be compared to the budget, the professional work hours available compared to the expected work hours, and the capacity to serve may be compared to the intended capacity.

A number of factors may have intervened, with the result that all did not appear to proceed as expected. Certain categories of staff may not have been transferred immediately; hiring new staff (particularly those in short supply) may take three to nine months; the stocking of materials and supplies may temporarily inflate costs; and other start-up expenditures or expenses may produce irregularities in monthly costs.

In such a clinical setting the ability to serve will depend on key professionals and the mix of those professionals. A particular service model may require that one receptionist, two physicians, six nurses, and one secretary be present 40 hours each week. If one physician is not present, the ability to serve clients may be cut in half. If one or two nurses are out, it may be possible (for a brief period) to serve the same number of clients but record keeping may suffer badly. The capacity of the service is therefore closely linked to particular professionals (the physician or the nurse) and less so to others. If a norm for a clinic service is assumed to be, for example, five clients per physician-hour, then the capacity can be computed as

$$2 \text{ physicians} \cdot 40 \text{ hours/week} \cdot 5 \text{ clients/physician-hour}$$
$$= 400 \text{ clients/week}$$

The number of clients who make appointments and come to the clinic, the mix of presenting symptoms, the experience and style of the professionals, the scheduling system, and other less critical factors will all affect the actual number of clients served in any week.

This form of input/effort analysis suggests what the clinic is capable of doing, indicates a commitment to a level of service, and provides information for control purposes (for example, we need to hire a seventh nurse because on the average only five are present in the clinic at one time and we need six). It does not guarantee that clients will be served at the capacity-to-serve levels; it does not look at quality of services directly (if in this example the norm were to be lowered to four clients per physician-hour, we might infer that the quality of services would be higher); and it does not consider treatment outcomes.

Performance Measurement Systems

Health service programs are more than a sequence of inputs that need to be monitored over time. As Chapter 4 indicates, health service programs involve a complex set of input, process, and output activities, along with a set of expectations as to what should be achieved by each of these activities. Performance measurement systems provide a technique for monitoring these various types of program activities and involve six steps (Hauver and Goodman 1980):

1. The analysis of program operations through the construction of a systems design. This step involves a careful analysis of the particular health service program in operation in order to divide it into its particular phases and activities.

2. The formation of explicit, quantifiable, time-limited objectives. *Objectives* are defined as statements of desired output—that is, definitions of desired changes in the status of target populations.

3. The development of indicators at appropriate program points to measure (a) activities performed, (b) progress of patients from target populations through the system to a desired end point, (c) costs incurred, and (d) indirect staff support activities. Indicators are established at specific points in the system to monitor program-related activities and their costs. For example, activity counts include the number of blood samples taken from patients; cost indicators are expressed in terms of allocated dollars or specific resources consumed by the program.

4. The construction of performance appraisal indicators that compare counts of patients from the target population who have reached specific points in the system to the number who should have reached that point.

5. The construction of staff support indicators that assess the contribution of the staff's indirect program services toward program objectives.

6. The construction of cost indicators that assess program costs in relation to program output. Cost-effectiveness indicators differ from activity efficiency indicators in that cost is related to actual program performance rather than simply to activities carried out.

On the basis of the systematic breakdown of a program into its constituent phases and activities, the pattern of patient flow through the system can be analyzed through the construction of four types of indicators: performance appraisal indicators measuring program progress toward attaining objectives; activity efficiency indicators measuring program costs in relation to activities; cost-effectiveness indicators examining cost in relation to activities performed by members of a predefined target population; and staff support indicators assessing indirect staff support activities for all patients processed, such as matching test laboratory results with the correct patient.

The approach has a great deal of potential and appeal to health service managers. First, it is comprehensive, providing managers with timely information about the various activities of the program. Second, because the approach is based on a firm understanding of the program and its specific components, it provides managers with specific intervention points and hence a mechanism to affect performance directly when problems are identified (Kotch et al. 1991).

Limitation

Many of the strengths of a performance measurement system are also its major limitations. First, the initial design and the establishment of explicit goals can be extremely difficult. The nature of health service programs and health professionals requires compromise, and so goals are often at a level of generality required to arrive at a consensus and are too general to be used to develop specific indicators of performance. Second, the amount of data collected and its level of detail are time consuming, and for many health professionals with an aversion to data collection, the effort required is overwhelming. Although the latter may not be a fatal flaw, for support systems may be introduced to gather appropriate data, the complexity of the system may adversely affect its adoption and ultimate use by critical decision makers within the organization. This point is particularly critical because many of these individuals are veterans of earlier versions of monitoring systems, such as Management by Objectives (MBO) or Program Budgeting System (PBS), and are skeptical, if not cynical, about the applicability of these approaches to health service programs. Finally, the quantification of goals limits the amount of improvement that can be achieved by the system (Deming 1986).

Quality Improvement Techniques

Monitoring provides an opportunity for not only assessing progress but also facilitating improvement. To see how quality improvement techniques might be applied, we will examine several such techniques as they might be applied to the delivery of noon meals in five hypothetical nursing units over a two-week period. The techniques discussed below include the run chart, the control chart, the checklist, the Pareto chart, the cause-and-effect diagram, and the flow diagram.

Run chart

A run chart is a simple display of the average time of the occurrence of the event of interest displayed over time. Table 5-2 shows the daily average delivery time of the noon meal for the five hypothetical nursing units for each day of the two-week period. These data may be converted to a run chart as illustrated in Figure 5-4. The run chart provides a very simple view of the average daily variation in the provision of food to patients in these nursing units. It is clear from the run chart that the last Sunday in the period was characterized by apparent late delivery of food. An examination of the run chart also reveals the less obvious fact that there is no clear pattern in variation of delivery time. For example, delivery on the first Monday was early, while on the second Monday it was late. Delivery on the first Saturday was also early, but on the second was virtually on the average.

Control chart

A control chart is an extension of the run chart that includes a statistically determined upper and lower limit for the normally expected variation. This was introduced in Chapter 4 as common cause varia-

Table 5-2 Food Delivery Process: Noon Meal Delivery Time

Day of Week	Delivery Time
Monday	11:30
Tuesday	11:35
Wednesday	12:00
Thursday	12:15
Friday	11:45
Saturday	11:32
Sunday	12:00
Monday	12:15
Tuesday	11:58
Wednesday	11:50
Thursday	11:45
Friday	12:03
Saturday	11:57
Sunday	12:56
Monday	11:35

Source: Data used with the permission of West Paces Ferry Hospital.

Figure 5-4 Food Delivery Process: Run Chart for Noon Meal Delivery Time

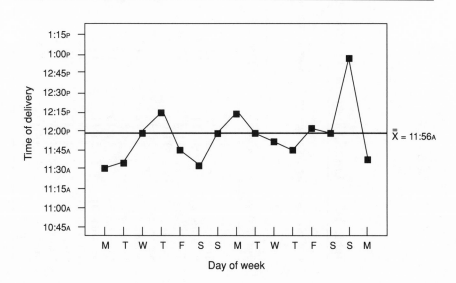

Table 5-3 Control Chart for the Process Average of Food Delivery Process: Noon Meal Delivery Time

1. Calculate the Average and Range of Each of the 15 Subgroups:

Day of Week	Floor 1	Floor 2	Floor 3	Floor 4	Floor 5	Average Time $\overline{X}$	Range R (minutes)
			Delivery Time				
Monday	10:45	11:01	11:27	11:55	12:22	11:30	97
Tuesday	10:45	11:11	11:41	12:05	12:13	11:35	88
Wednesday	11:11	11:37	12:02	12:30	12:40	12:00	89
Thursday	11:29	11:45	12:24	12:42	12:55	12:15	86
Friday	11:09	11:16	11:51	12:07	12:22	11:45	73
Saturday	10:46	10:58	11:39	12:02	12:15	11:32	89
Sunday	11:12	11:50	12:04	12:20	12:34	12:00	82
Monday	11:30	11:54	12:20	12:40	12:51	12:15	81
Tuesday	11:15	11:42	12:03	12:20	12:30	11:58	75
Wednesday	11:11	11:21	11:38	12:20	12:40	11:50	89
Thursday	10:59	11:25	11:48	12:10	12:23	11:45	84
Friday	11:17	11:39	12:04	12:30	12:45	12:03	88
Saturday	11:16	11:30	11:47	12:27	12:45	11:57	101
Sunday	12:10	12:46	12:57	1:17	1:30	12:56	80
Monday	10:48	11:13	11:38	12:00	12:16	11:35	86

2. Calculation of the Range Average ($\overline{R}$) and the Process Average ($\overline{\overline{X}}$):

$\overline{\overline{X}} = (11{:}30 + 11{:}35 + \ldots + 11{:}35)/15 = 11{:}56$

(Average of $\overline{X}$ column in 1)

$\overline{R} = (97 + 88 + \ldots + 86)/15 = 86$ minutes

(Average of R column in 1)

3. Calculation of Control Limits:

$UCL_{\overline{\overline{X}}} = \overline{\overline{X}} + (A_2)\overline{R}$ $LCL_{\overline{\overline{X}}} = \overline{\overline{X}} - (A_2)\overline{R}$

$\hphantom{UCL_{\overline{\overline{X}}}} = 11{:}56 + (0.577)86$ $\hphantom{LCL_{\overline{\overline{X}}}} = 11{:}56 - (0.577)86$

$\hphantom{UCL_{\overline{\overline{X}}}} = 12{:}46$ $\hphantom{LCL_{\overline{\overline{X}}}} = 11{:}06$

4. Table of Factors for $\overline{\overline{X}}$ Charts:

Number of observations in subgroup n	2	3	4	5	6	7	8	9	10
A_2 factors for $\overline{\overline{X}}$ chart	1.880	1.023	0.729	0.577	0.483	0.419	0.373	0.337	0.308

Source: Factors in section 4 taken from M. Brassard (1989, p. 289).

tion, which might also be reasonably assumed to be variation associated with random events. Variation that is outside the normally expected range might be considered to be variation that has been caused by some identifiable factor, and which might be controlled in the future if that factor is known. Construction of a control chart begins with the same data that used to create the run chart. The entire data set is shown in Table 5-3. Section 1 in Table 5-3 shows the actual delivery time of the noon meal for each nursing unit for each day of the two-week period, along with the average delivery time ($\overline{X}$) and the range (R) in minutes. Section 2 is a demonstration of the calculation of the process average ($\overline{\overline{X}}$) and the range average ($\overline{R}$). Section 3 shows the calculation of control limits based on these values and the factors shown in section 4.

Figure 5-5 presents the control chart for the noon meal delivery time with expected upper and lower limits included. This allows the assessment of the variations in delivery time relative to an expected level of variation. It can be seen in Figure 5-5 that all delivery is within expected limits except the noon meal on the last Sunday of the study period.

Figure 5-5   Food Delivery Process: Control Chart for Noon Meal Delivery Time

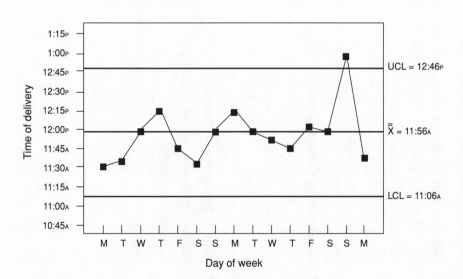

Checklist

The checklist is simply a form on which can be recorded all apparent reasons for the occurrence of a particular problem. For the food delivery situation, for example, a typical checklist might be as shown in Figure 5-6 for the nursing unit on floor 4 East. The checklist is completed by putting a mark in the appropriate category each time that a problem in food delivery occurs. Control and run charts provide data to track a process over time. The checklist provides information to assess why a particular run chart process may be occurring and what the important contributing factors are.

Figure 5-6   Food Delivery Process: Checklist

Date: 1/13/89 –1/19/89
Floor: 4 East

	M	T	W	T	F	S	S	TOTAL
Production sheet inaccurate	I	I				I		3
Menu incorrect	I		I		II		I	5
Diet order changed	I				I		I	3
Wrong order delivered	I		I		I	I		4
Patient asleep	III	I	ʼTHL	I	II	III	I	16
Patient out of room	ʼTHL	III	II	I	I	II	II	16
Doctor making rounds		II	IIII	I	I	II	I	11
Patient not hungry	I	I	II	I	III	I	ʼTHL	14
Cart faulty					I	I	I	3
Plate warmer broken	II	II	III	III	III	I	II	16
Heating unit broken	I	I			I		I	4
Thermometer miscalibrated	I					I		2
Nursing unavailable	III	II	III	III	III	III	III	20
Cart unavailable	II	III	II		II		II	11
Elevator malfunction			II	III		I		6
Tray mislabeled			I	I	I			3
TOTAL	22	16	25	14	22	18	20	137

Pareto chart

Data such as are provided by the checklist can be used to prepare a Pareto chart, a bar graph used to arrange information in such a way that priorities for managerial action can be established. Figure 5-7 presents a Pareto chart for the food delivery process showing the reasons that patients received cold food during a hypothetical January. The chart shows that nursing unavailability was the primary factor, followed by patients being unavailable. The Pareto chart includes a line graph that shows that all reasons for cold food are included in the chart.

Figure 5-7 Food Delivery Process: Pareto Chart

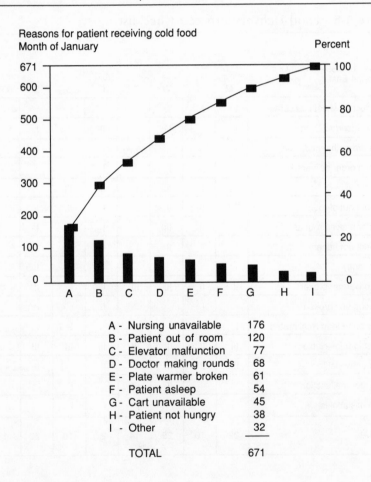

A - Nursing unavailable   176
B - Patient out of room   120
C - Elevator malfunction   77
D - Doctor making rounds   68
E - Plate warmer broken   61
F - Patient asleep   54
G - Cart unavailable   45
H - Patient not hungry   38
I - Other   32

TOTAL   671

Figure 5-8 Food Delivery Process: Cause-and-Effect Diagram
(Ishikawa Diagram)

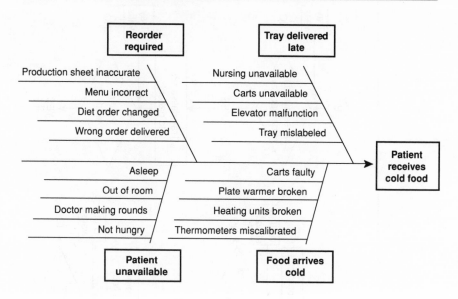

Cause-and-effect diagram

The cause-and-effect diagram is a graphic tool used to display all the factors that may produce a given effect. Often referred to as an Ishikawa diagram, this display provides information about the major contributing factors in any process variation. Figure 5-8 presents a cause-and-effect diagram focusing on food service delivery and outlines the major contribution factors associated with the patient receiving cold food. As can be seen from the diagram, major contributing factors include reorder required, tray delivered late, food arriving cold, and patient unavailable. Each of these is further broken down into subfactors.

Flow diagram

The flow diagram is a graphic representation of the flow of all actions involved in a given process. Such a diagram provides a detailed picture of specific activities involved in a process under study. Figure 5-9 outlines the flowchart for the food delivery process, providing insight into major events in the process.

Figure 5-9 Food Delivery Process: Flow Chart

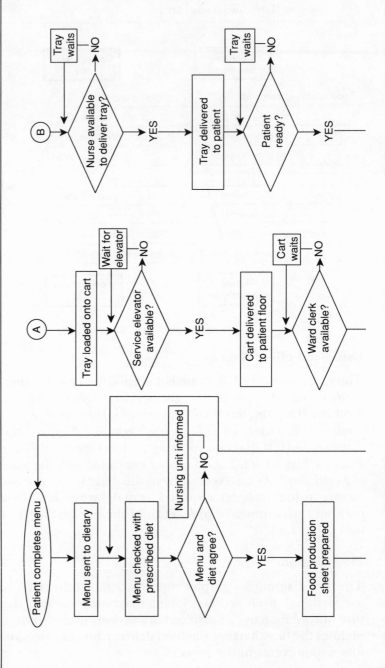

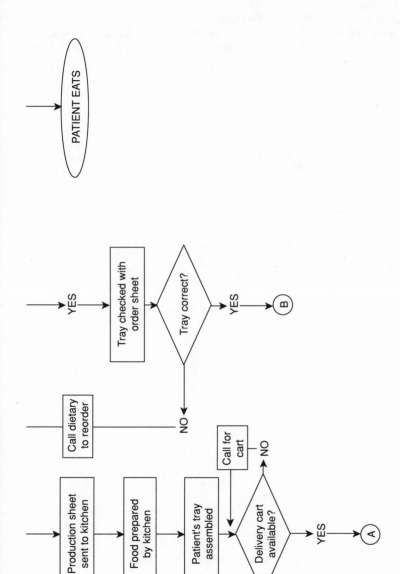

Discussion Questions

1. What are the similarities and differences between performance measurement systems and quality improvement techniques?
2. Select a health service program—or set of activities that you have been associated with—and develop a Gantt chart displaying critical activities.

Part III

Case Studies

6

Case Studies as an Evaluation Strategy

One of the most salient characteristics of the case study approach to evaluation is that it comes closer to being art than science. Although other evaluation strategies contain aspects that may be considered more rigorous, such as the use of sampling and statistical techniques for evaluation, case studies tend to rely more on the ingenuity, insight, and experience of the evaluator. The issue is not that other methods of evaluation are better than case studies, but rather that case studies provide a useful strategy for evaluation under certain conditions (Patton 1990). This chapter considers the appropriate settings for the case study, what can be learned from case studies, and what decisions can be made as a result of case studies.

What Are Case Studies?

A *case study* selects a single unique activity, organization, or entity for observation or selects one example from a number of entities, activities, or organizations for observation and bases conclusions on the observation of these items. This process greatly increases the amount and depth of information that may be collected over certain other evaluation approaches, but at the same time it limits the kinds of conclusions and decisions that case studies can produce. Even though case studies are essentially qualitative in nature, they use a variety of data collection methods and provide valuable insight to more quantitatively based evaluations. Here is a brief illustration of the case study as an evaluation tool.

Illustration: Cancer Control in the Rubber Industry

The design, implementation, and evaluation of a cancer control program at the worksite and the analysis of the factors that facilitate or impede that process is a complex undertaking. Using available material, memoranda, and correspondence as well as field interviews with program participants, a case study was devised to supplement the quantitative evaluation in two ways:

1. by describing program process and activities, that is, what actually happened at the work site
2. by identifying causes or determinants of program outcomes, that is, why things happened the way they did at the work site

Program

In 1983 the United Rubber, Cork, Lineoleum, and Plastic Workers of America (URW) was one of five unions selected by the National Cancer Institute to develop, implement, and evaluate cancer prevention education programs for their members. The URW subcontracted with the University of North Carolina to assist them in the development and evaluation of the URW-Developed Education Program (Kaluzny et al. 1987). The resulting educational project was named LIFE, an acronym for Labor and Industry Focus on Education. The LIFE program focused on the preventive actions workers could take to prevent cancer, which has a high incidence among rubber workers.

Evaluation design

The overall evaluation design was a prospective multigroup, pretest, posttest, experimental study of a sample of rubber-producing plants. A total of twenty-three plants were chosen for randomization into intervention and comparison groups. The plants were randomized into two groups based on work force size, product line, and company ownership. The plants within each were paired according to the size of work force; ten matched pairs of plants were obtained. One plant from each pair was randomly assigned to the intervention group; the other, to the comparison group. The remaining three plants were assigned to the intervention group—thus, thirteen intervention plants and ten comparison plants.

Program outcomes were assessed by mail questionnaires to a sample of labor and management personnel as well as by a series of tracking mechanisms designed to monitor the extent of participation in various components of the program. In addition, an in-depth case study was conducted in one intervention plant to focus on the following questions:

- To what extent did a project LIFE program actually occur?
- Specifically, what were the project LIFE activities during the one-year study period?
- Who were the key actors in conducting project LIFE activities?
- To what extent could the educational activities conducted be attributed to project LIFE versus some other factors?

The methods used to conduct the case study included

- three site visits, each lasting 2½ days
- participant observations of program activities
- interviews with key personnel
- analysis of a large number of documents

What can be learned?

The single case study provided important supplemental data to the overall evaluation (Steckler 1989). While the quantitative evaluation nicely documented that the LIFE intervention had relatively little impact on changing overall knowledge, attitudes, and belief on selected behavior patterns, the case study data provided insight into reasons for these minimal program effects. Each of these reasons can be viewed as threats to internal validity, with the first two being beyond the control of the project itself and the third suggesting that the program never really achieved a level of implementation sufficient to have an impact. Below is a brief discussion of each of these insights.

The first factor revealed by the case study was the fact that project LIFE occurred simultaneously with the implementation of the Occupational Safety and Health Administration (OSHA) Hazard Communication Rule. This rule required the creation of a federal standard for communicating information about hazardous chemicals to employees of chemical manufacturers and importers. In order to meet this federally mandated standard, the hazard communications training program totally consumed the energy and resources of the labor management representatives designated by project LIFE. In essence, the federal hazard communication activities precluded the union and management representatives from conducting the health promotion activities that had been anticipated by project LIFE.

The second factor revealed by the case study concerned the turbulence of the plant's environment itself. Many elements of the turbulent environment within the plant during project LIFE contributed negatively to health promotion activities at the work site including

1. the general decline of the U.S. rubber industry due to competition from abroad

2. the closing of several other rubber-manufacturing plants in the United States

3. a leveraged buyout of the parent company of the case study plant—and this was true of other plants participating in the study

4. rumors of the sale of the case study plant

5. sale of the chemical division of the case study plant's parent company

All these environmental factors preoccupied case study plant managers, workers, and union management representatives. As one worker said, "It is difficult to worry about lifestyle when you're worried about your job."

The third factor focused on the assumption of implementation, which in fact did not occur. The project itself used a "training the trainers" model; however, attendance and other monitoring data indicated that less than half of the intervention plants received full exposure to the various training events. The lack of exposure to training occurred because some labor and management representatives could not attend the training sessions; moreover, there was considerable turnover among both labor and management representatives. Lack of exposure to training, combined with turnover of plant representatives, led to great attenuation of the effects of training.

Appropriate Settings for Case Studies

The case study is a way of acquiring a great deal of information about a single program, either as a representative of a type of program activity or as the only one of a kind. In either instance, the case study will generally be carried out in a single organization or program. Case studies may be undertaken at any time. Unlike experiments or survey research strategies, case studies need not be planned or anticipated at the beginning of a program or started at the time of program implementation. A case study is a particularly useful tool when evaluators and practitioners want an insight into the entire working of a program. In this form the case study provides both detailed and extensive knowledge of selected aspects of a program or their operations and a broad overview of the total program.

A case study, unlike other forms of evaluation, is often exploratory. Very little may be known about a particular program by people or organizations that must make decisions regarding its level of funding, staffing, or even continuation. A case study can serve as a good source of initial information that may prove sufficient for decision making about the program itself or may provide the basis for the design of a monitoring system or for survey research, either of which may in the long run produce the evaluations of interest. A case study can even be the first step in setting up an experimental design to answer questions about the effectiveness, timeliness, adequacy, or impact of a program.

On the other hand, a case study does not necessarily need to be purely exploratory. The extensive, although often subjective, knowledge that a case study produces can be quite effective in providing an initial appraisal of the extent to which the program conforms to planning design and its overall impact and effectiveness. It must be remembered, however, that most of the information derived from a case study will be subjective, and decisions will be based on information collected in the absence of any control group.

Limitations

The case study approach has several problems that limit its use in a number of settings: lack of clear categories, selective perception, and interactiveness.

The lack of clear categories can be remedied fairly well by clear thought prior to the study about the issues that require decisions and the specific information that must be obtained to allow these decisions to be made. Once a series of questions has been established, the categories for information should follow.

Selective perception is not only a problem of how the answers to questions are perceived and recorded but also one of initial formulation of questions as well. To avoid the problem at the formulation stage, it is desirable to pretest the questions, along with the reasons for asking them, on a few people who can react to the appropriateness of the questions for producing the information desired. In the actual study situation, selective perception of answers can be avoided somewhat by the chance to ask for clarification, and sometimes even by restating the response in terms that the evaluator understands so that misperceptions may be corrected. Although this approach still leaves room for problems of perceptions, it is an effective data collection procedure.

Interactiveness is clearly a problem in the case study setting. Although observation is a means of obtaining data about program activity in a more or less natural setting, the observation itself immediately creates an unnatural setting. Because the case study creates an unnatural setting, evaluators must be very careful in interpretation of their observations. If so, knowledge gained in the case study approach may not differ markedly from the true situation.

A major problem of interactiveness is the difficulty of actually measuring its effect on study results. Except in highly controlled situations, most effects of interactiveness cannot be assessed. It is impossible to tell how much of an answer is real and how much was produced simply because the question was asked.

In a way, it might be easiest to discuss the appropriate setting for case studies as being inappropriate settings for other types of evaluation. Case studies are often carried out where no initial planning was conducted for evaluation before implementation of the program. No comparison groups were set up, or no criteria for inputs, process, or outputs were established by which to evaluate the program. The case study, then, frequently becomes the only strategy available for conducting an evaluation of a program. Other more positive statements that can be made about the case study approach are discussed later.

Appropriate Data for Case Studies

Almost any type of data is appropriate for case studies. The data collected in the course of a case study may include observation of program activity, reports prepared by the program, unstructured conversations with program personnel, statistical summaries of program activities, structured or unstructured interview data, or information collected through formalized questionnaires.

Because the case study as an evaluation strategy is most effective when its purpose is to provide information for decisions best made in the light of a general overall view of a program, any source of data may and can be used. Data collected through the case study approach are apt to be submitted ultimately to a subjective and impressionistic type of analysis, and so any type can be successfully incorporated.

A broad distinction in types of data that might be collected through the case study approach would be the classifications of subjective and objective data. *Subjective data* could include such information as might be collected through participant or nonparticipant observation and unstructured interviews. *Objective data* might include information collected from organization or program documents and records, or structured or closed-ended questionnaires and interviews. This distinction is not perfect. There is clearly a subjective component to questionnaire data no matter how rigorously collected and an objective character to nonparticipant observation at its best. Nevertheless, the general distinction is useful. Specific treatment of interview and questionnaire data, particularly of the structured and closed-ended type, is described in the chapter on survey research, for this approach depends almost entirely on these two forms of data collection even though they are applicable to the case study. Discussion of the use of organization documents and records, including organization statistical reports or program reports, appears in the chapter on time series analysis. The section here deals primarily with the subjective data of case studies—the informal and unstructured sources of data, such as participant observation, informal discussion, and open-ended questionnaires.

Participant and nonparticipant observation

Observation, whether participant or nonparticipant, might be thought of as the primary source of information. Participant observation is a strategy that received wide usage among anthropologists in the latter part of the nineteenth and early part of the twentieth century. It is essentially a strategy by which the researcher becomes a member of, and lives within, a given society. Such a strategy could be used for program evaluation when the evaluator assumes a working role within the program or organization being evaluated and collects data about it while working in the group.

Nonparticipant observation is a strategy seldom used in research per se but frequently used in evaluation. Under this approach a team of experts reviews and examines the workings of an organization or program for a period of time.

Although nonparticipant observation is more effective in serious evaluation work, both participant and nonparticipant observation have problems, some common to both and some greater problems for one or the other. These problems parallel the limitations of case studies mentioned earlier and are loosely characterized as three types. The first is the problem of cataloging and categorizing observations. The second is the problem of selective perception. And the third is the problem of interactiveness. Selective perception is a clear problem in participant observation. Interactiveness is a clear problem in nonparticipant observation. The problem of lack of ways for cataloging and categorizing observations is a general problem in both approaches.

If an evaluator comes to a particular problem on an exploratory basis, without much information about the program, it is probable that early observation will be largely unstructured and resulting data may not be easily classified in ways that will be useful to the evaluation. To avoid this situation, it is critical even in exploratory stages to have a clear understanding of what the evaluation is to accomplish, what decisions are to be made as a result of the evaluation, and what information must be obtained to make them. If not thought out in detail at the outset, the result is likely to be a random set of observations, all seemingly unrelated to one another or to the evaluation issue of concern.

The problem of selective perception is in many ways a mirror image of the problem of a lack of clear means for cataloging and categorizing observed activities. Under the best circumstances a set of selective categories to define needed data and classify observations is extremely useful to any evaluation study. It is natural for observers automatically to note actions or occurrences to which they have been sensitized by cultural values or learning and to classify them in preexisting categories. To a certain extent, this situation is desirable. It greatly limits the number of phenomena that need to be observed and permits rapid and fairly effective handling of those that do. Although selective perception permits conscious preselection of phenomena for observation, it has clear problems as well. It is often responsible for missing important aspects of program operation that do not fit predetermined categories. It may also contribute to interpreting program activities incorrectly. Possibly the most undesirable aspect of selective perception is that the preconception that a program may work in a certain way or be relatively successful or unsuccessful may produce what is known as the *self-fulfilling prophecy*. Consider a program evaluation concerned with a training program for health managers. The evaluator may believe—perhaps subconsciously—that a problem of such training programs is that they lack practical content. Here, the evaluator is likely to look for evidence of lack of practical content and to find it. The evaluator's initial perception becomes one of the findings of the evaluation, even though it might not have been true.

The self-fulfilling prophecy is an important source of invalidity in experimental evaluations and surveys, as well as in observations and structured interviews. But it should be noted that because the process of collecting data through observation and unstructured interviews is highly subjective, it is extremely difficult to avoid the problems of selective perception and self-fulfilling prophecy when data collection consists of observation or unstructured interviews.

A third problem of observation is interactiveness. It occurs because an observer, whether participant or nonparticipant, is rarely anonymous. While researchers or evaluators are observing and recording what is going on in the program, they are also, by their presence, affecting and shaping those activities. The results of an evaluation involving observational methods, especially over a long period of time, may be influenced as much by the observation technique as by the program itself.

This is not to suggest that other evaluation techniques do not also have some interactive characteristics. Both surveys and experiments can be interactive and will be discussed in subsequent chapters. The distinction, however, between interactiveness in case studies and other approaches is that it can be protected against in the case study or expert evaluation less easily than in other evaluation approaches. Surveys and experiments provide the quantitative basis for assessing interactiveness. Such a basis is not present for case studies, and thus the evaluator using case studies must be particularly careful.

Unstructured interviews

Observations and interviews can be used effectively together to obtain a great deal of information about a program. It is unlikely that a case study would be carried out that did not combine both observations and interviews, at least in practice if not by design. The same types of problems that occur with observation occur with unstructured interviews.

Even though this approach to data collection is referred to as unstructured, every effort should be made to determine before the interviews begin precisely what information is to be obtained. It may take the form of a checklist of specified items about which to ask or a series of roughly worded questions that can be paraphrased. At the very least, several leading questions to direct the conversation to the important issues should be determined ahead of time. It is probably best to have a brief checklist of points to cover and questions to raise arranged in a logical sequence and then to try to adhere to this sequence. Such a sequence may somewhat reduce spontaneity, but it will help to guarantee that all (or at least most) major points are covered. In an interview it is easy to get away from the main subject or to forget or skip points of importance, particularly for persons who are not highly experienced in the technique.

Data for Case Studies from Two Different Settings

To give additional specificity to the data appropriate to case studies, consider again the community clinical oncology program and the primary health care program discussed in Chapter 4.

Illustration: Community Clinical Oncology Program (CCOP)

While the CCOP evaluation was designed to monitor the ability of new organizational forms to accrue patients and to change physician practice patterns, an equally important function of the evaluation was to explain the dynamics of these organizations and their relationships with research bases and NCI—in effect, the why and how of what is happening.

The case study was a preferred strategy to meet this objective. Twenty CCOPs were selected along with five research bases for in-depth site visits. Each site represented a specific case study in which specific individuals were interviewed. A template outlining required data items was developed, which provided guidelines for interviewing the principal investigator, data managers, participating community physicians, administrators from participating hospitals, and representatives from relevant community organizations. Substantive areas that provided the organizational framework for each case study included CCOP goals, CCOP organizational structure, clinical trials, management procedures, physician relationships, component/ affiliate relationships, organization of cancer control research, research base relationships, NCI/DCPC relations, relationships with community groups, relationships with community physicians, environmental factors, and emerging issues and other significant factors.

Based on these site visits twenty CCOP cases and five research bases cases were prepared. For each group, the identified cases were reviewed comparatively in order to identify patterns for each of the substantive areas, for example, goals, physician relationships, etc. Exhibit 6-1, which follows the discussion questions, presents a listing of patterns that were identified based on the comparative review of selected case studies. These patterns were used to develop a series of hypotheses for testing based on data from the larger study and provided the basis for a dialogue with National Cancer Institute (NCI) program administrators about the various managerial actions to enhance program performance.

Illustration: Primary health care program

A case study of a community's effort to implement a primary health care program is an opportunity to evaluate the inputs, process, and outputs of an entire community's efforts. What we discuss here is in the traditional mold of case studies. If used as a primary evaluation strategy, a case study will probably be conducted by an external agency with some interest in the activity, such as an external funding agency or technical assistance agency. Probably, too, if the case method is the primary evaluation tool, evaluation will come after the fact, at least in the sense that the primary health care program will have been attempted and be under way before any evaluation is planned or carried out.

Despite the after-the-fact nature of the case study as opposed to a strict monitoring effort, all information appropriate to monitoring the implementation of primary health care would also be potentially useful in evaluating the program via a case study. It would be particularly useful, for instance, in a case study evaluation of the primary health care effort to know about the extent to which inputs of finances, personnel, transportation, space, equipment, supplies, and information were allocated to the program as it progressed. Such information might be collected directly from program records or acquired on the basis of structured or unstructured interviews with knowledgeable informants in the program. The same type of information might be useful for process and output data. Records of the sequence of activities and time schedules for implementing the primary health care program—those specifying the activities that primary health care personnel are expected to carry out and those on the expenditures of funds and use of resources—would all be of interest to a case study, as would systematic and recorded information and indications of the production of various types of services.

In addition to the information that could be acquired about general program aspects, appropriate to monitoring through the case study, other information acquired through the case study approach would bear on the success, adequacy, or effectiveness of the primary health care program. Simple observation of health service activities within the community could provide a great deal of data about the everyday working and effectiveness of the program. Such observation, of course, would be subject to the problems of selective perception and, more importantly, interactiveness; nevertheless, it provides substantial data for evaluation purposes. Of particular importance might be an assessment of the types of health service activities carried out by nurses and nurse practitioners, the volume of their work, the extent to which their work includes the full range of activities considered primary, and the acceptance of the program by physicians and other health providers in the community.

Extensive additional information about the primary health care program could be obtained through unstructured discussions and interviews with program personnel, community leaders, local physicians, and program clients. Such information could involve perceptions about the program's effectiveness, of problems and opportunities raised by its organizational structure, and about the expectations for the program's future success. Interviews or discussions with personnel directly involved could provide substantial and extensive information about the problems faced in delivering services, transportation, space and resources, community acceptance of services, and, again, the opportunities and advantages perceived for the future. Discussions with local clients themselves could produce information about the program's acceptability and accessibility and about the areas in which it is perceived to be most successful, requires additional effort, or is unacceptable. Such discussions and interviews could produce information about the things local people feel a primary health care program should do and not do, their perceptions of gaps in health care services, and a broad range of other types of similar information.

It would be possible to conduct highly structured interviews with primary health care personnel and community leaders as well as individuals served by the program. This information, too, would be valuable to the conduct of a case study. Because such information is discussed extensively under the heading of survey research, it is not considered further here.

Application to Decision Making and Types of Evaluation

Under the right circumstances perhaps more can be learned through the case study method than through any other evaluation technique. Because the evaluator is not bound by either a specific data collection methodology or a specific set of analytical techniques, the scope of a case study can range broadly across all aspects of program activity. The case study approach allows the evaluator to probe into areas of specific interest and obtain a wealth of detail about the operation of specific programs.

The major limitation of a case study in terms of producing knowledge is the absence of any technology for establishing the causal importance of a particular program. Because there is no comparison between settings in which a program does or does not exist, there is no formal way to assess its causal effect. Even when such evaluations are made in case studies, the number of factors that could be responsible for any apparent causal effect is quite large and uncontrollable. It is impossible in a case study to provide statistically a mechanism for the elimination for possible causal variables. There is no way to ensure that no other factor except the actual program itself was responsible for changes that may have taken place.

On the other hand, the case study is a relatively inexpensive way of acquiring information about how well a particular program works, plus subjective knowledge about whether it is performing according to expectations. The extent to which decision makers can have confidence in the kinds of results that a case study produces and can base decisions on such a case study lies very much in the realm of the extent or degree of their confidence in the objectivity, ability, and competence of the evaluators. Certainly, however, many important program decisions have been made on the basis of case study evaluations.

To consider the decisions that can be made on the basis of case studies and with what degree of confidence, it is useful to return to the five types of evaluation: relevance, progress, efficiency, effectiveness, and impact.

Relevance

The major issues raised in regard to relevance are as follows: Is there a problem that a particular program should confront? How clear is the problem if it exists? And how well defined is the problem? Examining the nature of the problem, determining whether it is of sufficient magnitude to warrant some type of program, and delineating the nature of the program needed to solve the problem are all issues amenable to the case study method.

Suppose, for example, that the health status in certain communities is low. A case study might be undertaken in one community or an area of a community to determine which factors lead to low health status and which programs might be useful in attempting to improve health status. Such an exploratory effort is an appropriate use of the case study approach. It should provide information about health problems and shortcomings in health systems and other systems that may lead to high rates of morbidity and mortality.

It is unlikely, however, that such a case study would point clearly to any specific solution. In primary care, for instance, the primary care worker would solve general health problems. It is more likely that a case study of this type would identify a broad range of factors leading to poor health outcomes, many of which would be related, others unrelated, some working in opposite directions to one another, and many about which nothing can be done.

For any conclusion from a case study to be an appropriate strategy for solving the problem it would need to be drawn from extensive information, including both the evaluator's initial subjective impressions and also perceptions grafted onto the study by the evaluator, community experts, or decision makers during the course of the work or afterward. In essence, a case study could identify a number of areas in which problems exist but would only coincidently lead to the conclusion that a primary health care program might be the appropriate mechanism for attacking them.

Progress

The case study approach can also provide information on the question of progress in a health services program. Progress, again, concerns whether inputs, process, and outputs meet some type of normative predetermined standards for their level of operation or success. Very often, however, if a case study is to be used to address the progress of a health services program as an alternative to uninterrupted monitoring, it probably means that the types of standards required for a good monitoring have not been thought through or determined at the outset. As a result the case study generally becomes both an examination of the program and an effort to set reasonable performance standards for the program as the examination is going on. Much can be learned from such an activity, but standards set as a study progresses are likely to be influenced by the actual performance of the project, thus removing the basic objectivity that could exist in the study situation.

Efficiency

The chief concern in an evaluation of efficiency is whether the results obtained by the program could have been obtained less expensively.

In the most rigorous sense, a case study cannot evaluate efficiency simply because there are no comparisons between what is produced under a given program and by a given process versus what it costs to produce the same results by using some other strategy. The fact is that a case study is the study of a single example of the program with no comparison group available. Still, it is possible for a knowledge-able person involved in a case study situation to make judgments about the extent to which the program is operating efficiently. These judgments, of course, must be based strictly on the experience and knowledge of the evaluator or evaluation team and cannot be based on comparisons with other operating programs. Yet such results can be useful in suggesting that a program is or is not operating efficiently and should or should not be modified in more efficient ways.

Effectiveness and impact

Effectiveness determines whether the program has produced what it is expected to produce, and impact determines the program's long-term consequences. It is quite possible, using the case study approach, to determine whether the aims of the program in the short run—the effectiveness aspect—have been met. It may be more difficult to examine the long-term consequences unless the case study is conducted at a time that allows a fair retrospect in regard to the program. If such is the case, then results accompanying the existence of the program can rather readily be perceived. The major problem, however, in evaluating either effectiveness or impact from a case study is that it is impossible to tell if major results of interest would have been obtained whether the program of interest had existed or not.

Discussion Questions

1. Why is a case study considered more an art than a science?
2. Under what conditions would the case study be an appropriate evaluation approach? An inappropriate evaluation format?
3. Why is interactiveness a particularly difficult problem in case studies? How might the problem be avoided or at least minimized?

Exhibit 6-1 Organization Patterns for Cancer Control Research among Four CCOPs

CCOP 1	CCOP 2	CCOP 3	CCOP 4
CCOP principal investigator, physicians, and staff believe that the current *structure is adequate* to deal with cancer control research. Do not anticipate adding behavioral scientists to Institutional Review Board.	*Organization for cancer control protocols* is essentially the same as for conducting clinical trials. Cancer committee reviews cancer control protocols (two have been approved), and executive director, ½ of data manager's time and protocol nurses are the mechanism for implementation.	With so few cancer control protocols available, *no one is sure what kind of organizational structure will be needed* for cancer control research. To date, the CCOP has only participated in a few cancer control companion protocols.	The *data management system in place for clinical trials could also be used for cancer control research.* Additional staff may be needed to maintain the longitudinal data necessary for patient follow-up.
Assume *nurse data managers would have a primary role* in cancer control because "they are better at educating patients" (yet current data management staff is overburdened with clinical trials work).	Expect future involvement in cancer control protocols to expand if protocols are "*nurse-driven*" and require little physician involvement (i.e., nurses will have to take major responsibility for identifying and enrolling patients and carrying out protocols).		
Both *hospitals* are involved in considerable cancer	*Hospitals* sponsor most prevention and screening ac-	*Component hospitals* have a history of involvement	Several of the *member hospitals*, as well as CCOP

control activity (e.g., free mammograms for employees, cancer education for employees, smoking cessation programs, breast exam education, colorectal screening). CCOP *physicians* are involved, but CCOP does not cosponsor.

tivities independent of the CCOP.

with cancer awareness programs, screening activities, and support groups that may help the CCOP to implement cancer control research studies. These programs have been conducted *independent* of the CCOP. Mobilization of primary care physicians for cancer control research may be facilitated by their previous involvement in hospital-based coronary heart disease studies.

physicians, have been involved with smoking cessation programs, screening mammography, and cancer support groups as well as activities jointly sponsored with the ACS. CCOP sponsorship of cancer control activities would require that all six hospitals be involved. This is not seen as feasible because it would interfere with individual hospitals' marketing plans.

Frustrated over *scarcity of cancer control protocols* from their research bases. Protocols that are available are specific to very limited patient populations.

Due to a *lack of available* protocols, the CCOP has put cancer control activities on the "back burner" waiting to see what will happen.

Very few protocols are currently available. The principal investigator indicated that the suitability of cancer control research for his CCOP depends on "good science and good questions." If both criteria are met, the CCOP will actively participate.

Two main barriers to this CCOP's participation in cancer control research: (1) lack of "appropriate" protocols, and (2) the physicians' dislike of the length of time for this type of research to demonstrate results.

Continued

Exhibit 6-1 Continued

CCOP 1	CCOP 2	CCOP 3	CCOP 4
IRB has approved three cancer control protocols for use at both hospitals. Also have eight open treatment protocols with cancer control credit of 0.1 that are appropriate for very limited populations.	IRB has approved *one* breast self-examination protocol.	One physician noted that the idea of cancer control research is still rather ambiguous and that their research base has committed itself to cancer control research on a "to be determined basis" (i.e., what constitutes cancer control will be determined as the program unfolds).	
CCOP *developed a cancer control concept* over a year ago. Research base keeps sending the draft protocol back for statistical adjustments. When they expressed their concerns about the slow implementation process to NCI, they were advised to "get out of the business of developing cancer control protocols" because there would soon be plenty available.			Nurses are developing a cancer control concept for one research base.

See low accrual credits assigned to cancer control protocols as a problem due to difficulties in finding patients and the minimum accrual requirements set by NCI.	Concerned about meeting NCI's cancer control accrual requirements because *so little credit* is assigned for each patient. Confused about how much credit they will receive for future cancer control protocols.	Principal investigator is concerned about low accrual credits for cancer control protocols. At 0.2 credits/patient, it would take 250 patients to get 50 credits.	
Hesitant to publicize cancer control research until they have something to offer.			
Changes in research base policies that would stimulate more cancer control research: More protocols that are relevant and involve large numbers of patients (e.g., primary care physicians see a lot of cervical dysplasia patients).	*Changes in research base policies that would stimulate more cancer control research:* There is a need for protocols that address "timely or critical questions."	*Changes in research base policies that would stimulate more cancer control research:* Need for "doable" protocols" (i.e., protocols that are scientifically valid, that ask good questions, and that have reasonable follow-up periods). Doubts that there will be enough "doable" protocols for all 52 CCOPs.	*Changes in research base policies that would stimulate more cancer control research:* Need protocols with interventions that are appropriate for community oncologists to implement.
The CCOP has just developed guidelines for off-site protocol participation to in-	*No preparatory work being done with community physicians or groups.*	*No contacts have been made with primary care physicians.* However, the PI estimates	The good relationships that CCOP physicians have with primary care physicians were

Continued

Exhibit 6-1 Continued

CCOP 1	CCOP 2	CCOP 3	CCOP 4
volve primary care physicians in future cancer control research. Their quarterly newsletter goes to all primary care physicians in the area. Steering committee is currently discussing how much emphasis to give to developing relationships with primary care physicians vs. more general public education efforts. Until more protocols are available, they prefer to concentrate on developing general community awareness of cancer prevention and control.		that ⅓–½ of the general internists at his hospital would be interested in participating in cancer control protocols. (An internist who was interviewed doubted that he would have time to keep the detailed records required.) *Incentives for primary care physicians:* (1) data management support, (2) opportunity to participate in research base continuing education, (3) coauthoring or receiving acknowledgments on publications. Financial inducements are *not* expected to be effective.	seen as a facilitating factor in the recruitment of subjects for cancer control research. Residents at one hospital attend presentations on the CCOP. Primary care physicians also learn about the CCOP at tumor conferences.

The CCOP has refrained from publicizing its activities so as not to appear to be advancing the special interests of any component hospital. This "anti-publicity" norm may make it difficult to inform area residents of cancer control research and to recruit subjects for cancer control studies.	Chairman of the local ACS chapter indicated that the ACS would be unlikely to cosponsor cancer control activities with the CCOP because of competition between the hospitals. Same is true for the local hospice. *Cancer control research is of "marginal interest"* to the high accruing physicians. Principal investigator and associate principal investigator were not particularly enthusiastic about cancer control research. Given the perceived lack of coordination from NCI and the lack of enthusiasm among the physicians, it appears that the CCOP would not participate in cancer control research without the RFA requirement.

Source: Working paper used to prepare McKinney (1989).

7

Case Study Techniques
and Interpretation

Because much of the data gathered through a case study approach is qualitative, analysis and interpretation tend to be highly subjective. Yet a few techniques are available to help the evaluator add structure to the data collection effort and analysis as well as guide the interpretation. Success depends on the evaluator's ability to fit endless bits of information into an overall picture that has meaning, relevance, and clarity. Perhaps more than any other evaluation approach, case studies depend on a multimethod approach to data collection and analysis. The objective of this chapter is to consider techniques that help structure the analysis and interpretation of data collected in a case study format.

Observational Techniques

When data from a case study are limited to unstructured observations or informal interviews, analysis also remains relatively informal. In general, analysis of data collected through observations and unstructured interviews requires careful sifting, cataloging, and recombining by the evaluator rather than application of specific analytical techniques. The evaluator must bring an objective eye and a creative mind to the interpretation of the data.

To increase objectivity and permit the application of simple quantitative techniques while maintaining the exploratory quality of the case study, it is possible and often advisable to use a variety of more structured forms of observation (Miles and Huberman 1984). One approach is *structured observations,* in which the evaluator develops categorical schemes during and after the observation. Using this technique, the evaluator is influenced in the coding process not by previous research or personal experience but by the events observed. The approach couples the flexibility of an open-ended or unstructured observation and the discipline of a structured evaluation. It provides an opportunity to understand things we may know nothing about. The approach is nicely illustrated by Bosk's (1979) study of surgeons.

Illustration: Controlling failure (Bosk 1979)

To determine how a group of general surgeons control deviance and failure, three types of data were collected over an eighteen-month period: (1) participatory observations, (2) written evaluations of house staff by attending surgeons included in personnel folders, and (3) interviews. The participatory observations were straight-forward, descriptive observations and provided the basis for the development of categories, interpretation, and hypotheses. They also provide the basis for returning to the field for further observations and the resolutions of problems identified in this initial analysis. Essentially the process included a series of iterations—involving the processing of raw field data, recoding, tabulating, coding and recoding, and analyzing these results until a conceptualization appeared. The laborious procedure provided a content that resulted in development of a meaningful and extremely insightful analysis of a process we know nothing about. The description challenges some of the most cherished beliefs about physicians in general and surgeons in particular.

Another approach is to a priori define the data categories based on some underlying conceptual model or theory. Consider the following example involving an evaluation of the implementation of a program in which a conceptualization guides a data collection process.

Illustration: Institutionalizing health promotion programs (Steckler and Goodman 1989)

By developing a model of institutionalization to explain the general processes by which health promotion programs become institutionalized, data drawn from interviews, observations, and program documents are used to examine how consistent each program operation is with the conceptualized model. The study examined ten cases of health departments involved with the implementation of a variety of health promotion programs. The data were applied to a technique termed *pattern matching*, in which the model was compared with the actual operations of the program. In pattern matching, empirically based patterns are compared with predictor patterns, and data from each case are assessed to determine if they support a set of theoretical propositions that are formulated as questions. If the case information matches the conceptualization, then internal validity is enhanced; the greater the number that match the conceptualization, the greater the external validity.

Use of Existing Information Systems

Programs routinely collect information about their operations. Much of this information is in aggregate form—number of clients served, number of visits made by type of people, and so forth. Many programs, however, collect information on patients' visits through the use of encounter forms. The specifics may vary, but information usually includes patient characteristics, diagnostic classification, treatment, and level of provider skill.

Because these data are collected routinely on all patients, they are generally available in standard form over a relatively long period of time. This availability permits a thorough and structured assessment of patterns and trends about a single program. The availability of this type of data, for example, permits the assessment of resource use and a detailed analysis of the types of patients served and their clinical problems. Consider the following use of existing data systems to facilitate evaluation efforts and enhance decision making.

Illustration: Joint Commission on Accreditation of Healthcare Organizations—Agenda for Change

By monitoring and evaluating selected patient care and support service activities using data routinely collected by the organization, it is possible to identify key tractable variables that influence the quality of patient care. The Joint Commission on Accreditation of Healthcare Organizations (JCAHO) through its "Agenda for Change" has initiated a program that identifies specific performance issues within a health care organization that requires more intensive review (JCAHO 1990).

Using a series of task forces, each was assigned the responsibility of developing indicators associated with various clinical areas and with the ongoing managerial operations of the organization. Clinical indicators included such areas as oncology, obstetrics, and anesthesiology. The organizational indicators task force developed measures associated with major functional areas of the organization, such as human resources, system processes, quality-of-care monitoring and evaluation activities, and financial resources. The indicators were based on data from major information systems. For example, within the area of organizational indicators, and specifically human resources, it is possible to track the following indicators thought to be related to quality:

- Nursing separation rate
- Stability rate: organizationwide for nursing and for ancillary, diagnostic, and therapeutic services
- Vacancy rate in selected key positions
- Turnover in selected key positions
- Unplanned absenteeism
- Nursing overtime rate
- Percent of nursing hours worked by contract nurses
- Nurse-patient staffing ratios

Similarly in the area of system performance, indicators include

- Turnaround time for selected diagnostic tests/procedures
- Average wait time in the emergency room for selected patient outcomes
- Turnaround time for selected lab tests ordered stat
- Average patient transport time to a more intensive level of care

Initially defined as separate from clinical indicators, organizational and managerial indicators have now been integrated into the overall clinical medical framework (Schroeder 1989). Obviously the critical challenge is to understand the relationship between organizational indicators and clinical outcome indicators. The JCAHO, as part of this program, is currently engaged in a rigorous pilot-testing scheme that will assess not only the feasibility of using these various indicators, but also their empirical interrelationships. While this is an extensive and ambitious project, use of existing information systems provides a convenient and relatively inexpensive assessment mechanism for ongoing operations. Because of the longitudinal nature of the data, the basis is provided for developing management strategies to continually improve organizational performance.

Illustration: Small area variation (Wennberg 1984)

By analyzing data contained in health insurance records such as Medicare, Medicaid, and Blue Cross–Blue Shield claims systems and hospital discharge facts, it is possible to monitor performance of health service providers/organizations in given geographic areas. The data should first be used to determine the geographic origin of patients who seek care at specific hospitals. Three kinds of reports are generated from this data base:

1. status of resource allocations to specific communities, that is, the number of hospital beds, expenditures, and hospital personnel, or the number of physicians invested per capita in the health care of the local communities

2. utilization of specific services for surgical and diagnostic procedures and for causes of admission

3. consequence of using particular treatments in terms of outcomes, for example, estimates of survival and complication rates following the use of specific treatments

These monitoring efforts based on existing information systems provide the basis for feedback on practice variations and outcomes targeted to critical decision makers within the communities, such as state medical associations, specialty societies, individual hospitals, and their physician staff. As a result of its visibility, this monitoring effort provides a unique opportunity to reassess decision making both at an overall policy as well as individual level and thus to reconsider the indications for specific services.

Existing information systems provide a convenient and relatively inexpensive assessment of resource use. Because of the longitudinal nature of the data, it provides the basis for developing management strategies to enhance performance.

The use of existing information systems is not without problems. Two problems need specific attention. First, whenever the evaluation is based on existing data, the evaluation is obviously limited to what exists. Often what exists is not directly relevant to the critical questions of the evaluation and what may be the intention of the decision-making process. Second, existing data are subject to coding or classification changes that further limit their utility. This latter problem is particularly critical, for often these classification changes become known only after considerable effort has already been invested in the evaluation process.

Tracer Methodology

To provide some focus to the case study format, particularly as it concerns program performance relating to the quality of care provided, evaluators may wish to structure the observation in data collection efforts around some particular disease entity. These particular disease entities are known as *tracers* and provide a framework for evaluating the interaction between providers and patients in their environment. The following criteria are considered appropriate for the selection of tracer conditions (Kessner, Snow, and Singer 1974):

1. A tracer should have a definite functional impact.
2. A tracer should be relatively well defined and easy to diagnose.
3. Prevalence rate should be high enough to permit the collection of adequate data from a limited population sample.
4. The natural history of the condition should vary with the use and effectiveness of medical care.
5. The technique of medical management of the conditions should be well defined for at least one of the following processes: prevention, diagnosis, treatment, or rehabilitation.
6. Effects of nonmedical factors on the tracer should be understood.

With few exceptions (Deuschle et al. 1982), the use of tracer methodology has had little application in the study of single programs or organizations. When it has been used, it has provided an opportunity to study thoroughly the provision of services within a particular organization. The approach, however, is time consuming, requiring a systematic effort to select the tracer and to designate criteria associated with the evaluation, diagnosis, treatment, and follow-up of patients with the tracer problem, as well as developing consensus among relevant providers in the program to the developed criteria. Once these criteria are developed and accepted, data are abstracted from the medical record to determine the extent to which actual care provided by the program matches that established by the criteria. Work to date indicates that use of tracer conditions is a feasible approach for the repeated assessments required in a thorough case study analysis of program performance.

A special application of the tracer methodology occurs in the development of sentinel events and its application to examining access to care in communities (Arnold et al. 1987). *Sentinel events* are medical conditions and stages of conditions that indicate a lack of access to acceptable quality primary care. These may be of three types:

- existence of the condition (for example, all children should be immunized against measles and should not contract the disease, yet occurrences of the disease reflect that there exist some barriers to accessing this particular immunization program)
- stage of the condition (for example, diabetes and hypertension)
- higher than expected rates (for example, the prevalence of low birth weight in infants, while never disappearing, can be reduced)

In a study designed to assess the utility of sentinel events four criteria were used for selection:

- The sentinel event is well defined and the condition can be easily diagnosed.
- Primary care patient management is effective in preventing, treating and controlling the conditions.
- The sentinel event must be observed in the population.
- Data are routinely collected on the condition and might be made available in many communities within reasonable cost and time constraints.

Using data from Maryland, Massachusetts, and North Carolina, sentinel event methodology was assessed to address two questions:

- Does the sentinel event method identify areas that are possible areas of underservice?
- Can sentinel events be used to target resources to specific at-risk population groups?

The results of testing indicate that this methodology has a great deal of utility: The method did identify areas with apparent health status problems and was an effective planning tool to help target resources and services to specific population groups.

Content Analysis

Case studies frequently use available memoranda, documents, and reports routinely generated by the program under study. Content analysis provides an unobtrusive and flexible method for studying and analyzing these types of communications in what can be a systematic, objective, and quantitative manner, although the technique is difficult to master and is seen by some observers to be as much an art as a science (Marshall and Rossman 1989). While few evaluations have used content analysis (for example, Kanouse et al. 1990; Wortman, Vinokur, and Sechrest 1982), it provides a useful technique for resolving the following types of evaluation questions (Holsti 1968):

1. *To describe trends in communication content.* For instance, what are the major clinical or managerial issues receiving attention in the program?

2. *To relate known characteristics of sources to communications they produce.* For instance, are individuals or programs with one set of characteristics likely to produce information with an orientation/content different from individuals/programs with a different set of characteristics?

3. *To analyze forms or styles of persuasion used within a program context.* For instance, was the implementation of a program the result of a coercive versus a more conciliatory attempt to influence behavior?

Perhaps the most critical problem in the use of content analysis concerns the selection and definition of categories, the pigeonholes into which content units are to be classified. There are many possible schemes for classifying content. A list of possible schemes for classifying data frequently used in content analysis follows. Because there are as many schemes as there are possible questions, they are neither exhaustive nor do they define the limits of content analysis (Berelson 1952).

"What is said" categories:

- *Subject matter.* What is the communication about?
- *Direction.* How is the subject matter treated (for example, favorable–unfavorable; strong–weak)?
- *Standard.* What is the basis on which the classification by direction is made?
- *Values.* What values, goals, or wants are revealed?
- *Methods.* What means are used to achieve goals?
- *Traits.* What are the characteristics used in describing people?
- *Actor.* Who is represented as undertaking certain acts?
- *Authority.* In whose name are statements made?

- *Origin.* Where does the communication originate?
- *Target.* To what persons or groups is the communication directed?
- *Location.* Where does the action take place?
- *Conflict.* What are the sources and levels of conflict?
- *Endings.* Are conflicts resolved happily, ambiguously, or tragically?
- *Time.* When does the action take place?

"How it is said" categories:

- *Form or type of communication.* What is the medium of communication (newspaper, radio, television, speech, etc.)?
- *Form of statement.* What is the grammatical or syntactical form of the communication?
- *Device.* What is the rhetorical or propagandistic method used?

It is difficult to discuss content analysis in the abstract, for the process is highly dependent on the particular problem under study. The following illustrates the use of content analysis to identify the variations in the content and style of a number of National Institutes of Health (NIH) consensus statements in order to determine what impact they have on subsequent dissemination.

Illustration: Content analysis of NIH consensus development statements (Kanouse, Winkler, Kosecoff et al. 1990)

As part of a much larger evaluation assessing the overall impact of the NIH consensus development program, an effort was taken to systematically examine the content and style of NIH consensus statements. The content analysis performed two functions:

1. Examining the variation in content and style of the actual statements provided an opportunity to select certain conferences for intensive study.
2. Examining how statements vary provided an opportunity to assess how this might bear on how the statements were in fact received by the physician community.

Content analysis was performed on 24 of the 30 conferences held between the beginning of 1979 and the end of 1983. Conferences covered a wide range of topical areas including antenatal diagnosis; estrogen use and postmenopausal women; cervical cancer screening: the pap smear; Reye's syndrome: diagnosis and treatment; liver transplantation; etc. Each of these were coded for selected attributes, including the treatment setting in which they were used, their physical nature, their medical purpose, and stage of development. Given this fairly macroclassification, attention was then focused on the content of the statement itself. Here each sentence of a consensus statement, beginning after the introductory material, was separately coded. The coding was on a multihierarchical basis as follows:

A. Recommendations
   1. Medical Care
      a. Global (applying to all patients) versus differentiating
      b. Concrete versus abstract
   2. Research
   3. Nonmedical
B. Declarations about Topic
   1. Research references
   2. Assertions
C. Contextual Comments
D. Other

In addition each item was separately coded and combined into a rating of consensus judgment. An agreement score was developed and assigned to each code item as follows:

1. *Unanimity.* All coders agreed on a coding category.
2. *Agreement about recommendations.* There was agreement that an item was a recommendation but there was disagreement which subcategory it fit into, or alternatively, there was agreement that the item was not a recommendation but disagreement as to whether it was a contextual comment, an insertion, or reference to research.
3. *Partial agreement.* Two raters agreed on a specific item but the third disagreed.
4. *Disagreement.* All three differed.

Analysis revealed a great deal of variability in both the characteristics of the conferences and the content of the consensus statements. Consensus conferences varied evenly between hospital-based and office-based medical procedures despite the office of medical research applications mandate to evaluate emerging technologies that focused on new expensive hospital-based procedures. Even more interesting was the analysis of the content of the consensus statements, which varied across content areas. Using a factor analytic approach, analysis revealed that it was possible to characterize the various statements on three dimensions: discursive, didactic, and scholarly. Discursive statements tend to be long and abstract and contain few specific recommendations for clinicians. Consensus statements characterized as didactic offer clinicians practical and detailed guidance, while scholarly statements offer up-to-date descriptions of the scientific evidence bearing on a topic and develop more attention than most statements (Kahan, Kanouse, and Winkler 1984).

Nominal Group Techniques

Individuals within a program are the most knowledgeable source of information on what a program is trying to accomplish and what activities have transpired to accomplish them. The critical issue facing the evaluator is to obtain a true representation of these objectives and activities and to channel individual contributions. The problem is difficult, for individuals have varying degrees of status, and one or two tend to dominate the program. The nominal group technique may be used to generate data systematically within a case study format.

The nominal group technique was first developed by Delbecq, Van de Ven, and Gustafson (1975). The technique involves a structured group meeting in which individuals are given a specific task. This task usually requires a judgmental decision characterized by a lack of agreement or incomplete state of knowledge concerning the nature of the problem or the components to be included in the solution. Participants are asked to respond to this task not by speaking to one another but by writing their ideas on a pad of paper. At the end of five to ten minutes all members of the panel present their ideas in a sequential process. These ideas are recorded so that the entire group can see them, but the ideas are not discussed as they are recorded. Once all ideas are presented, a discussion follows in which the ideas are clarified and evaluated. After the discussion there is a vote on the priority of areas, and the group decision is derived from the ranking of ideas on the basis of the vote.

The process provides a systematic basis whereby all individuals, regardless of their status, are able to present their ideas before the entire group. This ensures greater objectivity in the identification of issues or problems—but also increases the likelihood that individuals will identify with the process and thereby cooperate in and suggest evaluation activities.

The nominal group technique is particularly useful in initiating exploratory case study evaluation. The technique can be used to

1. identify and enrich the evaluators' understanding of a problem.

2. arrive at a set of hypotheses concerning the meaning of the effects of aspects of the problem.

3. focus attention on the major areas or types of problems amenable to evaluation, defined by knowledgeable individuals in their own language. These areas may be pursued in greater detail later by means of structured observations, interviews, or questionnaires.

The following illustrate the use of nominal group technique in the evaluation of health services.

Illustration: An application to quality assurance (Williamson 1978a, 1978b)

The nominal group approach is used to help establish priority areas where improvements of health or any other target outcomes will most likely be achieved. The nominal group technique involves a series of sequential tasks in which individuals are asked to list problem areas characterized as "achievable benefit not achieved" (ABNA). Such problems are listed on a flip chart in a series of rounds until ten or eleven topics are recorded. Following the listing of these topics, each is discussed by the group to clarify as precisely as possible the problems of patients and providers, and health care changes needed to affect improvement of the target benefit. Based on this discussion, the topics are scaled by each of the individuals according to their judgment of quality assurance and cost effectiveness. This weighting must be estimated in terms of

1. adequacy of evidence that the target benefit is achievable

2. necessity and practicality of quality assessment to verify current outcome deficiencies

3. likelihood that the improvement to be achieved would be worth the time and expense

Finally, the group considers each topic separately, analyzing priority weights in terms of ABNA. After the discussion each member records a final scale weight. The individual weights are collated to obtain an arithmetic total weight for each identified problem area. The total of each item represents cost effectiveness of the item for quality assurance activity.

The approach has undergone tests to assess its reliability (Williamson et al. 1978) and validity (Horn and Williamson 1977; Williamson, Braswell, and Horn 1979). Reliability in this context is defined as whether a given group judgment procedure will produce similar results when applied by independent groups within the same institution. Analysis for eight different institutions revealed

1. agreement on topic content
2. agreement on scaling of similar topics generated by the team independently
3. agreement by one team on scaling the topics generated by another team

Validity focused on the extent to which the approach

1. accurately identifies health deficiencies or strengths
2. properly identifies correctable causes
3. develops programs to improve health deficiencies
4. shows improvement attributed to the corrective action initiated by the assessment process

Analysis of data obtained in six medical institutions revealed that predictive validity was achieved for all criteria.

Illustration: Development and implementation of performance evaluation system for state and local health departments— Problem selection stage (Kotch et al. 1991)

Development and implementation of a performance evaluation system is not only substantively difficult but also politically challenging. The University of North Carolina School of Public Health, in cooperation with the Centers for Disease Control, the Association of Schools of Public Health, and the North Carolina Division of Health Services, expanded an existing performance evaluation system for state and local health departments. This developmental effort occurred in a process consisting of five distinct stages:

1. selection of a single maternal and child health problem judged amenable to performance evaluation
2. determination of objectives for a maternal and child health program designed to combat the selected health problem
3. definition of all activities necessary for fulfillment of these objectives
4. delineation of standards for all activities
5. development of an assessment mechanism to note and correct any problems in the overall system

To develop a performance evaluation system with relevance to public health personnel, a current maternal and child health problem was selected for use throughout the project. To select the problem, stage 1 above, a nominal group technique was used with public health personnel at the state, local, and regional levels. The selection involved the following steps:

1. Assemble the relevant providers and ask the question: "What maternal and child health problems exist in this state today?" Replies might include any condition proposed by any participant, such as
   - maternal and child health conditions negatively influenced by poor timing and spacing of children
   - post neonatal death rate due to accidents and poisoning
   - high rate of teenage pregnancies and related health and social problems
   - lead poisoning
   - prematurity
   - high incidence of genetically determined disease
   - low birth weight
2. Record each response in sequential fashion. Care should be taken to write down exactly the words used by the speaker. At this point no discussion of ideas is allowed except for clarification. The sequence continues until participants' ideas are all listed.
3. Eliminate overlapping items.
4. Determine ten items participants consider most important. Individuals rank and list the problems using two criteria:
   - how much positive change can be expected if an effective

performance system is implemented on an existing program designed to combat the problem

- the financial and personal cost of implementing the performance system on the already existing program

5. Arrive at consensus on the top ten problem areas based on consideration of individual rankings. Nominations are made by sequential procedure. Consensus on the top ten selections is reached by vote.

6. Discuss and clarify each of the selected ten problems. Participants consider agreements and disagreements within the group, analyzing the reasoning behind each selection and the appropriateness of each problem to development of the performance evaluation system.

7. Select from the top ten problems one problem for use in the project. Following discussion of each of the ten problems, each participant reconsiders his or her earlier vote in view of group analysis of the top ten selections. A final vote determines the single problem to be used in the project. (In the nominal group session, participants chose the prevention of prematurity and low birth weight as the problem most appropriate for development of the performance system for state and local health departments.)

Delphi Technique

The Delphi technique is usually associated with forecasting and large-survey strategies but has equal utility in providing structure to case study approaches. The primary objectives of Delphi is to

1. determine, develop, or arrange the set of alternatives
2. explore or expose underlying assumptions or information leading to different judgments
3. seek out information that may generate consensus on the part of the responding group
4. correlate informed judgments on a topic with a wide range of perspectives
5. educate the responding group about the diverse and interrelated aspects of the phenomena under study

The approach itself has a number of variations that basically involve a series of questionnaires and feedback reports to a desig-

nated panel of respondents. Researchers develop an initial questionnaire distributed by mail to the potential responding group. Respondents independently generate their ideas in answer to the first
questionnaire. The researchers summarize the responses to the first
questionnaire and develop a feedback report, along with a second set
of questionnaires for the responding group. Based on this feedback
information, the respondent panel members evaluate their earlier
responses. Based on the returns of the second questionnaire, the
researchers develop a second summary and feedback report to the
responding group.

This generic approach is having increasing utility in a number
of health services settings. The following is a description of a case
study approach using a modified Delphi methodology to assess the
appropriateness of a large number of detailed indications for the use
of selected medical and surgical procedures.

Illustration: Appropriate indications for selected medical and surgical procedures (Park et al. 1986)

What are the criteria that indicate whether certain procedures are in
fact appropriate? Using a modified Delphi technique, a panel of
expert physicians are convened to rate the appropriateness of indications for performing six procedures—coronary angiography, coronary artery bypass graft surgery, cholecystectomy, upper gastrointestinal endoscopy, colonoscopy, and carotid endarterectomy.

A panel was organized for coronary angiography and coronary
arterial bypass graft surgery; a gastrointestinal panel for indications
for cholecystectomy, upper gastrointestinal endoscopy, and colonoscopy; and a cerebral vascular panel rated indications for carotid
endarterectomy. Each of the three panels was conducted as follows:

- Project staff invited nine distinguished physicians to serve on
  the panel.
- Staff prepared initial list of clinical indicators for performing
  each procedure.
- The panelists rated the appropriateness of each indicator and
  mailed these ratings to a central statistical office, where staff
  tabulated them for use by the panel.
- The panelists met in a central location and reviewed these
  materials, discussed the indications, revised the indications
  list, and individually assigned final appropriateness ratings.
- Staff analyzed these ratings, resulting in a series of recommendations.

Exhibit 7-1 presents an example of the form used in the initial rating for indications for coronary angiography.

A central task in this procedure was to arrive at definitions of agreement and disagreement. For agreement, it was possible to arrive at two "conceptions." The stricter conception is, the raters agreed if all of the ratings for a particular indicator were within a single three-point region (that is, one to three, four to six, or seven to nine). Under these conditions all of the raters agreed to one of the

Exhibit 7-1 Example of Form Used for Initial Ratings

Indications for Coronary Angiography

Appropriateness Scale

1 2 3 4 5 6 7 8 9

1 = extremely inappropriate
5 = equivocal (neither clearly appropriate nor clearly inappropriate)
9 = extremely appropriate

	Rating of Appropriateness (circle one)
I. Asymptomatic Patients	
A. Coronary angiography (CA) is indicated in patients in high risk occupations if:	
1. No exercise ECG, no exercise thallium scan, and no exercise MUGA	1 2 3 4 5 6 7 8 9
2. Negative exercise ECG and	
a. No or negative exercise thallium scan regardless of MUGA results, if any	1 2 3 4 5 6 7 8 9
b. Reversible defect on exercise thallium scan and	
(i) No exercise MUGA	1 2 3 4 5 6 7 8 9
(ii) Negative exercise MUGA	1 2 3 4 5 6 7 8 9
(iii) Positive exercise MUGA	1 2 3 4 5 6 7 8 9
3. Positive exercise ECG and	
a. No exercise thallium scan regardless of MUGA results, if any	1 2 3 4 5 6 7 8 9
b. Negative exercise thallium scan and	
(i) No exercise MUGA	1 2 3 4 5 6 7 8 9
(ii) Negative exercise MUGA	1 2 3 4 5 6 7 8 9

Source: Reprinted with permission from R. E. Park et al., "Physician Ratings of Appropriate Indicators for Six Medical and Surgical Procedures," *American Journal of Public Health* 76 (1986): 767. © 1986 American Public Health Association.

following statements: the procedure should not be done, doing it is questionable, or it should be done.

A second conception is more relaxed: The raters agreed if all of the ratings were within any three-point range, even if that range straddles boundaries between two of the regions specified above. If all the ratings were within the range three to five, for example, there was agreement according to this more liberal interpretation, but not according to the first.

It was equally important that there be some definition of disagreement, and again this procedure resulted in two conceptions. The first conception is, raters disagreed if at least one assigned a rating of "one" and at least one assigned a rating of "nine." This is the most extreme polarization of disagreement.

A second conception is again more relaxed: raters disagreed if at least one rating fell in the lowest three-point region (one to three) and at least one in the highest (seven to nine).

This approach clearly demonstrated that the physicians can rate the appropriateness of large numbers of indicators for medical and surgical procedures. The technique provides an opportunity to evaluate the relationship between the appropriateness of care and the actual utilization of services under a variety of operational programmatic and geographical conditions.

Discussion Questions

1. How does the use of structured observation or an a priori classification scheme assist in gathering information?
2. What are the limitations of using existing information systems in case study evaluations?
3. Develop and analyze questions that are appropriate to the use of content analysis. What are the major advantages and limitations in using content analysis?
4. How does the nominal group technique differ from Delphi techniques as a case study methodology?

Part IV

Survey Research

8

Survey Research as an Evaluation Strategy

Survey research has long been the province of social scientists. As the need for evaluation has become more widely recognized and as social scientists have taken on the role of evaluator, survey research has become a common evaluation strategy. As such, survey research has been used primarily for summative evaluation of programs. But it can also be used for formative evaluation. As described later, survey research may overlap or be used in conjunction with monitoring, case studies, time series analysis, or even experimental strategies. The objective of this chapter is to define survey research, describe the context within which it occurs and the types of data collected, and illustrate its application in various health care settings.

What Is Survey Research?

Survey research is an approach to knowledge that uses information collected through questionnaires or interviews directed to a sample of persons drawn from some population of interest. In program evaluation a survey may be directed at any or all of the following groups: the recipients or potential recipients of services provided by a program, the service providers, or the program planners and managers. The purpose of these interviews or questionnaires is to obtain information about the perceptions and feelings of the recipients or providers of services on such issues as the adequacy, effectiveness, or continuity of a program's services.

Survey research may be mainly descriptive or mainly analytic. Although it need not be overstressed, the distinction should be made and understood because different types of evaluation questions are best considered by one or the other emphasis. However, there may not be descriptive components of analytic research and vice versa in any particular survey, but, in general, the research will have primary features of one or the other types.

Descriptive surveys are chiefly concerned with producing as accurate a picture as possible of a real-world situation. In the context of evaluation specifically, a descriptive survey might be concerned with describing a problem that requires some type of program activity, describing the program itself from the perspective of providers or service recipients, or describing results of the program or project from the perspective of providers or recipients. The following example illustrates a descriptive survey conducted to obtain a better understanding of the use and users of the Physician Data Query (PDQ) system. The PDQ is an information system developed by the NCI to provide community physicians and patients with the latest cancer treatment information.

Illustration: Evaluation of the Physician Data Query system (Manfredi, Czaja, and Nyden 1989)

A major objective of the evaluation was to describe who are the current users of the system, how and when they use the system, how they differ from nonusers, and what were the rates of awareness and use of the Physician Data Query (PDQ) system as of 1987. To answer these questions, data from several different sources were analyzed. In addition to using data from existing records of PDQ use, a telephone survey of current users of PDQ was conducted. Interviews were conducted with physicians who accessed the data base themselves, physicians who received information from intermediaries who search the data base for them, and intermediaries who conduct searches for physicians. From physicians, information was obtained on the characteristics of those who access the system themselves and of those who only received information through intermediaries. A survey also provided information on physician likes and dislikes concerning the PDQ system, the extent and manner of the use, the reasons for searching PDQ, the type of information sought, whether the information is used for clinical decisions, usefulness of the information, cost, how users became aware of the system, and whether they plan to use the system in the future. A total of 204 interviews were completed, 143 with physicians and 61 with intermediaries.

These data were combined with data collected from another NCI project that involved a panel study of physicians, which was part of a larger study to assess the effectiveness of the initial community clinical oncology program. These data were used as part of the PDQ evaluation to determine differences between users and nonusers among a general population of community physicians. These data were also used to assess the rates of awareness and use of PDQ at two points in time. Information about awareness and use was collected from a sample of physicians in 12 communities in 1985 and again in 1986. The analysis of these data indicates that awareness and use of PDQ were present to a limited degree among oncologists and other physicians with community involvement. However, awareness and use were practically nonexistent among physicians who were non-cancer specialists but had some involvement with cancer patients. Between 1985 and 1986 relatively little change occurred in either rate among physician specialities.

The descriptive analysis reveals that in 1987 awareness and use of PDQ within the medical community remained relatively low among physicians. Both awareness and use were higher for oncologists and especially for CCOP applicants but were very low for community physicians not in oncological specialties. Moreover, the highest use of the data base was by the Cancer Information Service (CIS), providing mainly information to the public, rather than by physicians and medical librarians.

Analytic surveys are concerned chiefly with describing relationships between real-world phenomena. An analytic-type evaluation survey, for example, might be concerned with (1) whether program recipients having different types of characteristics viewed a program more or less favorably or (2) whether there is some differential effect of the program on recipients having certain characteristics.

Clearly an analytic survey must have some relationship to reality; that is, the survey must be concerned with issues that exist in the real world. Although these surveys need not provide a true description of a given population, they must focus on the relationship between attributes of a person, a group, or set of organizations in the study population. Consider the following example.

Illustration: Evaluating the NIH consensus development program (Kanouse et al. 1990)

Some of the objectives of this large-scale evaluation project were to assess physician knowledge and attitudes concerning selected medical technologies that have been the subject of recent consensus conferences, gauge physician awareness of conference findings, and determine the degree of correspondence between conference recommendations and physician practices. To meet these objectives, the evaluation conducted a national survey of physicians. This survey was completed by 1,453 physicians from the specialities of general practice, family practice, general internal medicine, cardiology, oncology, general surgery, cardiac surgery, thoracic surgery, and obstetrics and gynecology, and involved measures of knowledge, attitudes, and practices with respect to both office-based and hospital-based technologies that had been the subject of consensus conferences. The survey elicited information about physicians' background characteristics and methods for keeping up with new medical developments.

Analysis revealed that physicians who had heard of the program were somewhat older; had practiced medicine about two years longer; were less likely to work in private group practice and more likely to work in a hospital, clinic, or other institutional setting; and were more likely to be members of the medical school teaching faculty and to report that they had responsibility for training students, residents, and interns. Moreover, their information habits and preferences were quite different. Physicians who were aware of the program reported spending more time reading journals, such as the *Journal of the American Medical Association*, where many consensus statements are published, and tended to talk informally with their colleagues about medical topics. They also reported spending over 30 percent of their time attending continuing medical education courses and tended to receive patient referrals from a larger number of physicians than those who were less aware of program recommendations.

Appropriate Settings for Survey Research

Survey research can be a powerful tool in various types of evaluation. Consider the use of descriptive and analytic survey research.

Descriptive surveys and program relevance

Descriptive survey research can be used prior to the establishment of any program to examine the nature of a particular problem that appears to warrant a program—in essence, to consider the relevance of a program. From this standpoint survey research can be used to define a problem as seen by potential program recipients and relevant personnel. In a rural community, for example, a descriptive survey of the general population and relevant provider personnel to determine their perceptions of primary health problems improves the effectiveness of any subsequent primary health care program developed. A comparison of survey results may reveal considerable discrepancy about perceived problems between provider and recipient groups. Designing the program to recipients' rather than providers' expectations could enhance both its use and its efficiency.

Descriptive surveys and program progress

A well-designed descriptive study can also provide information about how a program is actually progressing. This is, of course, the major function of monitoring, but survey research, particularly descriptive survey research, can shed substantial light on program progress. An example of survey research in this sense can be taken from the experience of an international agency that set out to identify personnel training needs in developing countries. The initial assumption of the program designers was that many developing countries needed continuing education for their national health service program managers. In one country that had agreed to participate in the effort to upgrade the health services program, the suggestion was made that perhaps training per se might not be the primary problem; instead an effort might be undertaken to determine the types of problems involved in the national health services administration and management, whether these problems involved training or lack of it, and what other steps, if any, might be taken to improve the system's management and administration. A survey of all health service managers at various governmental levels was then initiated to determine the extent to which problems existed and were attributable to limited training.

The actual survey was never carried out, but the pilot study and pretest indicated that although the lack of adequate training was a clear problem in the management and administration of the health services system, it was far outweighed by few resources, poor distribution of facilities, and simple lack of personnel—trained or untrained. This potential survey, directed at an ongoing national health services system, not only revealed how the system was working, but even in its formative stages also indicated that problems in its operation were not primarily those that introduction of a training program could solve. This survey, therefore, had the potential to define a problem to be addressed by one program and to evaluate the progress of another, much larger program.

Descriptive surveys and effectiveness

Descriptive survey evaluations are generally employed in a summative type of evaluation. In this type, the survey will be directed toward determining how the program worked, whether it was perceived as successful by personnel and clients, and what aspects of the program were perceived as making it more or less effective. Emphasis is on perception, for it is on this basis rather than on an objective accounting of program activity that individual actions rest.

Analytic surveys and formative evaluations

When an analytic evaluation is used, the objective is to compare the views of various groups about a program or health service activity and account for differing views rather than to describe the program or its operation per se. While the descriptive survey can be used to define a problem as seen by various audiences, including the potential program recipients and providers, an analytic survey compares views of a problem among different types of potential recipients and tries to account for these differing views as a first step in launching a useful program. Similarly, analytic surveys provide comparative information about how programs are currently operating or how a program has worked in the past.

Illustration

Analytic surveys often provide insight into problems of program operation. Suppose that a survey of program administrators and service providers indicates that, in general, recipients were satisfied with a primary health care program. Analysis reveals that even though administrators are satisfied with the program, many of the actual service providers are not. This result could be due to a number of factors, which a survey might indicate. Managers, for example, may be satisfied because they perceive the program to be operating according to plan. Further questioning may reveal, however, that they have little knowledge of actual day-to-day program operations. On the other hand, service providers' first-hand knowledge of day-to-day operations leads them to perceive the program as working less well. In essence, then, one variable that may be identified as contributing to a view that the program is or is not successful would be knowledge of actual program operations at the local level. On the other hand, the same survey might show that recipients are satisfied with the program because they are getting services that had never been available before, whereas providers are unhappy with the program because they realize that recipients (possibly because of lack of resources or time) are not receiving all the services that should be available to them. This analysis would indicate that satisfaction with the program is partly the result of the difference between expectations and reality.

Appropriate Data for Survey Research

Except for the limited case in which survey data are acquired from various physical measurements, such as height or weight (an aspect of monitoring), data appropriate to survey research are almost exclusively collected from people using some type of formalized questionnaire or interview schedule. As such, the data actually applied to evaluation via the survey research format are an amalgam of personal opinions, knowledge, and perceptions of people involved in the program or affected by it. When such information is used to describe a program, it is critical to make certain that the data sample represents the population of interest.

Questionnaires versus interviews

Because survey data are collected through either formal questionnaires or interviews, these two techniques deserve some discussion. The basic distinction is how each is used to acquire evaluation information. A *questionnaire,* in general, is an instrument or a schedule for collecting data that the respondent essentially self-administers. An *interview,* on the other hand, generally is an instrument or schedule for collecting data that an interviewer administers. This difference between questionnaire and interview is quite important for the design and structure of the two formats. Because an interviewer will administer the interview and usually will record answers in appropriate categories, an interview schedule can be substantially less formal and less carefully designed than the questionnaire. This does not mean that the interview schedule should not be well thought out. In fact, when the purpose of the interview schedule is to collect survey data for a systematic analysis, clear categories for recording responses to questions should be available for the interviewer ahead of time. What it does mean, however, is that the interviewer knows the structure of the interview schedule and is able to move through it with the interviewee without difficulty. A questionnaire, on the other hand, must be simple enough and have instructions that are clear and straightforward enough so that respondents can follow and complete it without assistance from the study directors.

Another difference between the questionnaire and interview schedule is that interviewers can deal with and record responses that do not fit predetermined categories. In the development of a questionnaire, particularly, it is necessary to ensure a possible response from everyone to whom the questionnaire is addressed. Consequently, both interviews and questionnaires are usually subjected to fairly extensive pretesting. The purpose of the pretest is to see that the interview or questionnaire schedule can be answered and that it provides the types of answers that the evaluator considers important to understand the situation.

Measurement

Whether a questionnaire or interview is used to acquire data for survey research, an important aspect of that data collection is the problem of measurement. Measurement is discussed in substantial detail in Chapter 14, but several important points should be mentioned here.

In survey research, measurement generally refers to the problem of acquiring data that will give both valid and reliable measures of personal opinions and knowledge of perceptions. One purpose of an evaluation activity, for instance, might be to determine the perceptions of program recipients about a primary care program. A strategy might be to ask the respondents directly whether they were satisfied or dissatisfied with the primary care program. But, in general, the survey researcher would assume that this question was attempting to tap too many dimensions of satisfaction or acceptability of the program. Instead the researcher would probably try to get an evaluation of the program through questions concerning satisfaction with the program or the acceptability of it in a number of more specific areas. Questions might be asked about satisfaction with information obtained from the primary care program, treatment of clients by the personnel, acceptability of hours of operation or physical facilities, acceptability of advice given, and numerous other aspects of satisfaction with the program.

The evaluator would probably have predetermined specific aspects of satisfaction that the various questions would raise. Several questions, for example, might refer to adequacy of physical plant and other physical facilities. Others might consider satisfaction with staff, treatment by them, and staff-client relationships in the agency. Yet another series of questions might concern the ease of scheduling access and hours of operation. After the data had been collected, it would be fairly common to construct measures of satisfaction in various areas, using a number of questions to tap each area or dimension. Five questions about physical facilities, for example, would be combined in some manner to form a single measure of acceptability of physical facilities.

How Data Are Acquired

As noted, survey data are acquired through questionnaires or interviews. Certain problems occur, however, in the acquisition of either type of data, particularly identification of respondents, access to them, and their willingness to cooperate.

Identification

Whether the strategy for collecting information is the interview or the questionnaire approach, legitimate respondents for the data collection instrument must be identified. If, for example, the survey wanted to determine client opinion about treatment received in a primary care clinic, it would be necessary to identify people who had used the clinic's services. If the clinic maintains good records of consultations and has, in addition, a record of addresses, it may be possible to identify potential respondents through clinic records. If, on the other hand, the clinic does not maintain names or addresses in its records, the only possible way to identify persons who have used its services might be to ask respondents who have been selected on some basis from the general service area of the clinic. Under these circumstances it may be necessary to interview five to ten times as many people as ultimately desired in order to find a large enough group of clinic users for purposes of analysis. In general, such an approach to acquiring a specific sample is so costly that it would not be used. In the conduct of any survey it is necessary to identify the population about which inferences are to be drawn either with some global statement, such as all people living in a given community, or by some limiting statement, such as all people who say on questioning that they have used the services of a particular primary care clinic.

Access

In order for data collection to proceed in survey research, access must be possible to people who are to serve as respondents. This aspect may not be too difficult for program personnel. In most instances, personnel can be reached through the program because the program must be able to contact them to pay them or give instructions and so on.

Clients may be much more difficult to reach. If a questionnaire is used, some information about clients' addresses or some other strategy for ensuring that they receive the questionnaires must be devised. If an interview is used, the interviewer must be able to find the respondents and gain their cooperation. The difficulty of gaining access to respondents is illustrated by the evaluation of a five-year health plan in a developing nation.

Illustration

The original study was conceived as a six-month effort beginning in December 1990. As such, data collection in the field was planned for March and April 1991. In fact, various delays, including a ten-week wait for the Health Ministry to process a request for funds to pay interviewers (though the funds were available from donor agencies), postponed the start of data collection to late June. Late June is when the monsoon starts, a time when roads in many parts of the country are completely unpassable. Data collection in most areas then became extremely difficult, and a number of areas had to be abandoned completely.

Monsoon problems were exacerbated in many areas by inaccurate information on the location of health post facilities and incomplete lists of households. A number of interviewers indicated that they would not agree again to undertake a task of this type during the monsoon.

There were numerous difficulties, some unavoidable, in interviewing at the household level. In two villages where murders had recently occurred, interviewers were mistaken for police and generally found people quite reluctant to talk with them. In one village they were mistaken for criminals who had raided the village earlier. In another area they were thought to be leprosy workers who, according to rumor, inject people with poisonous black serum and spread leprosy as a means of population control.

Even after gaining access to households, difficulties remained. There were problems of awkward questions and questions that were a source of embarrassment in the questionnaire, particularly in the family planning area. Also, some concepts, such as time (how long does it take to walk to the health clinic), were difficult for respondents to deal with. There is little conceptual difference in rural areas of the country between one hour and three hours, for example.

Nonresponse

Nonresponse refers to the unwillingness or the inability of persons selected for the sample to cooperate in answering either the questionnaires or interviews. The problem of nonresponse is most acute in the questionnaire situation. Unless some prior groundwork has been done to impress on potential respondents the importance of the questionnaire and the critical need to have it completed, it is likely that nonresponse to a questionnaire may run as high as 50 to 60 percent. If the questionnaire is addressed to busy professionals, such as physicians, nonresponse may run even higher. If questionnaires are simply received in the mail with a request to fill them out, they may well be ignored. There are numerous ways of improving on nonresponse in questionnaire settings, including the use of personally signed cover letters, follow-up letters and calls, self-addressed return envelopes, and partial payment for time spent completing the questionnaire.

Nonresponse is less a problem in interviews than in questionnaires. Fewer people are willing to decline to be interviewed than are willing to throw a questionnaire away. Nonresponse remains a problem since it is not reasonable to assume that those who refuse or fail to respond to a questionnaire or interview are essentially no different from those who do respond in regard to the subject of the survey. If, for example, a survey tried to elicit people's opinions about a primary care program as an evaluation of that program, those who are unwilling to respond to the questionnaire may be unwilling because they perceive the program to be irrelevant, undesirable, and unacceptable, whereas people willing to respond may do so because they perceive the program to be useful or valuable. Then analysis of the information supplied by respondents would substantially mislead the evaluators.

It is usually impossible to guard against all nonresponse. Generally, however, it is better to accept a smaller sample with a lower proportion of nonresponse than a larger sample with a larger proportion of nonrespondents. If evaluators set out to interview or obtain questionnaires from 400 respondents because they believe only 100 will respond and they desire 100 responses for the analysis, the results of that study are much less reliable than if they set out to collect data only from 100 people and made every possible effort to get those 100 people to respond. In fact, it can be shown that under certain hypothetical situations it would be better to interview 20 people and be certain to get all 20 than it would be to create a sample of 400 from which only 100 would be expected to respond.

Data for Survey Research from Two Different Settings

To discuss appropriate data for survey research on a somewhat more practical level, consider again the community clinical oncology program and the primary care program initially described in Chapters 4 and 6.

Illustration: Community Clinical Oncology Program (CCOP)

The evaluation was designed to monitor the implementation and impact of the program and to determine the characteristics of CCOPs and research bases, and how their interaction affects implementation and impact. As part of the effort to explain variation in implementation and impact as well as map activity within CCOPs and between CCOPs and research bases, a key informant survey was designed and implemented. Key informants were selected from all 52 CCOPs and 17 research bases and were selected from three strata: CCOP principal investigator/coprincipal investigator, physicians within the community who enter patients on NCI-approved protocols, and CCOP administrative staff. Prestudy telephone calls to each CCOP principal investigator requested his or her assistance in identifying one physician respondent from each of five specialty areas: medical oncology/hematology, radiation therapy, surgical oncology/general surgery, gynecologic oncology/gynecology, and pediatric oncology/pediatrics. The principal investigators also identified the two administrative respondents: a coordinator and a data manager. In the case of the research base survey, the research base principal investigators and chairpersons of the cancer control committee served as the informants.

These informants were mailed a survey instrument in which questions were specifically designed to address nine areas corresponding with the information gathered in the 20 in-depth site visits. Key informant questions included items on

- goals for the CCOP program
- CCOP internal structure
- CCOP principal investigator and physician attributes
- physician and staff relationships
- CCOP-hospital relationships
- cancer control issues

- CCOP—research base relationships
- CCOP and research base relationships with NCI Division of Cancer Prevention and Control
- CCOP relationships with community group

The analysis plan for the CCOP survey included both a descriptive and an analytic component. Many of the same questions were asked of respondents in the three strata. This provided rich descriptive data and allowed comparison of responses from the three respondent strata on such topics as the relative importance of various goals (relevance), CCOP success in attaining these goals (effectiveness), and policy changes that might enhance goal attainment (program progress).

The analysis component of the evaluation included an investigation of the association between both the individual respondent strata, and the combined respondent strata, responses and measures of effectiveness such as the number of cancer patients enrolled in clinical trials. The data also allowed the development of consensus variables that measured the extent of agreement or disagreement among the respondent groups in each CCOP on the topics addressed in the questionnaire. This made it possible to examine the relationship between the level of consensus among staff and CCOP effectiveness.

Illustration: Primary care program

To get some idea of the types of data that would be collected for an evaluation of a primary health care program implemented by a state department of human resources, consider the following summative-type evaluation using a survey strategy. Because the program was initiated at the state level but operated by individual local health departments, data were collected from relevant organizational levels of the primary health care program. These included the state department of human services, a district-level office responsible to the state and overseeing work of program staff in local health departments, the local health department itself at which services were provided, and local recipients of those services.

Data were collected on three categories of program activities: input and process, output, and impact. Input and process data included information about staff—total complement, attendance, training, and experience—supplies and equipment, budget and salaries, supervision, cooperation and communication, and planning. Output data consisted primarily of information about services provided and limited information about frequency and scope of services.

Impact data were concerned only with the approximate impact of services, including exposure to, knowledge of, and use of a limited set of health services activities and personnel, such as nurse practitioners and family planning techniques, as well as general knowledge of hypertension, PAP, and breast self-examination programs. To the extent possible, all these issues were considered relative to all levels of the study, including state, district, local, and recipients of care. Clearly certain questions were more appropriate to one level or another.

Data collection at the district and local level and among recipients of services involved a highly structured interview schedule. These interviews sought specific information about provision, training, service delivery, areas covered, specific programs provided, knowledge of these activities at both the district and local level, and agreement between district and local personnel on these categories of information. The questionnaires also sought detailed information about equipment and supplies, personnel, money, and the satisfaction of program personnel with the program's conduct. At the level of recipients the interviewers sought information about frequency, purpose, accessibility, and desirability of the treatment and perceptions of the extent to which treatment needs were filled.

An important factor in the success of data collection in governmental agencies is the support of the chief administrative officer at the state, district, and local levels. Official sanction is likely to represent the difference between successful interviews and a high nonresponse rate. Even with approval, however, problems arise, and the evaluator must be prepared for several follow-up efforts.

Survey problems

There were several problems in collecting data at all four levels. First, the problem of actually getting to interviewees among care recipients has been mentioned. Other problems included the time and effort involved in obtaining data, particularly at the district and local levels; problems in questionnaire construction and of consistency among interviewers; and the general size of the sample of service recipients.

Second, questions addressed to district and local respondents in the primary care program were extremely detailed and time consuming. Much of the information sought, such as number of leave days for staff in a year preceding the survey, staff training status, or specifics of budget preparation, was available only in office records. Often such records were difficult or impossible to locate. In other instances, data requested, such as total number of staff members, was a matter of record and accessible to survey staff at the central level. Both the extreme detail of the questionnaire and the lack of preparatory efforts in using available data, along with general skepticism on the part of the respondents, served to prolong the interviews to an average of about one per day. Nevertheless, the interviewers felt, in general, that the actual data were fairly accurate at these two levels. Opinion-and-attitude data were, in the view of the surveyers, more questionable. The respondents tended to give the administratively acceptable answer rather than their own opinion.

The issue of consistency among interviewers was a third problem not recognized until the analysis stage, but it should have been anticipated during data collection. About 25 different people were conducting interviews in the field, and despite the highly structured nature of the questionnaires, problems of consistency did occur. One series of questions, for example, involved information about the number of staff in various offices. In three offices the respondents reported for the entire district, whereas what was desired was the number specifically in the district office. Although this information was a matter of record at the central level and the inconsistency was truly glaring (the difference between the three misreported districts and the rest was on the order of five to one), the error was not realized until late in the analysis. By the time it was detected the conclusions based on the incorrect data had already been drawn and rationalized.

A final difficulty in data collection was the size of the sample of service recipients. The sample consisted of nearly 4,000 separate interviews. The rationale was that the analysis would require cross tabulations involving as many as 100 subgroups, each of which must have a sufficient number of observations for significance testing. In reality, a sample of 500 to 1,000 households would have been quite adequate. The question would almost certainly be raised as to whether such a sample would be representative of the state as a whole, but size per se does not make an adequate sample. Sampling procedures and the degree of variation in the data determine an adequate sample.

Application to Decision Making and Types of Evaluation

A number of insights can be gained about decision making as a result of survey research. They correspond to the various types of evaluation: relevance, progress, efficiency, effectiveness, and impact.

Relevance

On the descriptive side, survey research provides information about the perceived state of the system or the perceived nature of the problem with which a program is to deal. Although valuable information, it may not always be as accurate as desired. For example, there is increasing recognition of the importance of providing medical care services to the poor and near poor in the United States. It is likely that a survey of the relevant population would indicate that such people recognize a need for more medical care services. A close examination of the kinds of problems that these people deal with in regard to their health, however, would probably show that their major problems are problems of low income, poor housing (including lead-painted walls), malnutrition, poor sanitation, and lack of basic immunizations. Very few of these primary health problems would be affected appreciably by an increase in medical care services, although a survey of that population might reveal medical care services as the biggest perceived problem. This, in a sense, is the major difficulty with survey research. It invariably provides perceptions or beliefs.

Progress

Survey research can also provide information about how a program is operating and how well. When addressed specifically to managers and other program workers, it can offer insight into the progress and efficiency of a program. This kind of information can also be derived from responses of clients. Finally, on the more analytical side, survey research can shed light on how program effects occur, how different parts of a system work, whether certain strategies provide for more efficiency and effectiveness than others, and what the perceived impact of a program is among different groups of people.

Two additional points about the knowledge produced by survey research should be made. First, survey research provides information about perceptions or beliefs of respondents. Other strategies provide more objective data, but information derived from survey research emphasizes subjectivity—what informants perceive are the problems to which a program is directed, or what percentage of respondents perceives the program to have an impact. This is often considered a limitation of survey research; yet it is important to emphasize that decisions are made on subjective judgments rather than "objective" reality. Robert Sigmond, an early pioneer in health planning, says of hospital planning, "planning decisions are not made over 'hard facts,' they are made over 'hard liquor.'" This is equally applicable to the world of program evaluation.

A second point that must be understood is that in the analytical framework where cause-effect relationships are to be examined, survey research depends heavily on theory for the establishment of these relationships. Specifically, theory must be able

1. to establish time ordering between various aspects of the program being measured
2. to specify in enough detail those variables that need to be accounted for at the same time or ruled out to ensure that they are all measured as part of the survey and can be examined simultaneously with the relationships of interest

Some serious evaluation problems result with regard to the evaluation of efficiency, effectiveness, and impact. A brief discussion of these problems follows.

Efficiency

A survey could be addressed to personnel or service recipients to gain their impressions about the efficiency of the program or about alternative ways of operating it that might be more efficient. Comparisons could be made between those who feel the program is efficient and those who do not, and some causal statements drawn up about the characteristics of personnel that lead them to believe the program is more or less efficient. Yet, on the one hand, all that is available from such a survey is perceptions about efficiency; on the other hand, these perceptions are generally gained in the absence of any comparison between alternative strategies. The perceptions are formed only in the context of the existing program.

Effectiveness and impact

Effectiveness, of course, is the extent to which a program realizes its short-term or immediate goals, whereas impact is the extent to which the program changes the state of the world in some desired direction in the long run. Again, questions can be addressed to respondents about the extent to which they perceive the program to be effective or, at a later stage, perhaps the impact of the program. The questionnaire can also provide information for a causal analysis of the characteristics of program operation or respondents that are perceived to lead to greater effectiveness or impact. But, again, they will be mainly made in the absence of any comparison. This comparison—or lack of it—is particularly important with regard to effectiveness and impact because it is generally impossible to tell whether an alternative program or no program at all might have been more or less effective unless a specific strategy for alternative programs and control populations is set out in the beginning, which leads to the experimental model, or, alternatively, where a comparison is made between the time the program exists and a prior time when it did not exist.

Given some of these problems in survey research, the question of why it is used for evaluation is likely to arise. There are probably two reasons why survey research has been used as an evaluation format. First, despite the arguments against it, a great deal of information for program evaluation, particularly about the state of the system and of the program, can be acquired from survey research at any given time. Causal relationships can be inferred from survey research, particularly in the presence of a fairly good conceptual framework or theoretical perspective. Second, survey research is an approach to evaluation that is relatively well known to social and behavioral scientists who are often charged with responsibility for evaluation, and the skills and strategies involved in evaluation through the use of survey research—questionnaire design, sampling, questionnaire administration, and data analysis—can be passed on fairly effectively through didactic settings.

Discussion Questions

1. What is the difference between descriptive and analytic survey research? What type of basic evaluation questions are appropriate to each approach?
2. What are the limitations of using survey research in program evaluation? What precautionary steps are possible to increase the use of survey research as an evaluation format?
3. Consider a primary care program operating in a rural community. How might survey research help resolve problems associated with program relevance, progress, efficiency, effectiveness, and impact?

9

Survey Research Techniques and Interpretation

$\mathbf{B}$ecause the purpose of surveys may be either descriptive or analytic, the analysis of survey data must be appropriate to the survey's purpose. The objective of this chapter is to present some basic descriptive and analytic techniques and demonstrate their use in various types of evaluation.

Descriptive Techniques

Analysis techniques appropriate to descriptive surveys are concerned with assessing the parameters of a problem in a given area or population or with describing how a program operates as a means of assessing the effect of experimental changes prior to the initiation of full-scale programs. Frequency distributions and contingency analysis are two useful techniques. Their use requires little mathematical ability and yet provides important insights to evaluation questions.

Frequency distributions

A major analytical tool appropriate for descriptive purposes is the frequency distribution. Frequency distributions, depending on their subject matter, can provide significant information for evaluation purposes.

Table 9-1 is a simple example of a frequency distribution. This table shows a distribution of cases of motor vehicle trauma by road-use status of persons treated in hospital emergency departments in Rhode Island for 1984 and 1985. The primary information that can be immediately gained from the table is that the largest proportion of trauma victims, almost 75 percent, were occupants of a motor vehi-

Table 9-1   Number and Percentage of Resident Cases in a 25
Percent Motor Vehicular Trauma Sample by Road-Use
Status for Persons Treated in Hospital Emergency
Departments, and Associated Annualized Rates per
100,000 Population, Rhode Island, 1984–1985

| | Sample | | | 95 Percent Confidence |
Road-Use Status	N	%	Rate	Interval
Motor vehicle occupant	4,319	74.9	894	868–921
Motorized cyclist	318	5.5	66	59–73
Pedal cyclist	109	1.9	23	18–27
Pedestrian	273	4.7	57	50–63
Other/unspecified	750	13.0	155	144–166
Total	5,769	100.0	1,195	1,164–1,225

Source: Reprinted with permission from I. R. Rockett et al., "Age, Sex, and Road-Use Patterns of Motor Vehicular Trauma in Rhode Island: A Population-Based Hospital Emergency Department Study," *American Journal of Public Health* 80, no. 12 (1990): 1517. © 1990 American Public Health Association.

cle. The table is a typical example of a frequency distribution: The column "road-use status," on the left of the table, provides a category for every trauma case, in this example including an "other/ unspecified" category as a place to include 750 cases that do not fit into the other categories. Both the number in each category as well as the percent in that category are shown in the table. In addition, the rate per 100,000 persons in the Rhode Island population is also shown, along with 95-percent confidence intervals for these rates. These latter two components would be less commonly seen in a contingency table.

Limitations

Frequency distributions may leave many things unsaid. For example, the fact that nearly 75 percent of the trauma victims were occupants of motor vehicles may mean that being the occupant of a motor vehicle is very dangerous, or it may mean that most people using the roads are occupants of motor vehicles. Our experience would probably lead us to the second conclusion, but the table will not tell us, as it is constructed. Table 9-1 also does not give us any information about severity of the accident. It may be that all trauma cases are equally severe, or that one type, for example motorized cyclist accidents, is more severe than others, but the table does not reveal this.

An important aspect of Table 9-1 is that the categories of road-use status are both mutually exclusive (someone who was a motor vehicle occupant could not have been simultaneously a pedestrian, for example) and exhaustive. This latter characteristic is assured by the inclusion of the other/unspecified category.

Contingency tables

A simple extension of the frequency distribution, also useful for analysis in the descriptive mode, is the contingency table. Table 9-2 shows a contingency table taken from a survey study called the Survey of Income and Program Participation (SIPP). The paper in which the table originally appeared was part of a larger study of characteristics of people with long versus short spells without health insurance (Swartz and McBride 1990).

Table 9-2 shows the distribution of the duration of spells without health insurance from the beginning of the spell by income in the first month of the spell. This statement of the content of a contingency table reveals one of the important characteristics of contingency tables. They are always, at a minimum, presentations of one variable classified by another, a two-variable analysis. In some presentations a contingency table may include three variables, but almost never would a contingency table involve more than three variables. The complexity of such a table would quickly make it uninterpretable.

The two variables in Table 9-2 are family income in the first month of a spell without health insurance and the length of the spell. In a two variable contingency table it is often common to assume a causal direction. In the case of Table 9-2, the causal direction would be assumed by the reader to be from income to duration of spell without insurance, rather than the other way around. In general, contingency tables are designed so that the independent or causal variable is shown on the top of the table and the dependent variable is shown on the left side. Percentages are calculated by column, so that each column sums to 100. Percentages are compared, on the other hand, across rows.

The main purpose of a contingency table is to show the relation between the two variables. If a relationship exists, then the percentages in each row will be different from one another. As one example, the proportion of persons who had incomes of $2,400 or more in the first month of the episode and for whom the episode lasted more than 24 months is only 7.7 percent, while the proportion of persons who had incomes of less than $400 in the first month and for whom the episode lasted more than 24 months is three times as great as 22.8

Table 9-2 Distribution of the Duration of Spells without Health Insurance from the Beginning of the Spell: By Income in First Month of Spell

	Monthly Family Income in First Month of Spell (1983 dollars; 1989 dollars in parentheses)						
Spell Length	Less than $400 (< $498)	$400–$599 ($498–$746)	$600–$799 ($746–$995)	$800–$1,199 ($995–$1,492)	$1,200–$2,399 ($1,492–$2,986)	$2,400 or More (≥ $2,986)	Total
Less than 5 months	46.4	41.4	40.5	47.0	53.9	58.5	50.4
5–8 months	14.7	18.2	19.2	17.3	15.3	22.3	16.5
9–12 months	8.1	11.8	8.1	5.7	8.6	4.6	7.7
13–16 months	5.3	9.9	9.4	5.3	4.9	2.2	5.3
17–24 months	2.8	6.2	8.8	6.1	4.2	4.8	5.3
More than 24 months	22.8	12.5	13.9	18.6	13.1	7.7	14.8
Total	100.0	100.0	100.0	100.0	100.0	100.0	100.0
Sample size	869	408	436	811	1,537	1,172	5,233

Note: Other than for sample size, figures are percentages.
Source: Calculated from life table estimates of hazard rates calculated using a sample from the 1984 Panel of the Survey of Income and Program Participation (SIPP). Income adjusted to 1989 dollars using the Consumer Price Indices (CPI) for 1983 (99.6) and 1989 (124.0). Reprinted with permission from Katherine Swartz and Timothy D. McBride, "Spells without Health Insurance: Distributions of Durations and Their Link to Point-in-Time Estimates of the Uninsured," *Inquiry* 27, no. 3 (Fall 1990): 285.

percent. Other comparisons can be made from the table. A test of whether the number of observations in the various cells of the table are different from what would be expected if there was no relationship between the variables examined can be tested by the Chi-Square statistic. The Chi-Square statistic is applied not to the percentages in the table, but to the actual number of observations in each cell. In the example shown in Table 9-2, a Chi-Square could be calculated to determine whether there was a statistically significant relationship between monthly family income and length of a spell without insurance.

Continuous data

Often data that are essentially continuous are collapsed into a relatively small number of categories for presentation in a frequency distribution format. This is what was done for monthly family income and length of time without insurance. It would be impossible, or at best unwieldy, to present data that are inherently continuous in a contingency table format without reducing it to categories. The data in Table 9-2, for example, representing several thousand families, might involve several hundred cells if the data were not collapsed into categories.

How categories are chosen, however, may make a substantial difference in how it appears when arrayed in a table. The distinction between lower- and higher-income groups might have appeared much clearer and stronger if family income had been divided only into a low group and a high group at $1,200 and the duration of spell had been divided into short and long at five months. Had that been done, the result would have been as shown in Table 9-3.

The result in Table 9-3 is much clearer than the result in Table 9-2. Those with low incomes tend to have a higher proportion with longer spells without insurance than do those with high incomes. However, as we can recognize from looking at Table 9-2, many things are obscured by Table 9-3. For example, Table 9-3 does not tell us that there are a number of individual cells, which when examined on the basis of Table 9-2, do not follow the neat picture shown in Table 9-3.

The specific points selected as category boundaries can also have an effect on the results seen in a contingency table. If we had classified Table 9-3 into those with spells of 12 months or less and those with spells of more than 12 months, the result would have been 69 percent of the low-income group with short durations, compared to 83 percent for the high-income group. This is a difference of 14

Table 9-3   Distribution of the Duration of Spells without Health
Insurance: By Income in First Month of Spell

	Income in First Month of Spell	
Spell Length	Low (less than $1,200)	High ($1,200 or more)
Short (less than 5 months)	44.8	55.9
Long (5 months or more)	55.2	44.1
Sample size	2,524	2,709

percentage points, compared to only 11 in Table 9-3. So the relationship between income and length of time without insurance becomes stronger simply by how we choose to categorize the continuous variables.

Analytic Techniques

Survey data can also be examined from the standpoint of analytic studies, and analysis of such data can bear on analytic questions. Analytic surveys are concerned mainly with attempting to answer questions about why a situation exists, how it occurred, where it occurs (if, for example, it does not exist among one group of people but may exist among another), and what has caused this situation to arise.

The ultimate purpose of an analytic study is to look for cause-effect relationships: if X occurs, Y will follow. If a program is structured in a certain way, certain results in terms of success or failure will occur. Alternatively, if a program is structured in a certain way under certain circumstances—for example, in a rural area—the program will or will not be successful, whereas if it is structured differently and set in a different environment—for example, an urban area—a different success or failure outcome will result. Although the ultimate test of cause and effect lies only in well-designed experiments, and even then only through the accumulation of a number of such well-designed experiments, survey research can help to provide insights about cause-and-effect relationships. The analysis of survey research data from the standpoint of analytic evaluations is concerned almost totally with the question of cause and effect.

There are three criteria that—by the general agreement of a scientific community or by the rules of logic—must be satisfied if a cause-and-effect relationship is to be established:

1. time order of the events
2. association
3. elimination of other variables

Each deserves separate consideration.

Time ordering of events

By definition, cause must always precede effect. This issue would seem to require no elaboration, but in a survey setting where data are collected on the basis of interviews at one point in time, it is frequently difficult to establish convincingly the time ordering of perceptions, attitudes, or knowledge that a set of respondents has about a particular program.

If, for example, a survey finds that respondents who have a negative attitude toward primary health care personnel also fail to visit primary health care personnel, it would be impossible to determine, on the basis of the single survey, whether the negative attitude preceded the decision not to use the health workers' services or whether not using the services produced a negative attitude toward these people.

Certain personal characteristics, of course, can be listed in survey approaches for which time order is not a question or perhaps about which the question is irrelevant. It would be reasonable to hypothesize that as persons grow older they become more set in their ways and less likely to use new forms of services, thus making them less likely to use primary health care services. On the other hand, it would be unlikely for anyone to suggest that people who are less likely to use primary health care services will get older. Clearly age, along with a limited number of other variables, is uninfluenced by any other variables.

Apart from these uninfluenced variables, it is impossible to establish the time ordering of events in survey data on the basis of empirical evidence alone. What is required is the existence, availability, or development of a reasonable or plausible theory or conceptual perspective that indicates the time ordering. A very simple model of human behavior, for instance, would suggest that behavior follows attitudes. Thus, those people whose attitude is not to accept the primary health care worker would be less likely to use the services. It is not the only possible theory. An equally plausible theory of human behavior might suggest that people take on attitudes compatible with behaviors in which they engage. Thus, behavior would lead to a certain attitude.

In time series analysis, including panel surveys (those addressed to the same people regarding the same questions at more than one point in time), and in true experiments, time ordering of events is established by the evaluation format itself. In survey research, time ordering must be assumed on the basis of a reasonable theory or conceptual perspective.

Association

Basically, association refers to the notion that as one measure, phenomenon, or attribute changes, another measure, phenomenon, or attribute will change. As temperature increases from some low level, for example, ice will first melt and become water, and water will eventually boil and turn into vapor. A change in the state of the water is associated with a change in the temperature. In speaking of association, it should be clear that both phenomena of interest must, in fact, show variation. There can be no association (and hence no causal relation) between one phenomenon that changes (or varies) and one that remains constant. If, for example, temperature remains constant at 100°F but the water under consideration is gradually subjected to less and less atmospheric pressure, at some point before reaching a total vacuum it will begin to boil and change to water vapor. Now there is no association between the change in the water and the temperature because the temperature is constant. Here temperature cannot be seen as the cause of the change in the state of the water. A variable cannot be causally related to a constant.

In certain evaluation settings—especially in monitoring, time series analysis, and experiments—it may actually be possible to observe change occurring over time. In survey research, on the other hand, it is generally possible only to observe different levels of two phenomena that are to be related to one another. If the question is attitudes toward a primary health care program and the use of services provided by primary health care workers, for example, association could be established if both attitudes toward the program held by various people in the survey and their behavior about use of primary health care services differ from one another. Again, however, if there are no differences between the people in the survey either in feelings or behavior, there can be no association and hence no causal relationship between the two. It may, of course, be argued that measures of either attitudes or behavior in regard to this particular question of interest may be so gross as to obscure real differences among respondents. The evaluator's task in this type of setting would be to devise instruments for measuring either attitudes or behavior sensitive enough to detect differences that might be related to one another between these two variables.

Lack of variation in one or both measures under observation (for example, behavior and attitudes) is not the only, or even the most important, reason that the two measures may not be associated. It may be that even if both measures show substantial variation, the variation in one may be essentially random with respect to variation in the other. Under such circumstances association still may not be shown. Several analytical techniques—correlation, contingency analysis, regression, and analysis of variance and covariance—are capable of establishing the existence or lack of an association. These techniques are discussed in more detail in later sections of the book.

Elimination of other variables

If the time sequence is correct or can be established from a plausible theory or conceptual framework, and if association can be shown, the final task in establishing cause is to eliminate other variables as logical candidates for having caused the observed result, output, or effect.

In a survey situation, other variables can be eliminated in two ways. Other variables can be ruled out as likely causes of a phenomenon that has occurred or been observed, again, on the basis of a theoretical framework or conceptual perspective that makes them irrelevant to the process. If, for example, the concern is the relationship between attitudes toward a primary health care program held by potential care recipients and their use of primary health care services, it is unlikely that an evaluator, say, would consider that the height of interviewees was the real cause of the extent of their use of primary health care services. Height is a variable that would be simply considered irrelevant to the use of primary health care facilities in most concepts of how such use comes about. On the other hand, it might be quite reasonable to assume that one's perception of personal health status might be quite important to the behavior in regard to the use of primary health care facilities. Such a variable would need to be eliminated through analysis.

**Illustration: Attitudes and behavior
in a primary care program**

To clarify the issues of establishing cause, let us consider two hypotheses often examined in the evaluation of primary care programs:

H_1 = Attitudes of respondents toward the program are
the cause of their utilization behavior.

H_2 = Perception of personal needs for services are the
cause of the respondents' utilization behavior.

In terms of time ordering we have simply assumed, on the basis of
our conceptual framework, that attitudes precede behavior, that the
differential perceptions about services produce different use of services rather than the opposite. So we will not examine the alternative
possibility that behavior causes attitudes. We have essentially ruled
out the problem of time ordering.

Analysis of contingency tables

The problem of association can be resolved as indicated through a
number of mechanisms. To keep this example as simple as possible,
we will deal only with analysis of contingency tables at this point.
Regression and analysis of variance and covariance, as other analytic
techniques, are presented in later sections.

Assume that a sample has been drawn from people who would
normally use primary health care services in a particular organizational setting. Perhaps the initial sample is 200 people drawn on a
random basis. The evaluator has gone out to interview these 200
people and managed to get usable interviews from 190. Ten people
who were not interviewed, representing a nonresponse of 5 percent,
may have an effect on the results obtained from the evaluation, but
this nonresponse rate is very low even for an interview.

The evaluator, with a usable sample of 190 people who have
answered a series of questions, is able to construct three scales:

1. attitude toward the primary health care program
2. number of symptoms of ill health perceived by respondents
   that would be likely to require primary heath care services
3. use of primary care services

Assume that the evaluator has decided that the scales are so
gross that it makes sense to divide them only into two categories. For
attitude toward the program, the scales are divided into two categories: "favorable to the program" (containing 90 people who give the
most favorable response) and "unfavorable to the program" (containing the remaining 100 people). Use of services is divided into "high
use of services" (containing 80 people who use the most services) and
"low use of services" (containing the remaining 110 people). The first
question to be examined is whether attitudes toward the program are
associated with use of services, association being one of the three
criteria by which to judge the existence of a causal relationship.

Assume further that the evaluator has now examined a simultaneous occurrence of attitudes toward the program and use of services. The result of that examination might be as shown in Table 9-4—another example of a contingency table. In this table we can see that 38 of the 90 respondents who were favorable toward the primary health care program had high use of services and 52 had low use. At the same time, 42 of the people unfavorable to the program had high use of services and 58 had low use. This table indicates no relationship between attitudes toward the program, at least as measured on this two-dimensional scale, and use of services as measured on the two-dimensional use scale. Of those favorable to the program, 42 percent had high use of services; of those unfavorable to the program, 42 percent also had high use. There is essentially no difference between the two groups of people in their use of services. Thus if the evaluator were examining the question of whether attitudes toward the program resulted in subsequent use of services, he would, on the basis of Table 9-4, conclude that they did not.

Furthermore, from the standpoint of decision making about strategies for increasing the acceptance of services from the primary health care program, the evaluator would probably recommend that program managers not try to change the attitudes of people toward the program. If they wish to increase use, they should find an alternative strategy. It may not lead to any productive behavior for increasing use of services, but it could restrain the administrators from wasting time in education or attitude adjustment.

Table 9-5 presents an association between attitudes toward a program and use of services leading to a different conclusion. The categories remain the same, but the numbers have been changed within the cells for discussion purposes. In this case, of the 90 people

Table 9-4   Relationship between Feelings about the Primary Health Care Program and Use of Services: Alternative 1

	Favorable to Program		Unfavorable to Program		
	N	%	N	%	Total N
High service use	38	42	42	42	80
Low service use	52	58	58	58	110
Total N	90		100		190

Table 9-5 Relationship between Feelings about the Primary Health Care Program and Use of Services: Alternative 2

	Favorable to Program		Unfavorable to Program		
	N	%	N	%	Total N
High service use	50	56	30	30	80
Low service use	40	44	70	70	110
Total N	90		100		190

favorable to the primary health care program, 50 had high use of services. Among the 100 people unfavorable to the program, only 30 had high use of services. The difference in these two categories is 56 percent as compared to 30 percent.

This table shows a probable relationship between attitudes toward the program and use of services. Basically a higher proportion of persons favorable to the program had a high use of services. Those unfavorable to the program had a clear-cut lower use of services. If Table 9-5 had resulted from an examination of actual interviews with 190 respondents, the conclusion would be that the second criterion for cause (association) had been satisfied. A statistical test of significance of the data in Table 9-5 would also show that the relationship was not likely to have occurred by chance. The statistic used in this case would be the Chi-Square, which is discussed later.

The final step in the analysis is to eliminate other variables as possible causes of high use of services. The assumption is that we are working on a very simple theory. Either attitudes toward the program or perceptions of number of symptoms appropriate for treatment result in use of services. No other factors are assumed to cause use of services. Of course, this assumption is not reasonable. Other factors may contribute to use of services. Nevertheless, this premise will be accepted here.

To determine whether the number of symptoms perceived can be eliminated as an alternative causal explanation for use of services, it is necessary to examine all three variables simultaneously. One result of such an examination appears in Table 9-6. For this analysis, the 190 respondents have been grouped into eight categories, representing those with many or few symptoms, favorable or unfavorable attitudes toward the program, and high or low use of services. Two points about Table 9-6 should be noted. First, there are still 80 people who are classified as having high use of services and 110 people classified as having low use of services. Second, the four cells in Table 9-5 can be reconstructed from the data in Table 9-6. Those people with favorable attitudes toward the program and high use of services, for instance, are divided into those with many symptoms (45) and those with few (5). It totals 50 people in all, just as with that category in Table 9-5. The same can be said for all other categories in Table 9-5.

The importance of Table 9-6 is that there is no relationship between attitudes toward the program and use of services when this relationship is examined in conjunction with numbers of symptoms. For those people with many symptoms, attitudes toward the program had little effect on use of services. Of those with favorable attitudes, 64 percent had high use of services; 75 percent of those with unfavorable attitudes had high use of services. An opposite result occurs for those with few symptoms: 75 percent of those favorable toward the program and 81 percent unfavorable toward the program had low use of services.

The conclusion from Table 9-6 is that the relationship between attitudes toward the program and use of services as shown in Table 9-5 is not a direct causal relationship between favorableness to the program and use of services but is what we call a *spurious relationship;* that is, the relationship exists because both use of services and attitudes toward the program are related to numbers of symptoms.

Finally, Table 9-7 presents the same categories but demonstrates a situation in which attitudes toward the program have an effect on use of services. In the category of people with many symptoms, 60 percent of those with favorable attitudes toward the program use services extensively, whereas only 20 percent of those with unfavorable attitudes had similar patterns of use. In the category of few symptoms, 54 percent of those favorable toward the program also had a high use of services, and 33 percent of persons with unfavorable attitudes had a high use of services. In this case, attitudes about services cannot be ruled out as a cause of their use.

Tables 9-6 and 9-7 lead to substantially different conclusions and thus to different action strategies on the part of program managers. Table 9-6 would lead to the conclusion that the relationship between attitudes toward the program and use of services found in Table 9-5 was a function of the relationship of symptoms to both variables; these data would lead to the conclusion that efforts toward

Table 9-6 Relationship between Feelings about the Primary Health Care Program and Use of Services, Controlling for Reported Symptoms: Alternative 2a

| | Many Symptoms | | | | Few Symptoms | | | | |
| | Favorable to Program | | Unfavorable to Program | | Favorable to Program | | Unfavorable to Program | | Total N |
	N	%	N	%	N	%	N	%	
High service use	45	64	15	75	5	25	15	19	80
Low service use	25	36	5	25	15	75	65	81	110
Total N	70		20		20		80		190

Table 9-7 Relationship between Feelings about the Primary Health Care Program and Use of Services, Controlling for Reported Symptoms: Alternative 2b

| | Many Symptoms | | | | Few Symptoms | | | | |
| | Favorable to Program | | Unfavorable to Program | | Favorable to Program | | Unfavorable to Program | | Total N |
	N	%	N	%	N	%	N	%	
High service use	15	60	5	20	35	54	25	33	80
Low service use	10	40	20	80	30	46	50	67	110
Total N	25		25		65		75		190

education or other activities to improve attitudes toward the program would have relatively little effect in terms of increasing use of services. On the other hand, Table 9-7 has essentially ruled out numbers of symptoms as an alternative cause of the relationship between attitudes and use of services and would confirm the information of Table 9-5; that is, if use of services is to be increased, people should be given information that would improve their attitudes toward the program.

Approaches to Data Analysis

Several specific statistical techniques are appropriate and useful when survey research is the format for program evaluation. These techniques are presented under two headings, categorical data analysis and continuous data analysis. This approach may imply some distinctions in techniques that are, in other formulations, only artificial, but it is a useful division for a discussion of statistical techniques applied to program evaluation.

Categorical data analysis

Categorical data analysis involves techniques that may be used when important variables in the evaluation setting are measured on nominal or ordinal scales (for discussion of levels of measurement, see Chapter 14).

Every statistical analysis technique, whether using data of the categorical or continuous type, is basically a comparison between two measurements taken on set of objects that constitute the units of analysis. The "objects" may be people, geographic areas, political entities, organizations, or any other organizable units that may be subject to change because of the effects of a program under evaluation. The purpose of such a comparison is to determine whether the two phenomena being measured are associated with one another across the units of analysis to a degree that cannot be explained by chance alone. In general, one measure will be assumed to apply to an independent, or causal, variable while the other will be of a dependent, or caused, variable. This distinction, however, has no influence on the statistical or mathematical aspects of the analysis. Consider, for example, the almost classic illustration of a public television program that has been developed to increase mothers' awareness of the importance of polio vaccinations.

*Illustration: Evaluating public television efforts
to increase awareness of polio vaccinations
(Moser and Kalton 1972)*

To evaluate the value of the program, a questionnaire is sent out six
months after the program appeared to 1,800 households identified
when the program was aired as having children in a specified age
group who had not been vaccinated. Here are two questions asked in
this questionnaire: Did you (the mother of the household) view the
program? Has your child been vaccinated?

The two questions will both produce categorical results. It is a
minor point as to whether the results are measured on a nominal
scale—seeing the program is different from not seeing it—or an
ordinal scale—viewing the program or having a child vaccinated represents "more" of something than not doing so (see Chapter 14 for a
more extensive discussion of types of scales). Determining whether
the television program has been effective in promoting vaccination of
children can be made for categorical-type data by using contingency
table analysis. Table 9-8 shows the relationship between the television
program and vaccinations.

Of 1,800 women responding to the questionnaire, 800 reported
having viewed the program and 1,000 reported not having seen it.
Among those who viewed the program, 400 had their children vaccinated (50 percent) and 400 failed to do so. Of those who did not view
the program, 280 (or only 28 percent) had their children vaccinated,
whereas the other 720 failed to do so. Because the total number who
viewed the program or did not view it differs, it is easiest to compare
the percentages in a contingency table to determine the direction of
any possible relationship. In this case, half of those who viewed had
their children vaccinated and half did not, whereas nearly three-
quarters of those who did not view the program failed to have their
children vaccinated. It would seem to suggest that the program had
some influence on whether mothers had their children vaccinated.
Clearly it was not the only influence because only half the mothers
who saw the program had their children vaccinated; in comparison to
mothers who did not view the program, however, it appears to have
had some impact.

Statistical analysis becomes relevant when asking whether the
difference between mothers who viewed the program and those who
did not could be considered a chance occurrence. The question is:
Assuming that we were able to interview any 800 mothers who may
have viewed the program and any 1,000 who had not, what is the

Table 9-8 Relationship between Mother's Viewing of Program and Child's Subsequent Vaccination

	Mothers				Total	
	Viewed Program		Did Not View Program			
Children	N	%	N	%	N	%
Vaccinated	400	50.0	280	28.0	680	38.0
Not vaccinated	400	50.0	720	72.0	1,120	62.0
Total	800	44.0	1,000	56.0	1,800	100.0

Source: Reprinted from C. A. Moser and G. Kalton, *Survey Methods in Social Investigation,* Second Edition (New York: Basic Books, 1972), p. 448, with the permission of Dartmouth Publishing Co.

likelihood that the distribution we found would have occurred if we knew that there was no relationship between viewing and vaccination (or, more specifically, under the null hypothesis of no relationship)?

Calculating a Chi-Square. The statistical test used with categorical data of this type is known as the *Chi-Square.* The Chi-Square statistic is a powerful statistic for categorical data, particularly when a relatively few variables are to be considered. A Chi-Square statistic is calculated.

$$X^2 = \Sigma \frac{(O - E)^2}{E} \tag{9-1}$$

Here O represents the actual "observed" number in each cell and E the "expected" number in each cell. The expected number in each cell is simply the number that would appear in any cell if the values in the cells were distributed strictly proportionately to row and column totals. For example, 38 percent of all mothers have their children vaccinated. The expected number of families in the category "mothers viewed the program and children were vaccinated" would be 38 percent of the 800 families where mothers viewed the program. The easiest way to obtain expected values is simply to multiply the appropriate column total by the appropriate row total and divide by the overall total. The expected frequency in the first cell, then, would be $(800 \cdot 680)/1800 = 302.22$. Other expected values are obtained in the same manner.

Calculation of the actual Chi-Square value for Table 9-8 is

$$X^2 = \frac{(400 - 302.22)^2}{302.22} + \frac{(400 - 497.78)^2}{497.78} +$$

$$\frac{(280 - 377.78)^2}{377.78} + \frac{(720 - 622.22)^2}{622.22} = 91.52$$

(9-2)

Interpretation. The resulting Chi-Square value of 91.52 can be assessed on the basis of a table of the distribution of Chi-Square that appears in most elementary statistics books. Two things must be known to assess the Chi-Square: the actual value of the Chi-Square (91.52) and the number of degrees of freedom in the contingency table under analysis. The number of degrees of freedom in a contingency table analysis of this type is (the number of rows minus one) times (the number of columns minus one). On this basis, Table 9-8 has one degree of freedom. If the .01 level is accepted as a reasonable level of statistical significance, a table of Chi-Square distributions will show that with one degree of freedom a Chi-Square value as large as 6.6 has less than a 1 percent probability of occurring (.01) by chance when there is, in fact, no relationship between viewing the program and subsequent vaccination of children. Consequently, a Chi-Square with a value as large as that for Table 9-8 must, in general, be considered a result that did not occur by chance. The null hypothesis of no relationship between viewing and vaccination would be rejected. The conclusion that an evaluator draws on the basis of this information should be that a mother who views the program will be more likely to have her child vaccinated than one who does not view the program.

Analysis of the data shown in Table 9-8 satisfies two criteria for the establishment of a causal relationship between, in this case, mothers viewing the program and subsequent vaccination of children. It has satisfied the time ordering criterion by our knowledge that only families in which the children had not been vaccinated prior to the airing of the program had been surveyed subsequently. It satisfies the association criterion by virtue of the result of the Chi-Square analysis. The criterion of elimination of other variables has not been satisfied, however, and we will discuss briefly the use of contingency tables in considering this criterion. In doing so, we will continue with the example originally presented by Moser and Kalton (1972).

Spurious relationships. In any group of families with small children who have not been vaccinated there is some likelihood that over a six-

Table 9-9 Relationship between Class Status, Viewing of Program, and Child's Subsequent Vaccination: Example 1

	Mothers							
	Middle Class				*Working Class*			
	Viewed Program		*Did Not View Program*		*Viewed Program*		*Did Not View Program*	
Children	N	%	N	%	N	%	N	%
Vaccinated	360	60.0	120	60.0	40	20.0	160	20.0
Not vaccinated	240	40.0	80	40.0	160	80.0	640	80.0
Total N	600		200		200		800	

Source: Reprinted from C. A. Moser and G. Kalton, *Survey Methods in Social Investigation*, Second Edition (New York: Basic Books, 1972), p. 448, with the permission of Dartmouth Publishing Co.

month period some of the children will be vaccinated whether the program is viewed or not. It is possible that some variable other than viewing the program can account for the relationship found between seeing the program and subsequent vaccination of children. If such is the case, the effect or value of the program would be in question.

In Table 9-8, 800 mothers viewed the program and 1,000 did not. This is still true with Table 9-9. In addition, 800 mothers were classified as middle class and 1,000 as working class. It is also still the case that 680 children were vaccinated and 1,120 were not. Table 9-9, however, shows a substantially different outcome than Table 9-8. Looking at the percentages of those in the middle class who viewed the program and had their children vaccinated as opposed to those who neither saw the program nor had their children vaccinated, the percentages are precisely the same (60 percent). At the same time, the percentage of those in the working class who viewed the program and subsequently had their children vaccinated is exactly the same (20 percent) as those in the working class who did not see the program but did have their children vaccinated. Moreover, if a Chi-Square were calculated separately for those mothers who are middle class and those who are working class, it would be found that the Chi-Square value for either subtable would be zero. The conclusion that must be drawn, then, is that viewing the program has no relationship to subsequent vaccination of children; it is only social status that

Table 9-10   Relationship between Class Status, Viewing of Program, and Child's Subsequent Vaccination: Example 2

	Mothers							
	Middle Class				Working Class			
	Viewed Program		Did Not View Program		Viewed Program		Did Not View Program	
Children	N	%	N	%	N	%	N	%
Vaccinated	100	50.0	70	28.0	300	50.0	210	28.0
Not vaccinated	100	50.0	180	72.0	300	50.0	540	72.0
Total N	200		250		600		750	

Source: Reprinted from C. A. Moser and G. Kalton, *Survey Methods in Social Investigation*, Second Edition (New York: Basic Books, 1972), p. 449, with the permission of Dartmouth Publishing Co.

determines whether a child will be vaccinated. This is true even though the original table (Table 9-8) showed a significant relationship between viewing and vaccination. This relationship, when examined vis-à-vis class status, was found to be spurious, just as the relationship between attitudes and use of services (Table 9-6) was found to be spurious when symptoms were controlled. On the basis of this more thorough analysis, it would be concluded that the television program had produced no observable effect on the target population.

Three variable analysis

Table 9-10 shows that the number of mothers viewing the program continues to be 800 and the number not viewing it continues to be 1,000. The number of children vaccinated continues to be 680 and the number not vaccinated 1,120. But now the number of mothers considered middle class has been reduced to 450, and the number considered working class is 1,350.

The important characteristic of this table, however, is that it supports the conclusion drawn from Table 9-8. Half the middle-class mothers who viewed the program had their children vaccinated, whereas nearly three-quarters of the middle-class mothers who did not watch it failed to have their children vaccinated. The same result occurred among working-class mothers. The conclusion, then, that would be drawn from this table is that knowledge of class status does not eliminate the relationship between viewing the program and vaccination; an evaluator of the television program would conclude, at least on the basis of this information, that the program had been effective.

There are a number of other possible outcomes of three-variable analysis. It is possible, for example, to show a situation in which a relationship could exist between viewing the program and vaccination within one class that would be nonexistent in the other, or it would be possible to show situations in which the relationship actually reversed itself between classes. Any of these results would provide important information for the decision as to whether the television program was effective. Furthermore, many other factors or characteristics of mothers or families might theoretically account for the apparent relationship shown in Table 9-8. A thorough evaluation of the program should include measures on these other variables and appropriate analyses.

Analysis of contingency tables can become quite complex when a large number of possible variables must be eliminated before an apparent causal relationship can be accepted. The program evaluator in a survey situation should be aware of these other possible causal variables and make an effort to obtain measures on them before or during the course of the survey. If real causes of having children vaccinated were not measured in the evaluation of the television program, it would be impossible to eliminate them as possible causes in the subsequent analysis.

Limitations. If important variables can be specified in advance, analysis of contingency tables is a powerful technique for evaluating certain types of programs in survey situations. But it has two distinct methodological difficulties. One is the complexity of analysis when more than three variables are considered simultaneously. A table that involves four or more variables at one time may simply be quite difficult to interpret. Yet it is rarely the case in real applications that the results of an analysis involving more than two variables will be as straightforward as shown in Tables 9-9 or 9-10. These tables are ideal cases that would almost never occur in real life. When the distribution of data is quite complex in tables, it may be difficult to interpret the results adequately.

The second problem—loss of observations—can also be a major one in contingency analysis. The preceding example includes 1,800 families—a substantial sample size. On the other hand, the evaluation might have been based on a survey of as few as 180 households. Then the expected value in the first cell of Table 9-10 would have been approximately 7.5 for calculating the Chi-Square relative to the subtable middle-class mothers. It is possible to get a valid Chi-Square with an expected frequency of 7.5, but if the expected frequency goes below 5.0 and the table has more than four cells, the chi-square statistic is no longer strictly appropriate and there is no appropriate alternative. When expected frequencies in any cell approach zero (which is possible with small sample sizes and a large number of cells), the Chi-Square statistic may give a badly inflated view of the true relationship. Consequently, analysis of contingency tables using the Chi-Square must generally be limited to categorical data that take on a relatively few different values and to examination of no more than three or four variables at any one time.

Converting ratio and interval data: Independent variable. Thus far we have discussed data measured on all variables with essentially nominal or ordinal measurement. Various categorical data analysis approaches or strategies can also be applied to data in which the independent or causal variables are measured on nominal or ordinal scales but the dependent or caused variable is measured on an interval or ratio scale. It would be possible to convert the dependent variables in Tables 9-8 to 9-10 to a ratio scale by recording the proportion of mothers who viewed the program and had their children vaccinated compared to the proportion who did not view the program but still had their children vaccinated. In the former case, the proportion would be .5 or 50 percent and in the latter .28 or 28 percent. Acceptable statistical techniques are available for testing the difference between two proportions. Then it would be a test of the null hypothesis that the population from which the women came who viewed the program and the population from which the women came who did not see it both had the same probability of having their children vaccinated.

Converting ratio and interval data: Dependent variable. A second type of categorical analysis occurs when the independent variables are categorical but the dependent variable is a true interval or ratio measure (rather than simply a proportion generated from a nominal or ordinal dichotomy). Suppose that in our example, in addition to learning whether children had been vaccinated in the postprogram survey, the evaluators had also asked the responding women to rate on a ten-point scale, from very unimportant to very important, the value of the vaccination to the child's health. Assuming that this ten-point scale is treated as interval data for the purpose of analysis, it would be possible to calculate a mean value for the 800 women who saw the program in regard to the importance they placed on vaccination for the child's health and a mean value for the 1,000 women who did not see the program. These data could be analyzed in terms of the difference in the mean between the two groups, the null hypothesis being that the women come from two groups similar in their attitude toward the importance of vaccination. If the null hypothesis could not be disproved, it would suggest that the program has no influence on mothers' attitude toward the polio vaccine.

This type of analysis can be extended to include more categorical variables than simply having viewed or not viewed the program, such as social class (middle class or working class). Again, problems of numbers of respondents in each category will arise; in particular, it is frequently difficult to deal with different numbers of respondents in various cells. Partly because of this problem, analysis of this type (that is, categorical analysis of data where the dependent variable is either a proportion or a true continuous variable) is rarely carried out in survey analysis. Instead a different technique, essentially equivalent in terms of results but somewhat different in origin and approach, is generally used. This technique is known as *analysis of covariance*, which is essentially a class of regression analysis. The remainder of this chapter considers the analysis of both continuous and categorical data, using regression analysis and the particular techniques useful to program evaluation in this context.

A point should be made about the distinction between analysis of covariance or regression and analysis of variance. Regression, in particular, and analysis of covariance to a certain extent, developed from the survey research tradition of sociology, political science, and econometrics. Analysis of variance, on the other hand, developed from the experimental tradition of agriculture and psychology. The ultimate results of either analytical approach are essentially the same, but the mechanics of regression are somewhat better adapted to survey settings than those of analysis of variance. The mechanics of analysis of variance are somewhat better adapted to experimental settings. The application of analysis of variance is described in the section on analysis of experimental data.

Continuous data analysis

This section provides an introduction to certain regression techniques and analysis of covariance useful to program evaluation. These types of analyses are particularly useful to program evaluation when there are multiple causal variables and the dependent variable is an interval or ratio measure.

Regression

Regression is the primary analytical form for survey data in which the dependent variable can be expressed either as a proportion or probability or as a true continuous variable of the interval or ratio type. In general, independent variables in regression can be either categorical or continuous. To present regression in the simplest form, we consider the continuous independent variable first even though, for evaluation purposes, it is often necessary to consider categorical data as well.*

In its simplest form, regression is a technique for describing the relationship between two continuous variables related to one another in a linear fashion. This relationship between two variables is expressed in the form of

$$Y_i = b_1 X_i + b_0 + e_i \qquad (9\text{-}3)$$

Here Y_i represents the continuous dependent variable or caused variable, X_i the continuous independent or causal variable, b_1 the coefficient of the relationship between X and Y (often referred to as the *slope* of the equation), b_0 is an additive constant (often referred to as the *intercept*), and e_i is an error term that represents the difference between the actual and predicted value of Y.

In this simple two-variable case, X and Y are known values, and the problem is to estimate the values of b_1 and b_0. Estimates of b_1 and b_0 will then lead to estimates of the error, e_i. Ignoring the error term, Equation 9-3 is the equation for a straight line. If the joint distribution of X and Y is graphed with X on the horizontal axis and Y on the vertical axis, Equation 9-3 represents an attempt to put a best-fitting straight line through the joint distribution.

Illustration. To understand what these statements mean in somewhat more concrete terms, consider the graph of a relationship between a variable X and a variable Y as Figure 9-1 shows. The oblong shaded area represents a hypothetical set of a large number of points of the coincidence of the X and Y variables. When X equals 8, for example,

---

*For additional details, see Kleinbaum and Kupper (1978), Neter and Wasserman (1974), Wonnacott and Wonnacott (1979), Kerlinger and Pedhazur (1973), Theil (1971), and Gujarati (1988).

there are specific values of Y according to the shaded area between approximately 3 and 10. When X equals 4, on the other hand, there is no specific value of Y equal to 10, for this point falls outside the shaded area. The shaded area may represent any number of points that would correspond to the number of observations in the data set for which the measures X and Y are taken.

Regression is a technique for putting a best-fitting straight line through that set of points as indicated by line a. "Best fitting" in this case is generally understood to be the line that minimizes the squared difference between the actual value of Y and the predicted value of Y based on X. It is from this concept of the best-fitting straight line that the term *ordinary least squares*, often used to characterize regression, derives.

In Figure 9-1 line a crosses the Y axis at approximately 1.5 on the Y scale and slopes upward so that, as the line moves two units on the X scale, it moves one unit on the Y scale. Here, then, the value of b_0, the coefficient that represents the intercept, would be 1.5, and the value of b_1, representing the slope of the line, would be the distance traveled on Y as X moves one unit, or 0.5. In consequence, a formula for the relationship between X and Y based on the example of Figure 9-1 would be

$$\hat{Y}_i = 0.5X_i + 1.5 \qquad (9\text{-}4)$$

where $\hat{Y}$ represents the predicted value of Y ($\hat{Y}_1 + e_i = Y_i$).

Figure 9-1   Illustrative Graph of Relationship between a Variable X and a Variable Y

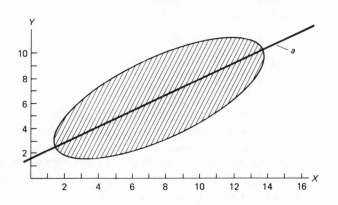

Calculating b *values.* In the simple two-variable case, the actual calculation of b_1 and b_0 are shown in Equations 9-5a and 9-5b. Because both values of X_i and Y_i are known and values of $\overline{X}$ and $\overline{Y}$ can be calculated from them, the value of b_1 can be computed from any set of variables X and Y that represents the slope of the relationships between those variables. The intercept term can be calculated by using Equation 9-5b so that any set of variables X and Y will allow the calculation of predicted values of Y.

$$b_1 = \frac{\Sigma (X_i - \overline{X})(Y_i - \overline{Y})}{\Sigma (X_i - \overline{X})^2} \tag{9-5a}$$

$$b_0 = \overline{Y} - b_1 \overline{X} \tag{9-5b}$$

Coefficients b_1 and b_0 calculated from Equations 9-5a and 9-5b are the coefficients that will produce the best-fitting straight-line relationship between X and Y as described by Equation 9-4. The question, however, is whether this best-fitting line actually represents a relationship between X and Y. The answer is based on whether knowledge of X is more useful in predicting values of Y than simple knowledge of the mean of Y itself. It is tantamount to the question of whether coefficient b_1 can be considered different from zero. There are various ways of testing whether coefficient b_1 or, for that matter, the intercept is different from zero. In one strategy for calculating the coefficients, both the intercept and the slope coefficients have standard deviations or standard errors. A test of whether the coefficient is different from zero can be made by dividing the coefficient by its standard error. The resulting value is a t-statistic with degrees of freedom equal to the number of observations (that is, the number of values of X and Y) less one. A second test of the likelihood that the coefficient of b_1 is different from zero is an F-test, which is carried out by dividing the average variance in Y that can be accounted for by X

$$\Sigma (\hat{Y}_i - \overline{Y})$$

by the amount of variance that cannot be accounted for by X

$$\Sigma (Y_i - \hat{Y}_i)$$

divided by appropriate degrees of freedom. If the value of either the t-test or the F-test is large enough so that the probability of its occurrence where no relationship actually exists in the population from which the sample of Xs and Ys was drawn would be less than some small number, such as .05 or .01, the general assumption is that a true relationship must exist between X and Y.

If the X_i represent a level of a continuous causal variable that can be directly manipulated by some type of service program and the Y_i represent a hoped-for outcome as a result of the manipulation of the X variable, evaluation of the program to change the values of Y by affecting the values of X can be assessed at least at the level of effectiveness.

Illustration: Evaluating the effect of environmental carbon monoxide (Levesque et al. 1990)

To illustrate regression as applied to a specific evaluation problem, consider an example taken from a recent study of the relationship between the environmental concentration of carbon monoxide and the alveolar absorption of carbon monoxide by athletes (Levesque et al. 1990). In this study, the authors were interested in determining whether the level of carbon monoxide in ice-skating rinks—generally associated with how well or poorly gasoline or propane-driven ice resurfacers operated (and thus how much carbon monoxide they gave off)—was related to the amount of carbon monoxide absorbed into the bloodstream of persons who were engaging in athletic events in the rinks. In particular, would increased levels of carbon monoxide lead to increased absorption of carbon monoxide?

One way of evaluating the effect of carbon monoxide levels on absorption would be examine the relationship between the level of carbon monoxide and the alveolar absorption rate using regression analysis. To do this, the authors measured the carbon monoxide exposure level for 90 nonsmoking hockey players playing on ten different hockey rinks and the absorption level of carbon monoxide for these same hockey players. Measurement techniques are described in detail in the article.

The result of the measurements on exposure and absorption are shown in Figure 9-2. Although the results in Figure 9-2 do not describe a simple oblong shaded area as in Figure 9-1, it is clear that there is a general linear relationship between the level of exposure and the level of absorption. In itself, this figure would suggest a relationship between the two variables.

If level of environmental concentration of carbon monoxide is taken as a logical causal variable in the level of absorption, it is possible to assess the degree of that relationship, as the authors have done, using regression. The data in Figure 9-2 were analyzed by the authors using regression analysis, with the following results:

$$\hat{Y}_i = 0.55X_i - 1.72$$

$$(.01) \qquad (.69)$$

$$(9\text{-}6)$$

Figure 9-2   Relationship between Aveolar
Absorption of Carbon Monoxide
among Players during a 90-Minute
Hockey Game based on Carbon
Monoxide Concentrations in Indoor
Skating Rinks (nonsmokers)

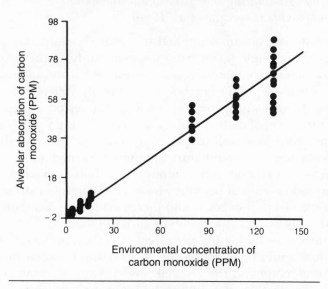

Source: Reprinted with permission from B. Levesque et al.,
"Carbon Monoxide in Indoor Ice Skating Rinks: Evaluation of
Absorption by Adult Hockey Players," *American Journal of Pub-
lic Health* 80, no. 5 (1990): 596. © 1990 American Public Health
Association.

where $\hat{Y}_i$ is the level of absorption and X_i is the level of exposure, and
the numbers in parentheses are the standard errors for the numbers
0.55 and −1.72, respectively.

Significance test. The values 0.55 and −1.72 are often referred to as
regression coefficients. One question often posed in regard to regression analysis is whether the regression coefficients are significantly
different from zero. A test of the significance of the regression
coefficients can be made by dividing the coefficient by its standard
error. In either case, the *t*-test with 88 degrees of freedom (90 observations minus one degree of freedom each for the two coefficients) is
significant well beyond the .01 level of significance for the coefficient
associated with *X*, and beyond the .05 level for the coefficient that
represents the intercept of slope at the origin. This means that the

coefficients can be judged to be different from zero, or in other words, that there appears from these data to be a real relationship between level of carbon monoxide exposure and alveolar absorption.

Proportion of variance accounted for: R^2. The extent to which knowledge of the relationship between X and Y can account for the variation in Y is also of interest. There are, as noted, two forms of variation in Y: (1) variation that is a function of X or is predicted by X and (2) variation that is not predicted by X or is essentially error variance. Their sum is the total variance in Y. If the predicted portion of the variance is divided by the total variance, it produces a statement of the proportion of variance in Y that is a function of X. This is the same as the square of the correlation between X and Y and is often referred to as R^2. For the data in Figure 9-2, R^2 is reported to be equal to .97. In other words, 97 percent of the variation in Y, absorption of carbon monoxide, is attributable to X, level of exposure.

Interpretation. A logical conclusion to be drawn from this presentation is that level of exposure to carbon monoxide determines the absorption of carbon monoxide. Indeed, there is little to make this a surprising conclusion. However, in making this conclusion, some caution would be desirable. Figure 9-2 does not contain the neat oval seen in Figure 9-1, but is rather a somewhat disjointed set of points, with several near the origin and several others farther from the origin, separated by a space where no points occur. This suggests that there may be more going on in this relationship than is easily assessed by examining only exposure and absorption without considering other factors. The authors themselves speak of the importance of variables such as age and pulmonary function.

A second aspect of Figure 9-2 makes the simple regression analysis subject to some question, as well. It is not unreasonable to believe that the variation in absorption might be related to the level of exposure (this can be seen because the distribution of points gets broader as exposure levels increase). In such a circumstance, the appropriate analysis may be more complex than simple regression, based on what is called ordinary least squares, and may rather be a weighted least-squares technique that takes into account the increasing variation in absorption with exposure.

Analysis of covariance

Analysis of covariance is an extension of regression that is particularly appropriate to program evaluation. It is especially relevant to those types of evaluations in which the persons receiving the benefits of a particular program, or the areas in which a particular program has been implemented, have not been chosen on a random or probability basis so that the evaluation cannot take the form of an experiment. In this case, it is still desirable to contrast the group of people or the areas that receive the benefits of the program with groups of people or areas that do not receive program benefits. Given such a situation, evaluation is often likely to be based on the survey approach. Still, the aim is to compare persons receiving the program or areas in which it is implemented to persons not receiving the program or the areas where it is not implemented. But doing so is difficult because it is never clear that the people or areas that the program is to affect were comparable at the outset. Analysis of covariance is a mechanism for comparing two groups or two areas, or sets of groups or areas, when the effects of differences in other characteristics of the groups or areas are held constant.

In this section we discuss such analysis of covariance only from the standpoint of mechanics and a hypothetical example. An example using actual data is given in the section on time series analysis, where analysis of covariance is also useful in evaluating program effects.

Multiple regression

To understand analysis of covariance, it is first necessary to have some exposure to multiple regression.* The discussion thus far has considered only a single dependent variable regressed on a single independent variable. The formulas for finding the coefficients of the regression equation were given in Equations 9-5a and 9-5b. *Multiple regression* is a technique for regressing a single dependent variable simultaneously on two or more independent variables where the equation is of the general type:

$$\hat{Y}_i = b_1 X_{1i} + b_2 X_{2i} + \ldots + b_j X_{ji} + b_0 \qquad (9\text{-}7)$$

In Equation 9-7 there are j different independent variables designated X_1 through X_j. There will be j different coefficients to be estimated for each of variables X_{ji}, plus a single coefficient b_0 for the intercept. It can be shown that the values of coefficients b_1 through b_j and b_0 can be found by solving a set of simultaneous linear equations

---

*For additional details, see Kaluzny and Veney (1980), Kerlinger and Pedhazur (1973), and Theil (1971). Actual operation is available through computer packages, such as SAS (SAS Institute 1988) and SPSS (Norusis 1988).

involving the dependent variable and each of the independent variables. There will be $j + 1$ of these simultaneous equations.

In Equation 9-7 variables X_{ji} may be continuous variables representing characteristics of the populations under study that are to be controlled, or they may be one or more dummy variables representing either control for the population or actual program characteristics. To illustrate its application to an evaluation problem, consider the following example.

Illustration: Evaluating a supplementary feeding program

Consider a supplementary feeding program for newborn children administered through a local public health department. The purpose of this program is to ensure better nutrition to newborns who otherwise would be in danger of inadequate nutrition. Assume that the program operates through the child's first year of life. One clear goal would be to increase the child's birth weight throughout its first year of life—and obviously at the end of its first year of life—over what might prevail if the child were not given additional nutritional supplement. Clearly it will be impossible to compare the child at any point in the first year of life with the situation that would have prevailed had the child not had the nutritional supplement. The child either has it or it does not. It might be possible, however, to compare the children who received the supplement to a similar population of children who did not in order to determine if weight at any particular point is different (and particularly greater) for the group receiving the nutritional supplement.

From an experimental standpoint it might be conceivable to begin with the population of all children born within a certain time period and randomly assign them to the group that receives a nutritional supplement and to a group that does not. In practical terms, however, such a strategy is all but impossible for program evaluation. First, a program of nutritional supplement would probably hope to provide the supplement to anyone who was eligible and could be reached on a continuing basis. Even then there would be a great deal of social stigma attached to a program so callous and calculating as to assign children to receive or not receive nutritional supplement on a random basis simply to determine whether that nutritional supplement made a difference in weight at any point in time.

But, for any program of this type, some children will receive the benefits (the nutritional supplement) because their parents are interested, concerned, willing to follow up and obtain the supplement, or because they are in an area where the supplement is readily obtainable, and so forth, whereas other children, for totally non–program-related reasons—and particularly for reasons not related to an experimental design propounded by the evaluator—will not receive these nutritional supplements. The question then is: Can a difference be detected between the children who received the nutritional supplement, even though not a random group, and another group of children that can serve as a control? The immediate reaction should be that the comparison is difficult because a number of items associated with a child's weight cannot be controlled or taken account of in a nonexperimental setting. This is precisely where analysis of covariance is useful.

The objective of the evaluation is to measure the effect of the program among children who have reached the age of one year. The evaluators realize that several factors could have influenced a child's weight in addition to having been in the program for a year—original birth weight, height, and some family predisposition to weight gain. Birth weight can be taken from the original birth record. Height can be recorded at the time of the one-year physical examination, and a family propensity to weight gain might be taken by measuring the mother's weight. An evaluation of the program based on analysis of covariance then could be constructed as

$$\hat{Y}_i = b_1 X_{1i} + b_2 X_{2i} + b_3 X_{3i} + b_0 \tag{9-8}$$

where $\hat{Y}$ = estimated weight at one year/height
X_1 = birth weight/birth length
X_2 = mother's weight
X_3 = program participation (1 if in program, 0 if not in program)

It should be noted that X_3 is what is known as a *dummy variable*. Unlike mother's weight or birth weight divided by birth length, X_3 (program participation) takes on only two values: one if the child participated in the program and zero if the child did not.

To be certain that the reader understands the nature of the data being presented, Table 9-11 shows a listing of the data to be analyzed for ten children, six of whom have participated in the program and four of whom have not. Table 9-11 represents very much what data arrayed for a study of this type might look like. Variable Y is the weight at one year in grams divided by height in inches. X_1 is birth weight in grams divided by birth length in inches. X_2 is mother's weight in pounds, and X_3 is a representation of program participation. Clearly

Table 9-11 Example of Data for Analysis of Covariance of Effect of Supplementary Nutrition Program

Child	Y	X_1	X_2	X_3
1	324	201	120	1
2	300	220	142	1
3	310	185	115	1
4	292	165	105	0
5	285	210	113	0
6	334	192	160	1
7	297	197	118	1
8	314	213	123	0
9	278	210	110	1
10	279	178	108	0

they may not be all the variables that could influence weight at one year. The variables have been restricted to two continuous variables and a single variable for program participation to keep the example simple.

Assume that the information indicated is available for 400 children who have participated in the supplementary diet program. A sample of another 500 children who did not participate but who came from the general area in which the program was operating and who will serve as controls has been drawn. Submitting the data for 900 children, 400 of whom have been in the program and 500 of whom have not, to regression analyses might produce a printout very much as shown in Table 9-12. (Remember that it is an entirely imaginary example.)

Calculating sums of squares. Table 9-12 is in three parts. The first shows the sum of squares that can be attributed to regression and the sum of squares attributed to error. A sum of squares that can be attributed to regression can be calculated from

$$SS_{Regression} = \sum_{i=1}^{n} (\hat{Y}_i - \overline{Y})^2$$

Essentially it represents the difference between each predicted value of Y as defined by Equation 9-8 and the actual mean of all values of Y.

Table 9-12   Example of Results of Regression Analysis on Type of
Data Shown in Table 9-11

	SS	MS	df	F
Regression	95,277	23,819.25	3	93.55
Error	228,133	254.61	896	
Multiple R	.5428			
Multiple R^2	.2946			

Variable	b	Standard Error b	t	Probability t
X_1	1.24	0.023	53.91	<.001
X_2	0.20	0.312	0.64	>.1
X_3	31.50	3.241	9.72	<.001
(Intercept)	20.26	1.796	11.28	<.001

This is the proportion of variance in the observed values of Y or the
proportion of variance in the child's weight to height at one year that
can be accounted for or attributed to the three variables—birth
weight to birth length, mother's weight, and program participation.
    The error sums of squares is also provided in Table 9-12 and is
defined as

$$SS_{Error} = \sum_{i=1}^{n} (Y_i - \hat{Y}_i)^2$$

The *error sums of squares* represents the difference between each observed value of the ratio between child's weight and height at one
year minus the predicted value for the same child. The second column in the first part of Table 9-12 shows the mean sums of squares
when degrees of freedom are taken into account. In order to predict
a regression line, four degrees of freedom (representing three variables and an intercept) are accounted for out of the total degrees of
freedom associated with 900 observations. The mean square for regression, then, is regression sums of squares divided by four degrees
of freedom. The mean square for the error is found by taking the
remaining degrees of freedom, 896, and dividing the total sums of
squares due to error, for a value of 254.61.

Significance tests. The final column in the first section of Table 9-12
represents a test of significance of the overall regression equation.

This is an *F*-test, as the column is labeled, with degrees of freedom 3 and 896. This *F*-test is simply the mean square due to regression divided by the mean square due to error. If the value of *F* exceeds a certain level (the level can be read from a table of the *F*-distribution, which can be found in the appendix of most statistics books), the overall regression is said to be significant in the sense that it represents something other than random chance. In fact, what it represents would be a nonchance relationship between some set of the independent variables and the dependent variable. With 3 and 896 degrees of freedom, an *F* of 93.55 would be significant far beyond the .001 level; that is, the probability that such a value would occur by chance when the predictor or independent variables have no real effect on the dependent variable is much smaller than .001.

Multiple R and R². The second section of Table 9-12 has two designations, multiple *R* and multiple R^2. The multiple R^2 may be slightly easier to understand than multiple *R*. The total sums of squares in the dependent variable can be found by adding the sums of squares attributable to regression and the sums of squares attributable to error. The sums of squares attributable to regression represent that portion of the total sums of squares that is predictable on the basis of the independent variable set. The multiple R^2 represents that proportion—in this case, .2946. In other words, 29 percent of the variance in the ratio of weight at one year in grams to height at one year in inches can be attributed to the independent variables under consideration.

Multiple *R* represents a multiple correlation between the dependent variable set and the independent variable set and, in fact, is simply the square root of multiple R^2. The multiple *R* is essentially the same as a correlation coefficient.

Coefficients. The last section of Table 9-12 shows the actual coefficients for the independent variables, the intercept term, and some statistical analyses of those coefficients. Here the coefficient for X_1, the ratio of birth weight to birth length, is 1.24; that is, as the ratio of birth weight to birth length changes by 1 unit, the ratio of weight at one year to height at one year changes by 1.24 units. The standard error of this coefficient is given as 0.023. A *t*-test for the significance of the individual coefficient is given by dividing the coefficient by its standard error, as shown in the column labeled *t*. Whether this ratio is significant is shown in the column labeled probability *t*. In this column the coefficient of X_1, the coefficient of X_3, and the intercept term are all significant (that is, they are all different from zero at some level of probability). The coefficient of X_2, 0.20, is not large enough relative to its standard error to show significance.

Because the coefficient of X_2—the coefficient of mother's weight—is not significant when considered along with birth weight and participation in the program, it would be reasonable to exclude mother's weight from the predictor variables and reestimate the coefficients of the other two variables—weight to height at one year and program participation. If this is done, there will be a slight change in the coefficients of the two remaining variables and in the intercept. When the coefficient is as small and nonsignificant as 0.20, the extent of change in the coefficients of the other two predictors and in the intercept will be quite small. Consequently, we will continue the discussion of the interpretation of the regression equation as shown in Equation 9-8 on the assumption that the coefficients of X_1, X_3, and of the intercept would not change at the second decimal level in a reanalysis.

If such a reanalysis were done, the resulting predictor equation for the ratio of weight to height at one year would be

$$\hat{Y}_i = 1.24X_1 + 31.50X_3 + 20.26 \qquad (9\text{-}9)$$

Here there is a significant coefficient for the continuous variable X_1 and a significant coefficient for the dummy variable X_3. These two coefficients mean substantially different things in interpretation, as can be seen when the two possible values for X_3 are substituted into Equation 9-9.

$$
\begin{aligned}
(\hat{Y}_i | X_3 = 1) &= 1.24X_1 + 51.76 \\
(\hat{Y}_i | X_3 = 0) &= 1.24X_1 + 20.26
\end{aligned}
\qquad (9\text{-}10)
$$

It is clear in Equation 9-10 that there are actually two regression lines. There is a regression line that represents the relationship between birth weight and weight at one year for those who participated in the program. There is a second, parallel regression line for nonparticipants, and these lines are exactly 31.50 units apart along their length. This 31.50 represents the increase in the ratio of weight to height at one year that can be attributed directly to the program itself, the program effect.

This example has considered only two continuous variables as controls that can be taken into account prior to examining the effect of the program (which, in this case, is a difference in weight of 31.50 grams per inch). The technique that it represents, however, can be used for any number of continuous or categorical variables that might be considered important to differences that must be taken into account before program effects can be measured. This approach to analysis of covariance represents a powerful technique for program evaluation when the basic data that must be relied on are essentially survey-type data.

Program interaction. The preceding section was based on the assumption that the effect of the program will be only to change the intercept of the regression equation but not to change any of the relationships between the continuous variables and the dependent variable. It is conceivable that the program will not simply influence the intercept but may have an effect on the actual relationship between the independent variables and the dependent variable themselves. This situation can be examined in terms of an analysis of covariance plus the possibility of an interaction between continuous variables and the program. Such a possibility can be taken into account through the estimation of coefficients in regression equations that involves an interaction term for the continuous variables.

Let us continue with the foregoing example and assume that we are concerned only with the ratio of birth weight to birth length as a continuous independent predictor that must be controlled before program effects can be assessed. But we are now interested in the possibility that the program may influence the relationship between birth weight and weight at one year. This issue can be evaluated by estimating the coefficients of the regression equation

$$\hat{Y}_i = b_1 X_1 + b_2 X_3 + b_3 X_1 X_3 + b_0 \tag{9-11}$$

where X_1 represents the ratio of birth weight to birth length; X_3, program participation; and $X_1 X_3$, the multiplicative product of the two. $X_1 X_3$ will be equal to X_1 when X_3 is one (when the child has been in the program) and $X_1 X_3$ will be equal to zero when the child has not been in the program. Solving for the regression coefficients in this equation will not only determine whether there has been an effect of the program but will also indicate whether that effect somehow interacts with birth weight to produce a differential effect on the relationship between birth weight and weight at one year.

Let us further assume that the coefficients in Equation 9-11 are estimated as shown in Equation 9-12 and that all four coefficients are statistically significant.

$$\hat{Y}_i = 1.15 X_1 + 17.23 X_3 + 0.32 X_1 X_3 + 20.54 \tag{9-12}$$

Under these circumstances there are two separate regression lines defined by Equation 9-12. These two regression lines are

$$(\hat{Y}_i | X_3 = 1) = 1.47X_1 + 37.77$$
$$(\hat{Y}_i | X_3 = 0) = 1.15X_1 + 20.54$$

(9-13)

Now it should be noted, however, that the coefficients of X_1 are no longer equal as they were in Equation 9-10, but, in fact, the coefficient of X_1 when X_3 equals one is larger and (if we assume that the coefficient of X_1X_3 in Equation 9-12 is significant) is significantly larger than the coefficient of X_1 when X_3 equals zero. The intercept terms also differ but only by 17.23 in this instance.

To further understand the contrast between the analysis of covariance as shown in Equation 9-10 when only the possibility of a difference in intercept term is considered and the analysis of covariance as shown in Equation 9-12 when the possibility of an interaction is considered, examine the graphs in Figure 9-3, which shows the two separate situations. Figure 9-3a shows the relationship between ratio of birth weight to birth length and ratio of weight at one year to height at one year when the possibility of an interaction is not

Figure 9-3   Relationship between Weight/Height Ratio at Birth and Weight/Height Ratio at One Year: (a) No Interaction, (b) Interaction

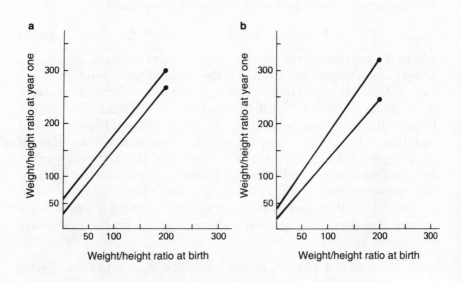

assumed, and Figure 9-3b shows the same relationship when that possibility is assumed.

The interpretation of the two separate graphs shown in Figure 9-3 follows. In the case of no interaction, the relationship between birth weight and weight at one year (standardized for height) is the same whether the child has been in the nutrition program or not. The only difference is the effect of the nutrition program itself, which at every point on the range of birth weight will add 31.50 grams per inch to the child's weight at one year. The interaction effect shown in Figure 9-3b, however, has a somewhat different interpretation. At every level of birth weight there is a differential effect of the program. This effect, however, is greater at higher birth weights than at lower birth weights for children in the program when compared to children who did not have the benefit of the program.

As indicated, analysis of covariance either with or without interaction effects can be a powerful tool for controlling for a number of extraneous variables when trying to assess the effect of a program itself. The examples given here represent only a few of the ways in which analysis of covariance can be employed. An additional discussion with regard to trend analysis appears in the next chapter.

Discussion Questions

1. What is the distinction between descriptive and analytic techniques? What is their relative utility in program evaluation?
2. What three conditions must be present in order to infer a causal relationship? How difficult or easy is it to achieve these conditions in program evaluation? Name factors that contribute to the ease or difficulty.
3. What are the distinguishing features of categorical versus continuous data? How does the evaluator handle the problem of spurious relationships in each situation?

Part V

Trend Analysis

10

Trend Analysis as an Evaluation Strategy

Trend analysis, sometimes called *time series analysis,* is a general evaluation strategy that combines aspects of monitoring with an effort to determine whether the introduction of a particular program can actually be viewed as having a causal connection to changes in the condition that the program was established to influence. Trend analysis provides an evaluation strategy for assessing such changes over time. The implicit assumption in the establishment of any program is that it will produce or cause some desirable changes. The objective of this chapter is to show how trend analysis can be used to assess such changes, to consider the settings in which it is an appropriate evaluation strategy and the types of data needed to use trend analysis effectively, and to present a health-related application.

What Is Trend Analysis?

Trend analysis is an evaluation strategy for examining the trends in performance indicators over a period of time. The strategy provides an opportunity to ascertain

1. whether changes have occurred in some measure of performance
2. whether such changes have occurred in association with a particular intervention program
3. whether such changes are outside the normal expected range of variation in the performance indicator(s)
4. whether possible explanations of the observed changes in

performance other than a particular intervention program can account for changes observed

The following illustration provides an example of trend analysis applied to the question of whether the introduction of diagnostic-related groups (DRGs) has an effect on the use and cost of medical care services and shows how each of the points above might be considered.

Illustration: The impact of DRG payment on hospital performance (Hsiao and Dunn 1987)

Debate persists about the most effective way to pay hospitals to limit health care cost inflation. The Medicare program adopted DRG-based payment in 1983, but according to Hsiao and Dunn (1987), the policy decision was not based on a completely informed choice about the relative efficacy of the DRG payment method. Using data from the state of New Jersey, which adopted its own DRG system beginning in 1980 (and phased in over a three-year period), Hsiao and Dunn present time series data for hospital cost per capita, expense per hospital admission average length of stay, and inpatient admis-

Figure 10-1 Expenses per Admission for New Jersey, 1971–1984

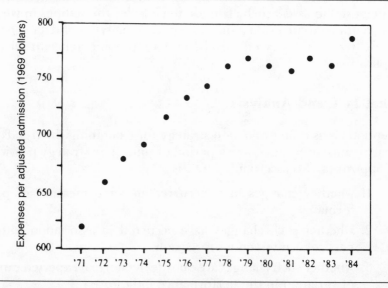

Source: Reprinted with permission from William C. Hsiao and Daniel L. Dunn, "The Impact of DRG Payment on New Jersey Hospitals," *Inquiry* 24 (Fall 1987): 215.

sions per capita from 1971 to 1984. The time series for expenses per admission is shown in Figure 10-1.

This time series actually represents two changes in the way in which New Jersey hospitals were reimbursed. From 1971 to 1975, hospital cost control in New Jersey was limited to voluntary budget review. In 1976, the cost control effort was changed to a prospective per diem payment under which New Jersey hospitals received a fixed payment per bed day for all Blue Cross Plan and Medicaid patients (approximately 45 percent of inpatient revenue). In 1980, the DRG-based payment was introduced. Based on the data used to produce Figure 10-1, the authors concluded that hospital expense per admission rose at a rate of 3 to 4 percent per year prior to 1976. With the introduction of prospective reimbursement in 1976, the rate of increase dropped to about 2 percent per year. When DRG-based reimbursement was introduced in 1980, the rate of increase in expenses per admission dropped to 0.5 percent per year.

The authors provide insight into why this occurred with the time series shown in Figure 10-2, average length of stay in New Jersey hospitals. As that figure shows, a slightly declining length of stay trend through 1979 begins to fall off precipitously from 1980 on, which accounts for most of the decline in expense per admission. On the basis of the data given in these time series, it is apparent that DRG-based payment has been effective in reducing expense per hospital admission, in large part, by reducing length of stay. Interestingly, however, Hsiao and Dunn show that there has been little effect on overall hospital cost per capita for the state, because admissions have gone up as length of stay has gone down.

This work by Hsiao and Dunn provides an opportunity to discuss the ways in which trend analysis can be used for evaluation. In viewing the time trends shown in Figures 10-1 and 10-2, it is clear that something occurred beginning at about 1980 that has changed hospital expense per admission and length of stay. In regard to the first point at the beginning of this chapter, trend analysis has demonstrated that a change has occurred in these two measures of hospital performance. Knowing that the DRG program was introduced in 1980 also provides the further information that the changes in hospital performance occurred in association with—that is, at the same time as—the introduction of this reimbursement scheme.

It is also possible from the two time trends shown to make an informal assessment that the changes that have occurred are outside the normal expected range of variation in these two indicators of

Figure 10-2   Average Length of Stay for New Jersey, 1971–1984

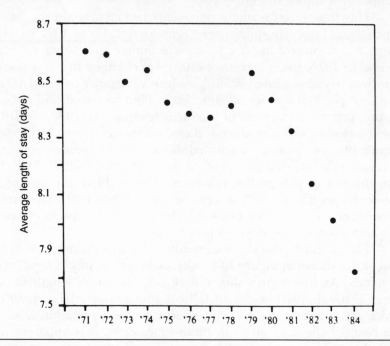

Source: Reprinted with permission from William C. Hsiao and Daniel L. Dunn, "The Impact of DRG Payment on New Jersey Hospitals," *Inquiry* 24 (Fall 1987): 216.

hospital performance, the third point made at the beginning of the chapter. For example, if average-length-of-stay data were available only from 1971 to 1980, it might be reasonable to argue that the drop in length of stay from 1979 to 1980 is not really outside the long-range general decline in length of stay. When that drop is viewed in the context of the data provided through 1984, however, it is clear that a real shift occurred between 1979 and 1980. This type of informal visual assessment can be confirmed using regression techniques that will be discussed in the next chapter.

The fourth point at the beginning of the chapter is that trend analysis can allow the examination of whether there are explanations other than the introduction of an intervention that can account for observed changes. The use of trend analysis in this context is not easily demonstrated from the Hsiao and Dunn article. If there was information available about other trends taking place at the same time that might affect length of stay or expenses per admission independent of length of stay, trend analysis could take that information into account in assessing the effect of an intervention. For example, trend analysis, again using regression techniques that will be discussed in the next chapter, could be used to rule out the possibility, for example, that the decline in expense per admission was caused by a general decline in the economic activity level for the state of New Jersey as a whole. In order to do so, however, annual economic data for the state would be required. All of these points will be discussed in further detail below.

Appropriate Settings for Trend Analysis

Trend analysis must be applied to information collected at more than one point in time and, in a sense, is quite similar to monitoring. At the same time, trend analysis generally tends to be concerned with the effect of a program's impact, which makes it more similar to experimental design in its major aspects.

Trend analysis can be effectively employed in conjunction with other evaluation techniques. Because it is similar in character to monitoring, trend analysis evaluations may be conducted by using data collected either primarily for monitoring purposes or in conjunction with monitoring effects. Consider the following hypothetical example.

Illustration: The case of high perinatal mortality rates

A reporter for *The Elmtown News* writes an article on the perinatal mortality rate in Greene County. He indicates that the perinatal mortality rate is high relative to other counties in the same area of the state. The mayor of Elmtown reads the article, as do the director of the local health department and several local physicians. These people regularly communicate with one another on an informal basis, and they now agree among themselves that something should be done to try to reduce the county's perinatal mortality rate. The health department director feels strongly that the high rate is primarily because of the lack of good and regular prenatal care for expectant mothers among the low-income population in Greene County. He points out to his colleagues that while the county health department has for some time provided prenatal care and consultation to low-income expectant mothers, reception of the services has not been overwhelming.

The mayor suggests that Elmtown allocate funds to launch an intensive and widespread publicity campaign to inform expectant mothers about the prenatal services available in the health department. This program is instituted, and Greene County leaders eagerly await the publication of the next year's state statistics for perinatal mortality. When these data become available, they see that the county's perinatal mortality rate has not only declined but, in fact, is now slightly lower than any other county in their immediate area of the state. The county leaders congratulate themselves on their wise use of resources in publicizing the availability of the prenatal counseling and treatment provided by the health department.

The illustration provides a classic example of the pretest–posttest–no control group design. A state of the system–that is, the perinatal mortality rate—was observed at one point in time. Subsequently a stimulus—publicizing the prenatal clinic in the local health department—was introduced into the system and, finally, a second measurement of the system was taken. On the basis of this design the decision makers, who also play the role of evaluators, decided that their program had been a success.

Sources of error

Although it appears from the one-year decline in perinatal mortality that the publicity campaign has had an effect, there are several possible reasons that such a conclusion could be in error. Four possible sources of error—discussed in some detail in Campbell (1969), Campbell and Stanley (1963), and Suchman (1967)—in the interpretation of these data are particularly worth noting.

Regression to the mean

Regression to the mean refers to the tendency for any time related data to "regress," or come back, to the long-term trend line. The perinatal mortality rate in Greene County became a matter of interest because it was higher than surrounding counties in the year in which it was observed and the newspaper article published. It is possible that this particular year represented an aberration in the rate that was on the high side of the long-term trend.

Figure 10-3 represents the two years in which Greene County was aware of the perinatal mortality rate as viewed in the long-term context. The figure shows a hypothetical set of perinatal mortality data for Green County for six time periods. The time period prior to the health department publicity campaign, designated t_0, and the period immediately following that campaign, designated t_1, are the observed rates, and four time periods, t_{-1}, t_{-2}, t_{-3}, and t_{-4} are prior unobserved rates. The solid line in Figure 10-3 represents the long-term trend line for the perinatal mortality rate. The broken lines

Figure 10-3   Trend of Infant Mortality over Time Showing
Regression to the Mean

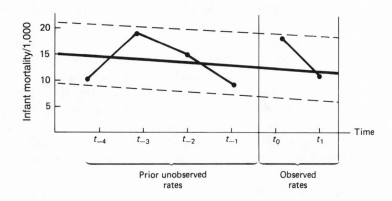

represent the limits that we would expect the perinatal mortality rate
for any given year to fall within with some probability—for example,
95 percent. In particular, the observed rates for the time periods t_0
and t_1 are both within the range that would be expected for perinatal
mortality by chance alone. Further, it is possible to observe that the
rate at t_0 was higher than the trend line and that at t_1 the rate has
regressed to a level below, but closer to, the long-term trend. Thus, it
is not possible to show that the publicity campaign was effective in
reducing the perinatal mortality rate because the change can be adequately explained by regression to the mean.

Reactiveness

A second possible source of error in the simple before-and-after
comparison of Greene County's perinatal mortality rate is the effect
of *reactiveness*—the effect of the first observation of perinatal mortality rates on the level of the perinatal mortality in the second time
period without regard to the program. In essence, reactiveness is the
effect of knowledge of a situation on subsequent measures of the
situation.

For example, it is possible that concern about the perinatal mortality rate associated with the original newspaper article, independent
of the publicity campaign launched by the public health department,
could have accounted for the decline in perinatal mortality. The concern of community leaders could have been manifested in many ways
that could produce a decline in rates. Various kinds of community
resources could be diverted from other applications and be brought

to bear on medical services for expectant mothers. The concern of community leaders could be reflected in different treatment of expectant mothers or newborn babies in county medical facilities. The concern could conceivably result in actual modification of the rates themselves through better or more selective counting.

Reactiveness, the effect of knowledge about a situation on subsequent conditions of the situation, is closely related to the self-fulfilling prophecy, the effect of expectations about how a situation will change on subsequent conditions of the situation. If community leaders expect the publicity program to influence perinatal mortality rates, they may be even more likely to make other changes in how expectant mothers are treated that will result in the reduction of rates, independent of the actual program. The power of reactiveness and the self-fulfilling prophecy should not be underestimated.

Consider the following brief example. Teachers in a selected group of classes were told that certain of their students, on the basis of IQ tests taken in the prior year, were likely to show significant improvements in school performance during the coming year. In fact, these students were simply selected at random by the researchers. At the end of the school year, these randomly selected students for whom the teachers expected better performance actually performed better than their nonselected classmates on a series of standardized IQ tests given to all students. The researchers ascribed the improvement in the selected students' performance to the expectation of the teacher about those children's performance (Rosenthal and Jacobson 1968).

This example clearly indicates the importance and effectiveness of reactiveness in producing outcomes of a desired type. Similarly, the expectation that the health department publicity program will make a difference in infant mortality rates produces a difference quite apart from the campaign's true effect because community leaders believe it will make a difference.

The difficult aspect of reactiveness or of the self-fulfilling prophecy is that we cannot successfully protect against it. In many research or evaluation settings the double-blind random clinical trial is the only research design that can successfully eliminate possible effects of reactiveness. This approach to evaluation is discussed in some detail in the chapter on experiments. Basically, the double blind random clinical trial is an evaluation in which two comparable groups are each given a treatment, one known to be ineffective or essentially a placebo, the other a new drug or technique to be evaluated. The person giving the drug or treatment and the person evaluating the outcome are unaware of which group received the treatment and which received the placebo. Although this is a powerful evaluation design and effective for eliminating reactiveness or the self-fulfilling prophecy, it is seldom, if ever, possible to apply this design to the problems of program evaluation. Unfortunately, for program evaluation, a double-blind random clinic trial stands as a good but unobtainable model.

Cohort and social structural change

Cohort changes refer to systematic changes associated with one particular age group of the population. A cohort change, for example, could be thought of as occurring if a large proportion of mothers with a potentially high risk for delivering children who would die in the first 28 days of life had moved from the county during the year. Although an unlikely occurrence, it could happen if, for example, a large group of migrant farm workers had left the area during that time period. Having data available for an extended period of time on population change would provide a means of evaluating this possibility.

Social structural change, in general, requires an extended series of observations for a successful evaluation. Such change can best be evaluated through some type of trend analysis. To consider how social structural change may have impact on the change in infant mortality rates in the county, consider Figure 10-4, which shows again the mortality rates for the six time periods of Figure 10-3 but

Figure 10-4 Trend of Infant Mortality over Time Showing Relationship to Percentage of Families Below Poverty Level

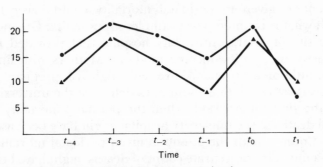

● Percentage of families below poverty level
▲ Infant mortality per 1,000

also plots on the same scale the percentage of population in Greene County with incomes below the poverty level. By looking at Figure 10-4, it becomes quite plausible to infer that the decline in infant mortality rates experienced in the county between t_0 and t_1 was in some way a function of the decline in the percentage of families with incomes below the poverty level. It is clear from Figure 10-4 that the two variables move through time quite closely to one another; in fact, a correlation calculated between these two variables would probably be close to .9. This information, which would not be nearly as obvious if viewed only at time t_0 and t_1, serves as an alternative to the publicity program itself to explain the decline in neonatal mortality rates for t_0 to t_1. This situation is much more easily demonstrated and perceived on the basis of a trend analysis than it would be on the basis of a simple before-and-after view.

Miscounting as measurement error

A last possible source of error in the conclusion that the Greene County education program was effective might come from the way in which mortality rates for the first and second time period were measured. It has often been observed that when a particular phenomenon begins to attract attention, the identification of incidents of the phenomenon are likely to increase simply because it is a current issue. After the first appearance of Legionnaires' disease, many new cases of the disease appeared that might have been diagnosed as something else had not Legionnaires' disease received publicity. The prevalence of AIDS, drug use, homicides, child abuse, and many other phenomena increase as attention is directed to them because they are better recognized and recorded.

It is not clear how miscounting could effect perinatal mortality in any given setting, but it is possible to imagine a situation in which the attention given to perinatal mortality could lower the rates through what is counted. For example, suppose that Greene County was the site of a large university hospital that provided relatively inexpensive care to low-income mothers. Mothers with limited resources, little or no prenatal care, and high-risk pregnancies come from several surrounding counties to deliver at the university hospital. In the first time period, when the perinatal mortality rate was high, all deaths in the university hospital might have been ascribed to Greene County. With the attention given perinatal mortality in the county, a much more accurate count of deaths might have been taken that would have the effect of lowering the rate because fewer high-risk births from other counties would be included.

This, of course, is only one possibility. A careful review of how perinatal mortality was determined in the first time period could rule this possibility out, but it is not always possible to be certain how data have been counted, after the fact. Time series analysis itself, however, would be of little value in detecting this particular source of error.

In summary, trend analysis can be an effective tool separating either regression effects or cohort or structural change effects from the effect of a program designed to influence some problem. Trend analysis is not an effective tool for eliminating the possibility that reactiveness or measurement error might have been responsible for the changes that may be observed either before and after, or over an extended period of time.

Appropriate Data for Trend Analysis

The single most important characteristic of data appropriate for trend analysis is that they be collected or maintained over a period of time. Frequently data on which trend analysis or time series analysis is based must be collected or maintained for substantially long periods of time. Such information as population change, change in average income, mortality rates by selected causes, and agricultural productivity has been maintained in the United States for many years. Information like infant mortality rates might be available for a selected community for a long period of time, making it a possible candidate for output measure status in determining the effect of some type of program or the effect of increasing or decreasing resources to a particular type of program.

The clear requirement that trend analysis or time series analysis be based on data collected and maintained over extended periods of time obviously serves immediately to require that data used in time series or trend analysis be collected on a routine basis. When a particular program is implemented, it may be relatively easy to ensure that various pieces of information about inputs and process are maintained routinely for the program. Monthly data on budget allocations, amount of space, number of people available to provide services under the program, specific quantities of services provided, or other program-specific information can be maintained routinely within a monitoring format like the one discussed in Chapter 4. But much information that may be of interest to the evaluators of the program may not be available on a continuing basis, making it necessary to consider an evaluation of program effectiveness or impact—

concerns associated with the outputs of the program itself—only on the basis of data routinely maintained and collected by existing government or quasi-government agencies. This requirement usually excludes from consideration within the time series framework of possible program results or expected results such entities as improvements in general perceptions of lifestyle, improvements in knowledge to carry out particular program tasks, or even declines or changes in morbidity status, to the extent that such morbidity data may not be routinely collected. Instead, the evaluation or assessment of a program in the time series–trend analysis framework will be much more likely to depend on such output measures as changes in mortality rates, in number of households with water-sealed latrines, in numbers of immunizations given, in number of houses sprayed for malaria, in the number of hospital beds available, or other data of an easily collected and quantifiable type.

To provide some concreteness to the notion of data for trend analysis, let us again consider the CCOP and primary care programs discussed in this same context in previous chapters.

Illustration: Community Clinical Oncology Program (CCOP)

One major objective of the evaluation is to monitor over time any change in physician practice patterns with respect to their treatment of breast cancer, bladder cancer, and colon and rectum cancer. The evaluation design requires a three-year data collection strategy based on determining whether there are any meaningful changes in the patterns of treatment of cancer patients. The changes are measured in terms of the proportion of patients treated according to protocol standards. This requires that patients be clustered by date of initial diagnosis and proportions drawn. To compare proportions between samples and determine if there is a change from one proportion to another, certain numerical requirements must be met. Since the impacts of the project on treatment patterns are to measured over a three-year period, the comparison periods should be as far apart as possible but covering a sufficient time period to produce enough cancer cases to assure that any differences in the proportions observed are not due to chance. To meet these requirements three annual aggregations of patients are proposed for the fundamental analysis of proportional differences. Proportional change will be tested for significance for year 3 minus year 1, year 3 minus year 2, and year 2 minus year 1. The addition of year 2 permits the determination of whether there is a steady pattern of change. The potential patterns in the trend analysis include the following:

Year 3 − Year 1	Year 3 − Year 2	Year 2 − Year 1	Characterization
significant positive	not significant	not significant	steady, low rate
significant positive	significant positive	not significant	late
significant positive	not significant	significant positive	early
significant positive	significant positive	significant positive	steady, high rate

Illustration: Primary care program

How would a primary health care program be evaluated within the trend analysis framework? An important set of data for evaluating the impact of the primary health care program would be to define a set of outcome measures. In general, it would be assumed that these outcome measures would be indicators of health status. The World Health Organization (1980) has proposed selected outcome indicators of health status that can be used to evaluate progress in primary health care.

Nutritional status can be measured in terms of birth weight: it can be expressed as the number of children per 1,000 births whose birth weight is below a certain norm—for example, 2,500 grams. WHO also recommends using nutritional status measures, such as weight for age, weight for height, and height for age of young children.

The infant mortality rate can be used as a sensitive indicator of the availability, use, and effectiveness of health services. The child mortality rate is the number of deaths between the ages of one and four in a given year per 1,000 children in these age groups. Child mortality excludes infant ·mortality. Although the infant mortality rate difference between developed and developing countries may be on the order of magnitude of 10 times, the difference between developed and developing nations with regard to childhood mortality may be as much as 250 times. This measure is a sensitive indicator of health from the standpoint of nutritional and environmental aspects. WHO also suggests life expectancy of a population at given ages and maternal mortality rates as measures of health status.

Clearly these particular indicators do not tap all aspects of health in any community. None of the measures refers to the health of adult males except for life expectancy at given ages. Moreover, life expectancy is relatively insensitive as a measure of changes in health status among those people who are and will continue to be alive. This situation indicates the difficulty of obtaining any measure of health status that can be uniformly or universally applicable to all aspects of health in a society. Nevertheless, the indicators mentioned are relatively good reflectors, or perhaps tracer conditions, for the health of the total society. It is possible that data on these characteristics could be used to monitor or evaluate the effect of a primary health care program in changing the health status of a population.

Regardless of whether the measures mentioned above are adequate reflections of health status, it is only part of the issue that must be resolved if they are to be used to represent the effectiveness of a primary health care program on the basis of a time series or trend analysis. Equally as important as the adequacy with which these measures reflect health status, is whether the data are available. In many rural areas, for example, it is difficult to collect accurate birth weight data. Weight-for-age and height-for-age data are particularly difficult to collect over periods of time because they require special surveys that must be conducted in the same way with comparable populations at multiple points in time. The infant mortality rate is perhaps the single best measure in terms of the availability of data over time, and yet it is certainly reported with differential quality in different countries. Civil registration of deaths is often incomplete or nonexistent, particularly in rural areas and particularly for infants dying in the first week of life.

In general, it would be even more difficult to find rural communities where good records have been kept over time on child mortality rates (deaths for ages one to four). Life expectancy at a given age is a useful indicator of health status, but, again, its calculation is not easy. It depends on life tables constructed from a knowledge of the makeup of a population at individual ages and from the deaths at such ages. Most communities will not have maintained this type of information over a long period of time. Moreover, many death registrations do not include accurate cause-of-death information, making the trend analysis difficult.

The same general criticism can be applied to other indicators. State and local registry data vary greatly in quality, and even those of adequate quality change definitions over time, making it difficult to measure change over time. So although a trend analysis or time series analysis of the effect of the introduction of a primary health care program in a community may be a conceptually useful strategy for evaluating such programs, practical problems of obtaining trend data that provide for an evaluation of effectiveness or impact make this strategy difficult to apply.

Application to Decision Making and Types of Evaluation

We have stated that the appropriate realm of evaluation is in the realm of cybernetic decision making, that is, the use of feedback of information about the state of a system to make decisions that can improve the state of the system in the future. In many situations it is likely that decision makers will want information on which to base decisions on a short-term basis. For example, it is likely that the state of New Jersey would have liked to have been able to show immediately that the DRG payment scheme had reduced aspects of hospital costs. The federal government, intent on finding ways to control costs, might have wished to learn from the New Jersey experience immediately so that they could structure their decisions accordingly. But as we have discussed, it may not be possible to determine with any degree of certainty whether short-term changes are a result of the intervention, or simply the result of random variation or regression to the long-term trend. It is often necessary to wait several time periods (whether these be weeks, months, or years) to be confident that observed changes following a program change are actually part of a new trend that may be ascribed to the program.

In a number of health areas, primary health care being a good example, it may be that the effect of changes may be detected only over a long period of time. Governments in developing countries may wish to know soon after the implementation of a new primary health care program whether it has been effective in reducing infant mortality, childhood mortality, maternal mortality, or several others among a list of possible health outcomes. But it is likely that the effect of a new program in primary health care will not have an obvious immediate effect on these health indicators, but will only appear in a cumulative manner over a period of time. The consequence of this is that trend analysis does not lend itself well to rapid day-to-day decision making. Nevertheless, it remains within the cybernetic decision-making mode to the extent that system outputs are quantified and measurable and information about these system outputs are used to make decisions about the nature of program inputs for the future.

Trend analysis provides important information for decision makers that corresponds to various types of evaluations. In terms of relevance, trend analysis gives important background information about the situation for which the program was designed to have an effect. Because trend analysis is usually based on an existing data system, it makes available a continuous source for defining the very nature of the problem.

More importantly, trend analysis gives information about program progress, effectiveness, and impact. Because data are available over a period of time, it is possible to assess the changes outside the normal expected range variation. This point is particularly critical to decision makers, for it offers an opportunity to initiate corrective action during the life of the program.

Finally, trend analysis, like experimental design (Chapter 12), gives managers the opportunity to assess effectiveness and impact. Because data are collected over time, it is possible to (1) observe changes before and after the implementation of the program and (2) hypothesize other explanations for the change and thereby clearly decide whether a specific program has had the desired effect.

Discussion Questions

1. Distinguish between monitoring and trend analysis. What are the similarities and differences between these two evaluation strategies?
2. Why is trend analysis so difficult to conduct and yet so important to health service programs?
3. Why is trend analysis appropriate to both summative- and formative-type evaluations?

11

Trend Analysis Techniques and Interpretation

In general, the approach to analyzing trend analysis or time series analysis data for evaluation purposes is to examine the trends or series over time. At the simplest level it may be done graphically, making inferences about the effectiveness or impact of the program on this basis alone. At a somewhat more complex level of abstraction, however, there are two primary ways in which data from the trend analysis can be examined: bivariate and multivariate regression. Bivariate regression involves time as the independent variable, and multivariate regression involves time plus a number of possible causes of change in program activity measures as independent variables. The objective of this chapter is to define these methodologies and illustrate their use in a health services setting.

Simple Graphic Approach

Figure 11-1 shows a trend line for an output measure of a health services program under three alternative program conditions. The output measure, undesignated in this case and strictly hypothetical, is measured on the left of the scale at 10, 12, 14, and 16. It is important, of course, to realize that whatever output measure is being examined in regard to trends over time would need to be quantifiable in terms of a scale of at least interval sophistication. A ratio scale would be even more preferable (scales of measurement are discussed in Chapter 14).

The trend data available for analysis (Figure 11-1) represent 15 years of the output measure in question. In year 10, as the figure indicates, a particular program was initiated and operated for a five-

Figure 11-1   Effect of Program on an Output Measure, Three
Alternatives: (a) Program Causes Change, (b) Program
Does Not Cause Change, (c) No Change Has Occurred

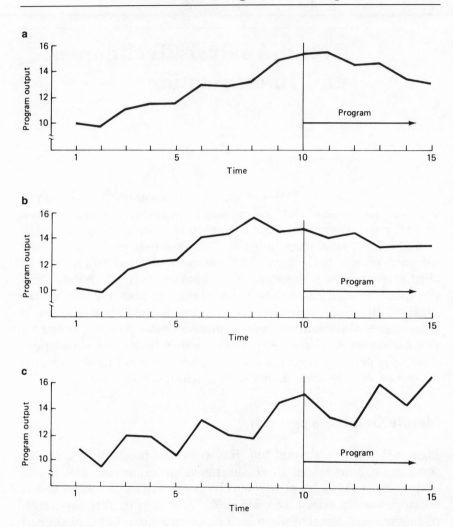

year period. The fifth year of the program is the year when an
assessment on the output measure in question is being made.

Figure 11-1a shows that the program has had an effect on the
output measure. The ten-year trend of the program output measure
has been steadily upward from the beginning of the recording period
to the time when the program was initiated (year 10). From years 10

to 11 the program output measure continued to increase slightly, but in the eleventh and subsequent years the trend line of the program output measure is a decreasing line. A reasonable conclusion to be drawn from this type of chart is that the program has been effective in reducing the program output measure.

The fact that the output measure has begun a fairly clear decline at the onset of the program can be taken as evidence of the effect of the program on it. It should be understood, however, that other activities may have been undertaken at the same time the program was initiated, which could account alternatively for the decline. Unfortunately, the simple graphic approach does not provide any information to conclude that some other factors occurring simultaneously with the program may have produced the change in program output measures—only that their decline occurred simultaneously with or were associated with the introduction of the program. Multivariate regression analysis of trend line data can, to a certain extent, rule out these other possible causes. This strategy is discussed further in the next section.

Although Figure 11-1a shows that the change in output occurred simultaneously with the beginning of the program, so that the program itself can be considered a possible cause of the change, the trend line in Figure 11-1b indicates that the program should not be considered a cause of the change that has occurred in the output measures. In Figure 11-1b the trend line is increasing from year 1 through year 8, but at year 8, two years before the initiation of the program itself, the trend line begins its downward slope. The program, introduced at year 10, is probably associated with this downward trend, but the fact that the downward trend started at a point prior to the initiation of the program would clearly rule out the program as a possible cause of the change.

Figure 11-1c is another alternative trend line related to the program output measures and introduction to the program. In Figure 11-1c there is a steep decline in the output measure from year 10 to year 12. Given the general nature of the trend line in Figure 11-1c, however, including the large degree of variation in program output measures from one year to the next and the fact that the output measure increases from year 12 to year 13 and again from year 14 to year 15, it would be reasonable to conclude that the program has no discernable effect on the measures.

This figure particularly shows the importance of long-term trend data in any type of serious trend analysis effort. If data had been available only for years 8, 9, 10, 11, and 12, a logical conclusion would have been that the steep increases in the output measures over the two years prior to the program were reversed by the program, and the desired decline in the output measure was realized. It is only when data are available for a longer period that it becomes clear that no real effect in the output measures has been produced.

The examples in Figure 11-1 are fairly clear because the hypothesized or illustrated effect of the program on the output measures is quite substantial. It is often the case, however, that the shift in trend line that the evaluator is trying to detect or assess is not nearly as visually apparent as in Figures 11-1a and 11-1b. Under those circumstances it is possible to use a regression technique known as *regression discontinuity* to examine the possibility that the program in question has had an effect on the output measure of interest.

Figure 11-2 shows two different possible effects of a particular program. The first is a change in intercept. What this means essentially is that while the program may not have changed the rate at which a particular output measure is actually increasing, the program's introduction at a particular point has served, at least for that brief introductory period, to shift the general trend line of the increase in output measures downward, so that the trend line continues to increase from an essentially lower starting point. This notion can be seen in Figure 11-2a, where there is a discontinuity at year 10— when the program was introduced—in the broken line that represents the long-term trend of the output measure.

Another possible way that a program may affect the general trend line and some output measure is through a change in the slope of the long-term trend line. Figure 11-2b shows this possibility. The long-term trend line for program output is basically an increasing one, where the slope of the trend line prior to year 10—when the program was introduced—is greater than the slope of the line after the introduction of the program. Regression discontinuity analysis can test whether this change in slope is one that could have been considered to have occurred by chance or one that is of too great a magnitude for this assumption to be made. If the downward shift in the slope was great enough to be assumed not to have occurred by chance, it would represent an effect of the program that could be revealed by regression discontinuity analysis.

It should be noted in regard to Figure 11-2b that the change in the trend line is not qualitatively different from the change in the trend line in Figure 11-2a. In the case of Figure 11-2a, however, it was clear that the trend line was increasing before introduction of the program and decreased after its introduction. In most real-life set-

Figure 11-2   Effect of Program on an Output Measure,
Regression Discontinuity: (a) Change in Intercept,
(b) Change in Slope

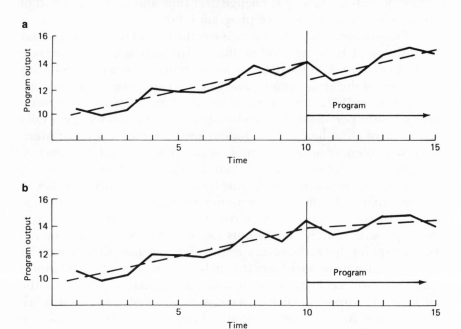

tings the effect of a program will probably not be as marked as that in
Figure 11-2a. It is much more likely that the program will (if it is at all
effective) be successful only in shifting long-term trend lines rather
than completely reversing their direction. In circumstances where
visual examination of the data does not reveal a shift as obvious as
those in Figure 11-2, regression discontinuity analysis can be extremely useful in determining whether slight modifications can be
seen as real effects of the program or as only chance occurrences.
The actual techniques involved in the application of regression discontinuity analysis will be described later in the chapter.

Multivariate Applications of Trend Analysis

Thus far, the discussion of trend analysis as an evaluation technique
has dealt only with the examination of the output measure itself, and
the assessment of whether that measure has shown a change in slope

or intercept with the introduction of the program. It may, however, be desirable to carry out a somewhat more sophisticated analysis of trend data, including an examination of input factors other than the program itself as these may change over time and an examination of changes in the actual level of program inputs.

Output measures selected to assess the impact of a program may be influenced by factors other than introduction of the program itself. Consider child mortality as an example of an output indicator to represent the effect of a primary health care program in a developing nation. WHO indicates that the child mortality rate (the number of deaths per 1,000 children between ages one and four) is a valid indicator of child health for a nation and reflects the level of nutrition, sanitation, control of communicable diseases, and accidents.

It is reasonable to assume that the child mortality rate in any society will be influenced over time by a number of variables. Let us assume that only the gross national product (GNP) and average caloric intake for persons in a country are under consideration—perhaps because they are the only two variables measured. The important point here, however, is the general analytical principles rather than specific variables. It may be assumed that the child mortality rate will be influenced in some substantial way by both the financial resources available to persons in the country and their nutritional status. As a measure of financial status, it may be acceptable to use the country's GNP as measured over time, and to use the number of calories consumed per person per day as a measure of nutritional status. In explaining the method, we will consider only these two variables as independent or causal variables in relationship to changes in child mortality over time.

A second set of factors making it desirable to carry out a sophisticated analysis using trend data concerns information about the program itself. In examining the trend data relative to time in the preceding discussion, we considered only the point when the program was initiated and subsequent time periods. It is possible that all program activities will not be put in place or begin operating at the immediate point when the program is initiated. It is conceivable, for example, that the amount of funds going to a primary health care program might begin at some relatively low level at the onset of the program and increase over a period of time. Certainly the number of personnel trained or in place to provide services is likely to increase over time as a function of program development.

Figure 11-3 is a composite of a number of different trend data measures. The child mortality rate is the heavy solid line in the fig-

Figure 11-3   Trend in Child Mortality, Caloric Intake, Gross
National Product, Money to Primary Care, and
Primary Health Care Workers in Place

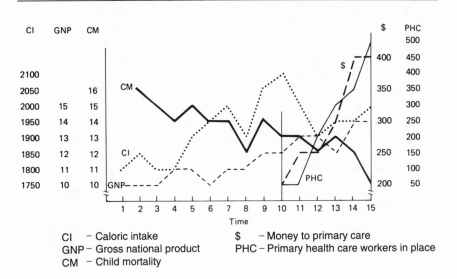

CI   – Caloric intake $ – Money to primary care
GNP – Gross national product   PHC – Primary health care workers in place
CM   – Child mortality

ure; child mortality declines from 16 per 1,000 to approximately 11
per 1,000 in 14 years. Over the 15 years for which the rest of the data
is recorded, gross national product for the country in question increases from 10 to 14 billion dollars. Daily caloric intake per capita
increases from 1,800 to 2,000 calories. All represent hypothetical
trend data for the entire 15-year period.

The solid vertical line at year 10 represents the initiation of the
program. The line represented by long dashes shows the amount of
resources going to the program in thousands of dollars from its onset
in year 10 through year 15. As the line shows, there is a sharp increase
in the amount of money over this time period. The thin solid line
shows the number of primary health care workers actually in place in
the country over the five years of the program. Again, there is a
sharp increase from a low of 50 primary workers to 500 over the five-
year period.

Visual examination of the data in Figure 11-3 may suggest several things. First, the downward trend line in child mortality is generally matched by an upward trend line in GNP and calories consumed.
If GNP and caloric intake can be thought of as causally related to
child mortality, then it should be clear that a portion of the decline in
child mortality is a function of the increases in the measure of finan-

cial status and nutrition. The primary health care program is being introduced in a situation of declining child mortality as a function of improving living conditions within the country. The result is that any effect of the program itself is likely to be more difficult to detect than if conditions in the country were remaining basically constant.

The introduction or onset of the program in year 10 is not clearly or immediately associated with a greater or more obvious decline in child mortality. It is clear from Figure 11-3, however, that the substantial gains in program funding and workers in years 14 and 15 are associated with a fairly steep decline in child mortality for those two years. This situation may be evidence that the program itself has begun to have some effect on child mortality rates.

Nonlinear trend lines

The examples of trend line data discussed so far are all trends that are primarily linear. Not always—or even frequently—do trend line data follow a linear pattern. The trend line in Figure 11-4 could be considered an example of a nonlinear trend. Through year 10 the

Figure 11-4   Effect of Program on an Output Measure, Nonlinear Increase

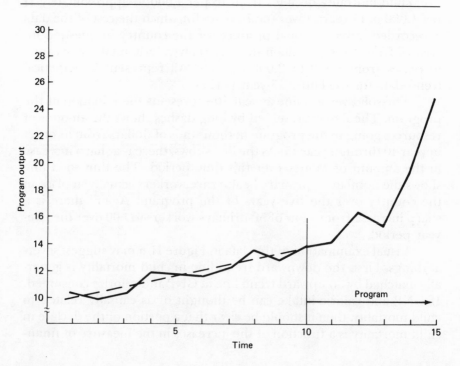

data appear to follow a more-or-less linear pattern of very slight increase. In year 10 the pattern seems to change to a much sharper rate of increase and by years 14 and 15 the trend appears to be growing at an increasing rate. Such trends may be difficult to analyze visually unless program effects are of a high order of magnitude. If the nonlinear aspect of the trend is not too great, analysis can adhere to the basic linear assumptions of regression. If the nonlinear trend is substantial, however, analysis should not proceed directly with regression techniques because the regression approach automatically assumes that the relationships under examination are linear. Clearly in Figure 11-4 the relationship between time and the level of program output or the measure being considered is not linear. It is possible to rescale such data, however, to make it compatible with the regression requirement for linearity in the data. A general discussion is beyond the scope of this particular section, but extensive discussions of rescaling appear in most econometrics books—for example, Kmenta (1971), Theil (1971), and Gujarati (1988).

A common rescaling technique would be to convert the dimension on which a particular trend is changing most rapidly to its logarithmic value. If a trend like the one in Figure 11-4 is developing, the transformation of the measure on the vertical axis to the log of that measure will substantially flatten the trend line and make it more adherent to the basic linear assumptions of the regression. If, for example, in the case of the data in Figure 11-4, the approximate value of the output measure at year 1 was 10.5 and at year 15 was 27, the difference between the two is on the order of magnitude of approximately 2.5. Converting both to logs would give a value of approximately 1.02 for the log of 10.5, and 1.43 for the log of 27. Now we can see from this conversion that the difference in order of magnitude between the output at years 1 and 15 is less than one. Conversion of this type will help to make nonlinear relationships more amenable to the assumptions of linear regression.

Regression Analysis

Two different regression approaches can be used to analyze time series data involving a one group pretest-posttest design in which data are available for a number of times before and after program implementation (for an introductory discussion of regression analysis, see Chapter 9). One is to consider the primary independent variable to be time itself. In this approach the evaluator examines the trend in the series as a function of time per se and attempts to assess the effect of the program intervention in light of possible changes in that series. A clear advantage of this approach is its conceptual simplicity, particularly the ability to visualize a change in the series over time.

Although the use of time as the predictor variable against which program change is evaluated is conceptually attractive, it has the major drawback of misspecifying the predictor model; that is, in most situations time per se is not the primary causal variable but a surrogate for other causal factors. In this case, coefficients of variables in the model will not be theoretically correct and conceivably might lead to incorrect conclusions.

An alternative strategy is to assess the effect of the program intervention in a time series by taking into account its true causal structure. Under this strategy attention is given to various causal variables relevant to the overall context or situation under evaluation.

Illustration: Impact of 55-mph speed limit on automobile deaths

In 1974 the federal government mandated a 55-mph speed limit throughout the United States. This speed limit remained in effect until early 1987, when the government made it possible for the states to raise speed limits to 65 mph on limited access highways. A question of interest in regard to the original reduction in speed limits is whether there was an associated reduction in automobile deaths. A question of interest in regard to the subsequent potential increase in speed limit is whether it was associated with an increase in automobile deaths.

An examination of a time series of automobile deaths by month in North Carolina from 1964 to 1980 (Veney and Luckey 1983) showed that there was a reduction in deaths of as much as 30 to 40 deaths per month following the introduction of the 55-mph speed limit. Figure 11-5 shows the same time series (automobile deaths) averaged across all months by year from 1964 to 1988. The additional eight years of data allows us enough observations so that it is possible to carry out analysis of the time series of fatalities by year rather than by month, substantially simplifying the analysis, and it also allows us to examine the possible effect of the permitted increase in speed limits on limited access highways that occurred in 1987.

The time series in Figure 11-5 does seem to indicate a substantial decline in automobile deaths in 1974 and continuing thereafter. Even disregarding the two-year decline in deaths that occurred in 1982 and 1983, the average number of automobile deaths per month be-

Figure 11-5 North Carolina Traffic Fatalities, 1964–1988

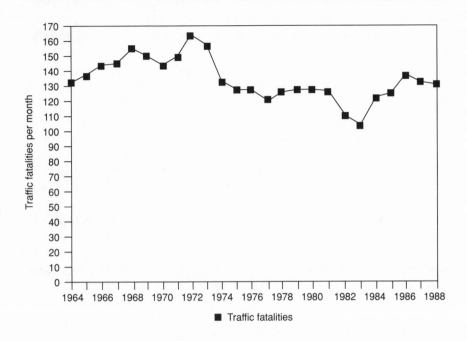

■ Traffic fatalities

fore 1974 appears to be about 150, while after 1974 it appears to be about 125 to 130. The series does not, however, suggest that there has been an increase in automobile deaths associated with the increase in speed limits beginning in the summer of 1987. Deaths in both 1987 and 1988 were lower than 1986. Future data may show automobile deaths beginning to increase, and the increase may then be attributable to the increase in speed limits. But at the present time, no such increase in automobile deaths can be documented.

One simple way of assessing the existence and extent of an effect of the speed limit reduction in 1974 is to compare the average number of deaths per month before 1974 with the average number after 1974. If this is done, the average deaths per month prior to 1974 is 148, and after 1974 is 125. Using a simple *t*-test, it is easy to show that the difference between the two means is statistically significant.

But a simple *t*-test ignores at least three important things. First, if the average number of deaths per month on an annualized basis was increasing or decreasing either before or after the introduction of the speed limit law, that is, if there was a secular trend in automobile deaths, the simple mean of deaths before and after will almost certainly present an over- or underestimate of the real effect of the change in speed limit. A second problem is the possibility that the difference in deaths can be accounted for by some factor other than the speed limit law that is not being examined, which when taken into account might reduce or eliminate the effect of the change in the speed limit.

A secular trend or other, unexamined factors are substantive issues. A third problem, which is purely methodological, is serial autocorrelation of errors over time. Serial autocorrelation of errors results in artificially inflated tests of statistical significance, so that if a *t*-test was applied to the difference between 148 deaths before 1974 and 125 deaths after, it may show that these two levels were statistically different from one another when, in fact, the *t*-test was misapplied because of autocorrelation. We will deal with all three of these issues in the material that follows.

Let us first examine the apparent reduction in deaths that followed the speed limit law in 1974, attempting to account for a possible secular trend. A good first attempt would be to use ordinary least-squares regression to predict automobile deaths from the two variables, time and the introduction of the 55-mph speed limit:

$$D_t = b_1 T_t + b_2 Y_t + b_0 \qquad (11\text{-}1)$$

where D_t = average annual deaths per month
   T_t = time in years from 1974 (1973 = -1; 1974 = 0; 1975 = 1; etc.)
   Y_t = 0 if time is prior to 1974 and 1 otherwise

This is the simplest possible model for assessing the effect of a change in the speed limit law. Using this model, predicted deaths are a function of the year and the change of the speed limit to 55 mph. The model results in two separate regression lines, as shown in Figure 11-6. It can be seen that there is a predicted line (1964–1973) that is relevant to deaths before the introduction of the speed limit law, and another line, with precisely the same slope but with a different intercept, that is relevant to deaths after the introduction of the speed limit law. With ordinary least-squares regression this model produces

$$D = 0.674T - 31.705Y + 151.667$$
$$(0.473) \quad (6.959) \quad (3.855)$$
$$(11\text{-}2)$$

where the numbers in parentheses represent standard errors.

This model indicates that there may be a slightly increasing secular trend in deaths over time (the coefficient of time is not statistically significant), but that the introduction of the speed limit law

Figure 11-6   North Carolina Traffic Fatalities, Model 1 Predictions

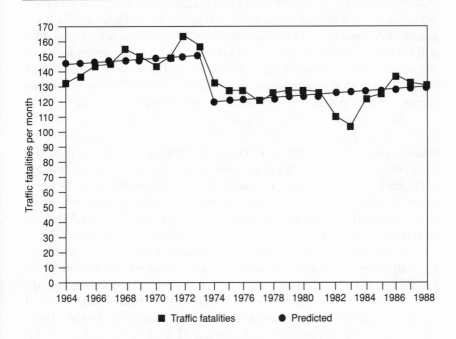

resulted in a one-time drop in the annualized average monthly deaths of approximately 31. Moreover, the standard error of the coefficient for deaths is small enough that this drop could be viewed as statistically significant.

As a result of this analysis, then, it might be concluded that the change in the speed limit law did have a statistically significant one-time effect on deaths. Moreover, as this decline is about 20 percent of the level of deaths before the speed limit law, it would certainly be considered substantively significant. Certainly on this basis the speed limit law must be seen as an important intervention.

Limitations

There are several shortcomings to the analysis at this level, however. These include the possibility that the secular trend has not been adequately modeled, and hence the one-time decline may still be depicted as too large or too small; that we have not examined the possibility that other variables may have accounted for the decline; and finally the potential continuing methodological problem of serial autocorrelation of errors.

It may be most useful to address the methodological problem of serial autocorrelation of errors first. Ordinary least squares assumes that error terms in the dependent variable (that is, the difference between the predicted value of the dependent variable, in this case automobile deaths, and the actual value of the dependent variable) will be uncorrelated in any serial fashion; that is, any given value of the error will not be more like some specified preceding value of the error than it is like any other value of the error. Where the error terms are correlated, the condition is termed *autocorrelation*.

An example of what this means can be fairly easily seen in Figure 11-6. The predicted values of deaths are all higher than the actual values for the years 1964, 1965, 1966, and 1967. Thus, the difference found by subtracting the actual from the predicted for each year, the error terms, would all have a positive sign. But the signs for the next two years are negative; the next two, positive; the next nine, with one exception, negative; and so on. This serial change in sign of the errors is strong evidence of autocorrelation.

Even though the coefficient estimates found using ordinary least squares on autocorrelated data are unbiased, they tend to be inefficient because they are likely to have large variances—while appearing to have small variances—so that tests of significance applied to the coefficients will generally overestimate the extent of the effect. Thus, it is possible, relative to Equation 11-2, that the indicated decrease of 31 deaths per month may not, in fact, be a significant reduction relative to its standard deviation. This would indicate that the apparent reduction in deaths is not a true consequence of the change in speed limit laws but only the result of correlated errors.

A test for autocorrelation

The question, then, is whether autocorrelation does exist in the data and, if so, what to do about it. A common test for autocorrelation is the Durbin-Watson test, which is calculated by

$$
d = \frac{\sum_{t=2}^{n} (e_t - e_{t-1})^2}{\sum_{t=1}^{n} e_t^2}
\tag{11-3}
$$

where e_t is the difference between the observed and predicted value of the predicted variable. The confidence limit for the Durbin-Watson test is not easily established, but any econometrics text will give confidence limits for samples usually up to size 100—see, for example, Kmenta (1971), Wonnacott and Wonnacott (1979), and Gujarati (1988). In general, total lack of autocorrelation will produce a Durbin-Watson d of 2. Any value greater than about 1.75 would be evidence of no serial autocorrelation of the positive type, or a value of less than 2.25 would be evidence of no serial autocorrelation of the negative type. Positive autocorrelations are most likely to result in inefficient estimates of the coefficients of the model and inappropriate tests of significance.

The Durbin-Watson d-statistic for Equation 11-2 predicting deaths from time and the year of implementation of the speed limit law is 0.821. This is strong evidence of positive serial autocorrelation and casts doubt on the apparent effect of the change in the speed limit law as indicated by a coefficient of -31. The problem, then, is what can be done about such serial autocorrelation in attempting to assess the effect of a program intervention.

Adjustments for autocorrelation

One possible adjustment for autocorrelation involves a two-stage process for eliminating the effect of autocorrelation on the coefficients found from regression and on the significance tests performed on such coefficients. This can be examined using the model shown in Equation 11-2.

Serial autocorrelation in the error means that the value of the error at time t is some function of the value of the error at previous time periods. Frequently the simplest possible error structure is assumed. This error structure is essentially as shown in Equation 11-4, where the error term at time $t(e_t)$ equals ρ times the error term at time $t - 1$ (e_{t-1}) plus a constant. The value of ρ and the constant can be determined by regressing e_t on e_{t-1}, using ordinary least squares.

$$e_t = \rho e_{t-1} + c \qquad (11\text{-}4)$$

The value of ρ is then used to adjust the original variables in the model in Equation 11-2:

$$
\begin{aligned}
D_t^* &= D_t - \rho D_{t-1} \\
D_1^* &= \sqrt{(1 - \rho)^2}\, D_1 \\
T_t^* &= T_t - \rho T_{t-1} \\
T_1^* &= \sqrt{(1 - \rho)^2}\, T_1 \\
Y_t^* &= Y_t - \rho Y_{t-1} \\
Y_1^* &= \sqrt{(1 - \rho)^2}\, Y_1
\end{aligned}
\qquad (11\text{-}5)
$$

It is necessary to use the alternative adjustment for time 1 because there is no value before the first observations. In addition, it is necessary to adjust the intercept term by transforming it to $1 - \rho$ (by analogy to Equation 11-5, to $\sqrt{(1 - \rho)^2}$ for $t = 1$).

Efficient estimates of the coefficient for time and for the introduction of the speed limit law can be calculated by regressing the adjusted value for deaths on the adjusted values for time (T^*) and the dummy representing the speed limit law (Y^*) and an adjusted intercept term (it is necessary to use a regression package that allows the specification of the intercept). When this is done, the result is quite similar to the result shown in Equation 11-2:

$$D^* = 0.703T^* - 29.314Y^* + 149.769$$
$$(0.623) \qquad (8.095) \qquad (5.148)$$

$$(11\text{-}6)$$

This adjusted equation shows the decline in deaths to be about 29 per month, rather than 31, following the introduction of the speed limit law. The standard error for the variable Y^* is small enough so that it is still statistically significant, and the Durbin-Watson statistic for this equation is 1.66, which indicates that there is no serial autocorrelation in the error term. Thus, using an adjustment for autocorrelation in the error term, it has been possible to estimate the effect of the speed limit law on automobile deaths on the assumption that there is no secular trend in deaths (a nonsignificant coefficient for time), but that there was a one-time drop in the level of deaths at the time the law was introduced (a significant coefficient for the year dummy). But there may still remain problems with this estimation procedure, including misspecification of the model and the absence of important independent variables other than time and the speed limit law, as we will see below.

Types of autocorrelation

How the problem of autocorrelation might be handled in the presence of an effort to assess program effect may depend in large part on the nature of the autocorrelation itself. Basically two different types of situations may show evidence of autocorrelation in error terms. The first is the result of true autocorrelation between the dependent variable and its lagged values. What such autocorrelation would indicate is that any value of the dependent variable at time t is causally influenced by the value of the dependent variable at time t minus 1. The second type of autocorrelation that might be found in error terms results from misspecification or inadequate specification of the model. Then there is no true causal effect of the dependent variable at t minus 1 or at any other lag on the value of the dependent variable at time t, but certain real causal variables have been left out of the model so that there appears to be autocorrelation.

An example of the first type of autocorrelation—that is, a real relationship between the dependent variables over time—might be the level of salaries of nonphysician hospital staff (nurses' salaries, orderlies' salaries, and so on). Clearly the level of salaries at time t will be causally related to the level of salaries at some past time period. Salaries are not created *de novo* at each time period. If we were to try to assess the effect of the initiation of collective bargaining on salaries by using time series data for average salaries over a period of many months, it would be conceptually reasonable to include a lagged value of the dependent variable as a predictor of the current value of the dependent variable. Under such circumstances of true autocorrelation, regression coefficients are both biased and inefficient. If such an analysis is to be carried out, it is appropriate to employ more sophisticated methods of analysis, such as the Box-Jenkins model of the autoregressive integrated moving average (ARIMA) type.

The second type of autocorrelation in the error term occurs when the model is essentially misspecified. For example, in predicting the number of highway deaths per month in North Carolina, there is no logical direct causal link between the number of deaths occurring in any month and deaths occurring in any subsequent month. Although the level of deaths may appear to be autocorrelated when viewed in the context of the model in Equation 11-2, such autocorrelation is not logically due to a true causal relationship. In fact, it is probably due to inadequate specification of the model. So, what may be done to specify the model in a way that may result in a better assessment of the effect of the speed limit law?

Model specification to eliminate autocorrelation

Examining the time series in Figure 11-5, it might be concluded that the secular trend modeled in Equations 11-2 and 11-6—that is, that the slope of time is the same both before and after the introduction of the speed limit law—is not the best possible representation of the trend. It might be suggested that the slope of the time trend is steeper before the introduction of the law than after. This possibility can be modeled according to the following equation as one possible way of eliminating autocorrelation through a more appropriately specified model.

$$D_t = b_1 T_t + b_2 Y_t + b_3 T_t Y_t + b_0 \qquad (11\text{-}7)$$

where D_t = average annual deaths per month
$\quad\quad T_t$ = time in years from 1974 (1973 = -1; 1974 = 0;
$\quad\quad\quad$ 1975 = 1; etc.)
$\quad\quad Y_t$ = 0 if time is prior to 1974 and 1 otherwise
$\quad\quad T_t Y_t$ = the product of the time and Y variable

An examination of this model will reveal that the inclusion of the TY term in the equation allows for what is known as "interaction," that is, the possibility that the slope of the time line may differ before and after the introduction of the speed limit law. This is one way to better specify the model to attempt to eliminate autocorrelated errors.

When this model is estimated using the original data, the results are

$$D = 2.718T - 38.728Y - 2.645TY + 162.906$$
$$(0.878) \quad (6.714) \quad (0.999) \quad (5.500) \qquad (11\text{-}8)$$

This equation indicates that there is a statistically significant positive slope for time before the introduction of the speed limit law of 2.7 (for each year, the number of deaths increases by 2.7 per month), a different slope of 2.7 − 2.6 after the introduction of the speed limit law (2.7 − 2.6, or 0.1, is statistically different from 2.7, but probably not from 0) and an effect of the speed limit law of a decline of about 39 deaths per month (also statistically significant). The graph of the predicted line using this model, which is shown in Figure 11-7, appears to fit the actual data better than the predicted values in Figure 11-6. If one accepts this model of the effect of the speed limit law, one would conclude that not only did the law result in a one-time decline of about 39 deaths per month, but also that it had the effect of eliminating a secular increasing trend in deaths. If one considers the possibility of autocorrelation, however, it is still possible to see several years in a row when the sign of the residuals are either all positive or all negative. This graphic evidence of autocorrelated errors is confirmed by a Durbin-Watson statistic of 1.12, which is evidence of positive autocorrelation.

It would be possible to adjust this new, more complex model for autocorrelation just as the model in Equation 11-2 was adjusted. But such an adjustment would only result in continuing to assess the effect of the speed limit law using a model that might be essentially

Figure 11-7   North Carolina Traffic Fatalities, Model 2 Predictions

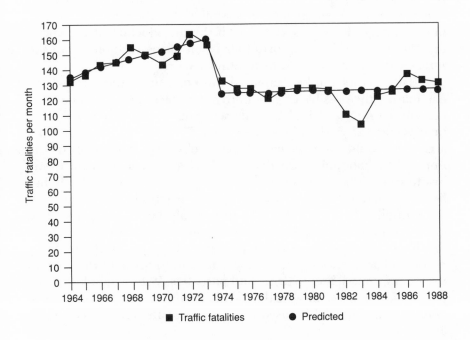

■ Traffic fatalities   ● Predicted

misspecified. Further, neither of these models has yet provided an assessment of the possibility that there may be other forces at work that could have accounted for the apparent reduction in deaths associated with the speed limit law. Finally, neither model examined thus far adequately accounts for the large dip in deaths in 1982 and 1983.

There may be a number of factors that could account for the number of automobile deaths. The number of automobiles on the road might be one of these. Another might be the level of alcohol consumption. Willingness of people to take risks with their automobiles might be a third. If it could be shown that a factor such as these was highly correlated with the number of automobile deaths during the time period under consideration, it might call into question the effect of the change in the speed limit as a causal factor in the reduction of automobile deaths.

Since this is basically a discussion of a method for assessing the effect of a program intervention using time series data, it is not necessary to assure that all possible factors that might affect automobile deaths need be considered. It is sufficient, perhaps, to examine two factors that might be logically related to automobile deaths to demonstrate the general method of improving the specification of the causal model, both for the purpose of eliminating autocorrelation and as a means to eliminate the possibility that the apparent decline in automobile deaths associated with the introduction of the speed limit law may be simply a fortuitous result of the relationship of the number of automobile deaths to other factors.

Two factors will be examined to demonstrate the method for eliminating the possible effect of other variables. These are the average annual number of automobile accidents per month and the annual average state unemployment rate. The number of automobile accidents would seem to have a fairly obvious relationship to the number of automobile deaths and does not seem to require any justification. The unemployment rate may be less obvious. It has been suggested that highway deaths are negatively correlated with the economy. It is not clear why this should be so, but perhaps in good economic times people are more likely to take risks, perhaps drink more and party more, or perhaps are simply on the highway more. In bad economic times they may tend to be more cautious, to drive fewer miles, and to drink and party less. Without explaining or justifying this possibility further—this is only an example—the unemployment rate will be used as a proxy for the level of economic activity.

If the unemployment rate and the accident rate are to be used as examples of a way in which the possible confounding effect of variables other than the program change of interest may be assessed and eliminated as important variables, it will be useful to look briefly at the time series of these two variables relative to automobile deaths. Figure 11-8 shows the three variables, automobile deaths, automobile accidents, and unemployment rate for 1964 to 1988. The graph is presented in standard score form (that is, as variation about a mean of zero) because the three variables have values that are so different in absolute size; the level of automobile deaths varies from about 100 to 170 per month, the level of automobile accidents from about 6,000 to 15,000 per month, and the unemployment rate from about 3 percent to 12 percent per month on an annual basis. The standard scores for these three variables puts them all on essentially the same distribution.

Two things are immediately apparent from Figure 11-8. The first is that the accident rate has been generally increasing slightly each year since 1964. This alone would suggest that it is not likely to be the cause of a change as dramatic as the apparent decline in

Figure 11-8   North Carolina Traffic Fatalities, with Accidents and Unemployment

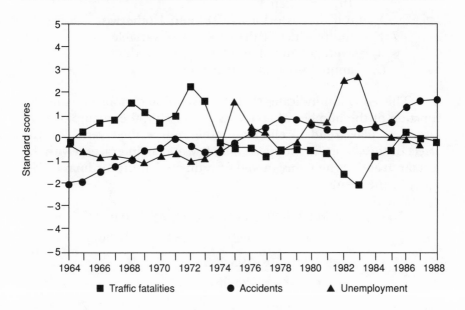

■ Traffic fatalities   ● Accidents   ▲ Unemployment

automobile deaths that began at the time of the introduction of the speed limit law. Second, the unemployment rate shows two dramatic peaks, both associated with a drop in the automobile deaths—one in 1974 and 1975, and one in 1981 to 1984. Interestingly, though, the first increase in the unemployment rate seems to have occurred after the reduction in automobile deaths, so it is probably not a cause of that decline. The second increase in unemployment may have occurred prior to or simultaneously with the drop in deaths in the interval 1981 to 1984 and might, on this basis, be considered a causal factor. The question, then, is how these relationships can be explored statistically and, at the same time, possibly eliminate the problem of autocorrelated errors.

Retaining the idea that there is probably an interaction between the introduction of the speed limit law and the level of automobile deaths, the beginning point is the model given in Equation 11-7. To this are added a term representing the number of accidents and a term representing the unemployment rate:

$$D_t = b_1 T_t + b_2 Y_t + b_3 T_t Y_t + b_4 A_t + b_5 U_t + b_0 \qquad (11\text{-}9)$$

where D_t = average annual deaths per month
T_t = time in years from 1974 (1973 = -1; 1974 = 0;
1975 = 1; etc.)
Y_t = 0 if time is prior to 1974 and 1 otherwise
$T_t Y_t$ = the product of the time and Y variable
A_t = average annual accidents per month
U_t = annual unemployment rate

This equation indicates that the level of automobile deaths is a function of the number of accidents per month, the unemployment rate, a secular trend to eliminate other unspecified variables, the effect of the change in the speed limit law, and an interaction with the secular trend. When this model is estimated using ordinary least squares, the result is

$$D = 3.166T - 27.160Y - 2.925TY - 0.002A$$
$$(1.066) \quad (5.022) \quad (0.842) \quad (0.002)$$
$$+ \ 3.416U + 193.296$$
$$(0.693) \quad (25.062)$$

$$(11\text{-}10)$$

The standard error of the terms in the above equation is small enough so that they would each be considered statistically significant at the .05 level except the coefficient for accidents. Further, the Durbin-Watson statistic for this model is 1.84. This is quite large enough to assure that there is no serial autocorrelation in the error term, so that the standard errors are accurate representations of the true situation.

Essentially, this results in the following conclusion. The number of automobile deaths is associated with the level of unemployment (a significant coefficient on U). This may or may not be a causal relationship, but if it is, it may account, particularly, for the large drop in automobile deaths in 1982 and 1983. Even taking into account the unemployment rate, there remains a secular increase in automobile deaths before the introduction of the speed limit law (a significant coefficient for T) that is significantly different after its introduction (a significant coefficient on TY, which may produce a slope after 1974 that is not different from 0). Finally, there remains a one-time drop in automobile deaths of about 27 per month that is—assuming there are no other variables that could have caused this drop—a result of the introduction of the 55-mph speed limit (a significant coefficient on Y). When the model in Equation 11-10 is used to predict auto-

Figure 11-9   North Carolina Traffic Fatalities, Model 3 Predictions

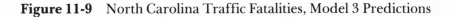

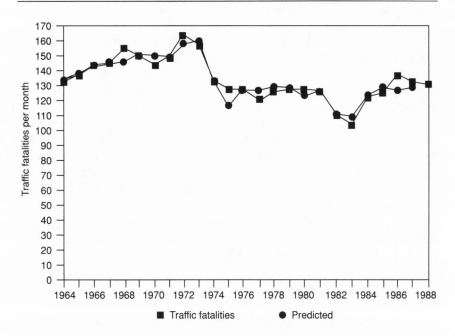

mobile deaths, the result is a surprisingly good fit to the actual number of deaths (Figure 11-9). The model in Equation 11-10 accounts
for 87 percent of the variance in automobile deaths.

   The purpose of this example is not to prove that the introduction of the 55-mph speed limit in 1974 was the reason for the decline
in the automobile deaths in that year, although it is convincing evidence. It is rather a vehicle to demonstrate a powerful tool for assessing the effect of a program intervention when time series data are
available. Further, the approach demonstrated here is only one of
several different ones that may be employed to reach essentially the
same goal. In a classic article, Gillings, Makuc, and Siegel (1981) have
demonstrated a variety of strategies for analyzing time series data
that allow the assessment of more than one intervention point in the
time series, an issue that is not yet of consequence for the automobile
deaths problem, but that may be in a few years when data on automobile deaths following the recent increase in the speed limit are
available. Most econometrics texts—for example, Gujarati (1988)—
have a section on the analysis of time series data and can be used to
guide the analysis of data to detect a program effect.

Application to Decision Making and Types of Evaluation

The primary value of trend analysis or time series analysis is in making decisions about the effectiveness or impact of a program. Although aspects of trend data analysis may concern monitoring and assessments of progress, trend analysis is not basically aimed at assessments of progress per se. To the extent that a trend analysis shows that a program has been effective or has had an impact, this factor leads to an assessment of relevance in a sense. But, again, the chief purpose of trend analysis would be to evaluate effectiveness or impact. Efficiency is not easily or well addressed by trend analysis because usually there is no comparison between alternative program strategies that may be more or less efficient.

Trend analysis would be generally most effective with regard to decisions about continuation or noncontinuation of a program. The evaluation that is most likely to be made with trend analysis is an evaluation of the summative type: Did the program have an effect? Was that effect as expected? And if the program did have an effect or is having a continuing effect, should we continue with it?

In a more limited sense, if trend analysis or time series analysis shows an increasing program effect as more resources are provided to the program over time, a logical conclusion might be that continuing to increase the amount of resources available will continue to make the program more effective or to provide a greater impact on health outcomes. Given the fact that there may be some lag time between program initiation and effect, however, such a conclusion would be tentative at best. Trend analysis, under the right circumstances, provides a rigorous test of program effect on specified and measurable outputs desired as a consequence of the program in a situation in which multiple program strategies are present.

One example of the use of trend analysis in such decision making is as follows (Campbell 1969):

> In the mid 1960s, the state of Connecticut instituted a crackdown on speeding and drinking drivers. In the first year of the program, highway death rates fell off dramatically. The result was the wide belief in the efficacy in the Connecticut program. When the data were later examined from the standpoint of trend analysis, a different perspective arose. When the deaths occurring in the first year of the program were contrasted simply to those deaths which had occurred in the previous year, a substantial decline was noted. When, on the other hand, the deaths occurring the first program year were seen as repre-

senting one year in a long series of years, it was evident that the first program year could not be seen as different enough from previous years to be certain that it might not have been a chance occurrence. The variation in death rates from year to year was large enough that the extent of decline in the first program year could have been attributed to chance itself. Furthermore, in subsequent years of the program, rates continued in a pattern which fit the general preprogram trend line.

On the basis of a short-term examination of the program, it would appear that the crackdown had been effective in reducing accidents and deaths from accidents in Connecticut. On the strength of this information, two things are likely to occur. First, the state of Connecticut is likely to continue the crackdown, with the concomitant problems that would entail, such as probable higher costs and some expenditure of political capital. Second, other states looking at the Connecticut experience might be inclined to undertake similar crackdown programs of their own.

When the data are examined on a trend basis, however, it becomes evident that the Connecticut program has not, in fact, been effective in reducing the number of traffic accidents but that the decline seen immediately after the program was implemented can be accounted for as a chance occurrence. With this better information, it is possible that the state of Connecticut might see the financial and political costs involved in the crackdown as too great to merit continuation, and other states that are contemplating a program similar to Connecticut's might recognize that it would be unlikely to solve the problem of traffic fatalities. Moreover, there is always the possibility that the phenomenon of interest is simply affected by larger events. In highway safety, for example, the reduced speed limits nationwide apparently have had some impact on traffic deaths on a national basis, complementary to any state and local effort.

Discussion Questions

1. What is the difference between bivariate and multivariate regression in the analysis of time series data? Give an example of each type.
2. What is autocorrelation? How might it be avoided or at least handled in the analysis of trend data?
3. Define the term *model specification*. What does it mean when a model is "misspecified"? How might "misspecification" lead to inappropriate decision making?

Part VI

Experimental Design

12

Experimental Design as an Evaluation Strategy

Experimental studies have long been viewed as the pinnacle of evaluation research efforts. This is not without some justification. Under the proper circumstances, an experimental study can provide an unequivocal answer to the ultimate evaluation question: Did the program make any difference? There is no other evaluation strategy that can do so. The objective of this chapter is to describe various types of experimental designs and the settings in which they are appropriate and to illustrate their use in different health service settings.

What Is an Experiment?

In its simplest form an experiment can be characterized by the following sequence of events. Some indicator of a system state is observed. Following this observation, some modification (the experiment) is attempted on the system, and finally, a second observation of the indicator of the system state is made. The difference between the first and second observation determines whether the modification had an effect.

Illustration: A training event

Does a training event make a difference? The answer must be yes, because training events are held by the thousands. But the question could be treated in an experimental manner. If we remain with the very simple characterization of an experiment given above, it is possible to view a training event as an experiment. In this experiment, the state of a system (level of knowledge or ability of a group of potential trainees) is assumed or measured at one point in time. Then an intervention, the training event, is introduced (the trainees attend the training event). Finally, the state of the system (level of knowledge or ability of the group of trainees) is measured at some point after the training event.

While it may be enough to assume the level of knowledge or ability before the intervention, it is critical to measure the level of knowledge or ability after the training for the activity to constitute an experiment. The basic *sine qua non* of an experiment is that an outside agent introduces an intervention into a system and that the expected results of that intervention are measured in some manner after the event. Without these two components, an experiment has not been carried out.

To remain with the simplest possible example in the training context, perhaps a group of family planning personnel from a national family planning program attend a two-week training session on management of family planning programs. At the end of the training event they are given a four-page multiple-choice examination on material covered during the course. The ability of the participants to answer the questions then becomes an assessment of the effectiveness of the course. If the participants can answer the questions at a satisfactory level, the conclusion might then be that the training event made a difference in knowledge. Further, while it would be a stretch to make the leap of logic to the conclusion that training events in general are effective, that inference may be drawn by many.

The training event is an experiment in the most rudimentary sense. But there are some significant, and generally obvious, problems with conclusions either about the actual training event itself, or about training events in general. First, it is not clear that the ability of the participants to answer the questions on the final examination (assessment) was a function of the course or something they already knew, because they were not assessed before the event. This illustrates the importance of prior assessment. But prior assessment also carries the risk of sensitizing the participants to the materials on which they will be tested, which adds to the difficulty of showing that the course per se, rather than sensitization to specific material to be contained in the assessment, made a difference.

Failure to measure knowledge levels at the outset is only one type of problem associated with assessment of the training event. A second, which is really two problems, has to do with measurement of any type, whether it is prior to the training event or after the event.

This is the dual problem of measuring the right thing and of measuring it well. If the assessment of the training event is to be a test of knowledge, then it is critical to devise some type of test (the assessment tool) that will effectively measure the knowledge that is to be gained from the training. But frequently the knowledge that might be gained is not easily assessed, especially if it is knowledge designed to improve decisions and actions rather than simple rote learning of facts. And this leads to the dual nature of the measurement problem. In the case of this event, it may be that the ultimate aim is to improve management skills. To carry out an assessment that will test management skills may be a long-term and high-cost endeavor. So knowledge may be used as a proxy. But there may not be a clear relation between the ability to parrot expected answers in a written test and the ability to manage well in a real-world situation. The results of the training event may be too subtle and complex to be measured by a test, and the ability to answer test questions may be trivial compared to the skills that are expected to be gained.

This last point is, in fact, a major problem of program evaluation. It is all too often the case that what we can assess objectively tends to be only trivial or minor aspects of the program. This can be seen in regard to the WHO definition of health: "complete social, mental, and physical well-being, and not simply the absence of disease." But WHO acknowledges that some of the only useful measures of health as an outcome are such relatively insensitive measures as mortality rates.

The problems of measurement are only one set of problems that plague the attempt to use experiments to assess programs, and they are actually problems for all types of assessment. Measurement issues will be discussed in detail in Chapter 14. There are other issues as well that are important to the success or failure of an experiment. These include design issues, study site and sample selection issues, adequate observations for effective decision making, and economic and political realities.

Experimental Design

In program evaluation the conduct of an experiment is a complex undertaking, but the basic pattern is relatively simple. The state of a system at a given time is observed, an experimental variable or stimulus is introduced, and the state of the system is again observed after the fact. But this straightforward statement does not do justice either to the complexity of launching a good experiment in a program evaluation setting or to the number of different alternative strategies that might be used to structure such experiments. While there are a range of experimental designs, for the most part many of the designs are too complex for reasonable application in health program evaluation. Below are descriptions of several experimental designs feasible and appropriate to health care settings. (The designs are based on material in Campbell and Stanley 1963.)

Pretest-posttest design

$$t_1 \qquad t_2$$
$$E \quad O_1 \quad X \quad O_2$$

In the pretest-posttest design the only group considered is the experimental group (represented by E in the illustration). At time 1 a first observation (O_1) is made. From the standpoint of program evaluation this may be an observation of a number of characteristics of a system state. It may, for example, include information about current infant, child, and maternal mortality; population; number of cases of malaria; families without a safe source of drinking water; or whatever other important classes of information may characterize the system.

Between time 1 and time 2 an experimental intervention, indicated by X, is introduced. The experimental intervention may be an entire program, such as providing primary health care services, or a more limited activity, like exposing personnel to a particular type of training program. Finally, at time 2 a second observation (O_2) of the system is made, and the effect of the program is considered to be the difference between the measure of the system state at time 2 and time 1.

Illustration: The effects of fluoride mouth rinse on dental caries (Leverett, Sveen, and Jensen 1985)

In the fall of 1975 in an unfluoridated community in upstate New York, 1,915 children in kindergarten through grade eight began a school-based program of supervised weekly rinsing with 0.2 percent aqueous solution of sodium fluoride. At baseline and annually thereafter, a random sample of children in kindergarten through grade eleven received clinical dental caries examinations. The prevalence of dental caries by grade at each of the follow-up dental examinations was compared to the grade-specific prevalence of dental caries at baseline. Overall, there was a decline of 57.8 percent in prevalence of caries in permanent teeth after seven years of rinsing. Among children in kindergarten through grade five, there was a decline of 35.4 percent in the prevalence of caries in primary teeth during the same time period.

Design problems

This study could be considered to be a time series study since it covers seven years. But the authors treat it in the article as a pretest-posttest design with no control group. The purpose of the study (experiment) is to assess (or perhaps to demonstrate) the efficacy of a fluoride rinse in preventing cavities. Without taking any stand with regard to the efficacy of fluoride, it is possible to use this study to demonstrate the several design problems inherent in a pretest-posttest design with no control group, and to show how these design problems may negate the value of the evaluation.

Extraneous variables. Because there is only one group under examination, the experimental group itself, it is impossible to eliminate any real effect of the program (the experimental variable) from other simultaneously occurring factors. In the course of the life of a major program, such as primary health care, family planning, or any other major program effort, there are likely to be a number of factors other than the program itself influencing the observation at time 2 and producing a difference between the two observations. Resources generally available may change, attitudes of relevant populations about a particular problem may shift, and so on. The design described here cannot eliminate the effect of these other possible factors.

The importance of possible extraneous variables is recognized by the authors of the fluoride rinsing study themselves. They point out that a decline in the prevalence of caries in primary teeth among kindergartners about to come into their study suggests that factors in addition to the mouth rinse program may have contributed to the decline in caries prevalence (p. 95).

Particularly in a pretest-posttest assessment of the duration of the fluoride rinsing study, one category of extraneous variable, *history*, cannot be overlooked. History refers to secular trends during the course of the study that might produce the same results as the intervention. In the same issue of the *Journal of Public Health Dentistry* that contained the fluoride rinsing article, other authors warn of the possible overstatement of effectiveness of preventive dentistry demonstrations based on the pretest-posttest design with no control group. They point out that historical comparisons automatically incorporate changes such as those associated with secular decline into treatment results, and thereby bias treatment effectiveness (Bohannan et al. 1985). With a study that lasts seven years, secular decline cannot be ignored.

A final aspect of extraneous variables that must be considered in a study such as the fluoride rinse study, and that is particularly important in any situation where the study compares different subjects over time, is the possibility of cohort change that is unrelated to the study intervention. In the fluoride rinse study, the comparison was between different groups of students at given grade levels; that is, persons in each grade at time 1 were compared to other persons in the same grades seven years later. It is possible that the cohorts of children themselves might have been different due to some factor, such as the influx of new people to the community following the opening of a factory or out-migration due to closing of a factory. While the authors of the mouth rinse study do not mention any factors that might lead one to suspect a cohort change, it is always a possibility in a study that extends over a number of years.

Regression to the mean. If the first observation were off the trend line relative to the system state under observation, the second observation could be expected to shift back toward the trend line, either a higher or lower value, without regard to any effect by the program that had been introduced. With the pretest-posttest design, there is no way to assess whether the original observation was on the trend line, above it, or below it. In consequence, this effect cannot be separated from any apparent program effects.

While there is no reason to suspect that the communities selected for the fluoride rinse study were selected because there had recently been high levels of dental caries identified there, it is nonetheless a source of error that the pretest-posttest design with no control group cannot control for.

Sensitization. Recognition that one is participating in an experiment may, by itself, have an effect on assessment outcomes. This recognition of the experimental situation, or *sensitization* to it, may result in a change between two observations that is, strictly speaking, not a function of the program or experiment at all, but simply of the fact of being in the experiment. This phenomenon is referred to as the *Hawthorne effect,* first recognized in conjunction with studies by Roethlisberger and Diskson (1939) at the Western Electric plants in Hawthorne, Illinois. What they observed, essentially, was that when workers in the plant knew they were the subject of experiments, they acted differently than they would otherwise, and this difference was substantial enough to obscure the expected effects of the interventions.

It may be difficult to imagine how the Hawthorne effect could have an influence on dental caries. But the fluoride rinse program involved supervised use of the rinse weekly in all classrooms. It is likely that parents of the children knew the study was being conducted. All this attention to their teeth might have led many students to put in more time brushing, may have led parents to schedule more frequent dental appointments, and may even have resulted in changes in eating patterns that could have been possible causes of changes in dental caries levels. The critical point is that the design used in the fluoride rinse study cannot control for the possibility of this sensitization.

Reactiveness. The expectation of the observer or the one measuring the system state may also have an effect. Actually, this effect may not simply be the evaluator's expectation but may also be bound up with the expectations of those people involved in providing the program itself. This problem of expectations is sometimes referred to as the *self-fulfilling prophecy.*

There may be reasonable doubt as to the importance of the self-fulfilling prophecy in an evaluation of program effectiveness or impact. If fairly objective measures of the system state at the two time periods are taken, it may legitimately be argued that the evaluators' expectations are not likely to have an effect if they are honest in their assessment. On the other hand, the expectation of the people introducing the program, if it were high, is likely to be a legitimate aspect of program implementation rather than a confounding factor to protect against. Consequently, the self-fulfilling prophecy may be of less concern here than in certain other types of settings. It should be realized, however, that if a program is introduced on an experimental basis and if desirable results actually occur because of the program implementers' expectations, rather than because of the program itself, the results may be quite misleading for the establishment of the same type of program on a routine basis by people less committed to it than those involved in the initial experimental situation.

In the fluoride rinse study, there are two points where the self-fulfilling prophecy might be of importance. The first is quite similar to the problem of reactiveness. If the experimenters conducting the study, the technicians monitoring the rinsing, and the teachers expected that the intervention would reduce cavities, they may have passed on to students and parents, in an inadvertent but powerful way, the expectation that the students should improve their general dental hygiene, that more frequent visits to dentists should be scheduled, and that improvements in diet should be made. In this case, the self-fulfilling prophecy has the same effect as reactiveness and results in a real improvement, independent of the rinse itself.

The second aspect of the self-fulfilling prophecy is the expectation by the experimenters that a change should have occurred. All children in the study were examined by three dentists—the authors. Given that they had an expectation that the fluoride rinse program should have an effect, it is not unreasonable to expect that they might have assessed dental health differently at the posttest than at the pretest. It is likely that they would assess a missing tooth the same way at both times, but some early cavities might have been assessed as cavities at the first point in time, and not as cavities at the second. This is not to say the dentists were trying to create the result they expected, but simply that they may have unconsciously erred in favor of their expected result in situations of doubt.

Again, the single pretest-posttest design will not protect against the self-fulfilling prophecy. In fact, no experiment will protect against the self-fulfilling prophecy unless it is of the type known as *double-blind*. We will discuss this experimental strategy when we introduce the next design.

Relative efficiency of program inputs. Because the pretest-posttest design involves a single experimental variable (that is, a single program structure), there is no way to assess the efficiency of alternative strategies for providing the same services or of alternative ways of organizing those same services within this design.

Pretest-posttest with a control/comparison group design

$$
\begin{array}{ccc}
 & t_1 & t_2 \\
E & O_{E1} & X & O_{E2} \\
C & O_{C1} & & O_{C2}
\end{array}
$$

This design includes both an experimental group, E, and a control or comparison group, C. At time 1, observations are made on both groups. Between time 1 and time 2, an intervention is introduced to the experimental group. At time 2, second observations are made on both the experimental and control/comparison groups. The comparison of interest in such an experimental design is $(O_{E2} - O_{E1}) - (O_{C2} - O_{C1})$. Essentially this formula indicates that the observation taken on the experimental groups at time 2 minus the observation taken of the same group at time 1 is compared to (subtracted from) the observation on the control group taken at time 2 minus the observation for the same group at time 1.

Consider the following illustrations involving the evaluation of several different types of interventions. Interventions may be a priori designed or may capitalize on ongoing events within the field, such as the implementation of contract management within hospitals or the implementation of prospective reimbursement at the federal level. All use a pretest-posttest with control group (comparison) design.

Illustration: Contract management and hospital performance (Kralewski et al. 1984)

What are the effects of contract management on hospital performance? To answer that question this evaluation assessed changes in performance measures of matched contract-managed and traditionally managed not-for-profit hospitals before and after the contracts were executed. Hospitals were matched on the basis of size, geographic location, population base, average per capita income in the population base, ownership or control, and presence of a medical education program. Data were collected on 20 matched pairs of not-for-profit community hospitals distributed across the United States. Each pair consisted of a hospital managed by an externally controlled firm under a contract and a hospital managed traditionally. Data were collected on each hospital for a six-year period, including the three years before initiation of contract management and the first three years that the contract was in effect. Data for this analysis were obtained from the American Hospital Association tapes.

Analysis revealed that among 12 performance indicators, such as gross patient revenue/total expenses, net profit, occupancy, etc., only occupancy rates differed significantly in the two samples in the years before contract management. Occupancy rates were lower on average in hospitals that later became contract managed. During the three years following the onset of contract management, the contract-managed hospitals showed no improvement in productive efficiency but did show changes in the way services were priced. The ratio of gross patient revenue to total expenses increased substantially in the contract-managed hospitals relative to their matched institutions.

Illustration: Comparing investor-owned and not-for-profit system hospitals (Friedman and Shortell 1988)

The introduction of the Medicare prospective payment system (PPS) was a major event in the operation and delivery of health services in the United States. This study focused on the degree to which PPS has affected hospital cost and profitability, whether effects observed for investor-owned hospitals differed from effects for not-for-profit hospitals by location and related sociodemographic characteristics of communities served, and extended to which hospital strategic responses—and type of responses—played a role in the financial outcomes.

To answer these questions a group of approximately 300 hospitals were studied for fiscal years 1983 and 1985, the years bracketing the initiation of PPS. The hospitals were owned or leased members of three investor-owned systems and five not-for-profit systems. The hospitals were located in 45 states and were not considered representative of all short-term hospitals in the nation nor of all hospitals in multi-institutional systems.

Participating hospitals responded to an intensive standardized internal hospital survey on cost, revenue, assets, and volume of care as well as providing data on structure and process indicators. Quality of care was assessed on the basis of data obtained from the Joint Commission on Accreditation of Healthcare Organizations. Case mix was measured by the 1984 unpublished HCFA case-mix index for each hospital.

Analysis revealed that in both 1983 and 1985 competitive environment, case mix, age of facility, and scope of diversified services were important determinants of average cost, while a process measure of quality was not significant. The independent effect of ownership type was not significant for cost. Moreover, the effects of HMO competition in hospital strategies was stronger in 1985 than in 1983, and operating margins for all types of hospitals showed increases, with a somewhat greater increase for not-for-profit system members. Significantly greater declines in volume of care occurred for investor-owned system members than for not-for-profit members.

Design problems

How does this new design deal with the confounding effects in the pretest-posttest design? Consider the evaluation of a primary health care program.

Extraneous variables. Can the addition of a control/comparison group eliminate the effect of other factors occurring simultaneously? Basically if it can be assumed that the experimental and the control/comparison group will be subjected to the same type of other factors, this design will essentially control for their effect.

If, for example, a primary health care program is being implemented in a rural community and there is some desire to determine its effectiveness by using an experimental design, the pretest-posttest design with a control/comparison group will control for any other forces active in the community at the same time as the program if it can be assumed that these factors affect all areas of the community in the same way. If the control/comparison and experimental groups have the same basic health problems, social structure, and geographic characteristics, probably any other simultaneously occurring factors that could confound the results of the experiment will be effectively controlled by the comparison between the two groups. If, on the other hand, the experimental group is influenced by different factors from the control group, if it is in a different geographical region or has different surface characteristics—such as being in the mountains as opposed to a control group in the lowlands—if it has a different social structure, or if the government is treating the experimental area differently in terms of other resources apart from the program, then the comparison between the experimental and control groups will probably not be effective in eliminating these other factors and in demonstrating the true results of the program itself.

One particular factor that may create difficulties in separating the program effect from confounding factors is how the two areas are chosen to act as the experimental or the control group. For example, if the experimental area is selected because the type of problems that primary health care would be expected to address are particularly acute there, then the comparison between experimental and control groups is at best questionable, and apparent program effects would be debatable. In order for the pretest-posttest with a control/comparison group design to be truly effective in controlling for simultaneously occurring factors outside the actual experimental variable, it is absolutely necessary to select two areas or groups that are matched as nearly as possible on relevant characteristics, such as geography, region of a country, language style, and social characteristics, and then to select one of the two by chance (randomly) to be the experimental group. This is the only truly effective way of deciding which group should serve as the control and which as the experimental.

Regression effects. Will the pretest-posttest with a control/comparison group design solve the problem of regression effects? Again, if it can be assumed that the experimental group or area and the control group or area are both essentially identical with regard to the problem under consideration or, more specifically, factors affecting the problem, then it can be assumed that regression effects will be essentially equal for both groups or areas between time 1 and time 2. It may, of course, be a relatively weak assumption, but without time series data to measure the trend line for the two areas or two groups over time, no other assessment of regression effects can be made. In any case, the control group design provides a better assessment of the program effect than the pretest-posttest design without a control group.

Sensitization. The control group design is not entirely effective in controlling for the problems of sensitization—the Hawthorne effect. Both the experimental and the control group are observed at time 1, so that any difference occurring between them cannot be attributed to the observation or the measurement because the groups are equal on this aspect of the experiment. Sensitization to a particular characteristic, such as mortality rates, or some other impact measure being evaluated, however, may result in a different effect when an experiment follows immediately—for example, the provision of a program—than a similar observation would produce if a program did not follow. In a sense, it may be called an interaction effect between the observation and the experiment or experimental variable. There is relatively little information on the magnitude of this effect, but its possibility should be recognized.

Reactiveness. The pretest-posttest design with a control group will not control the possible effect of expectations on the part of program evaluators or program personnel. As noted, one major problem of expectations—or the self-fulfilling prophecy—is that the expectations of committed program providers might produce a result under experimental conditions that would not be produced on a routine basis by the same type of program provided by people less committed to the program.

A second problem of expectations is that evaluators, if they have some stake in the program's outcome, may unconsciously and with the best intentions observe the results of the program differently. This situation would be rather unlikely when before-and-after measurement is taken in some fairly objective manner, such as comparing morbidity or mortality rates. But there could be a substantial problem if before-and-after observations were more subjective.

Controlling expectations: Double-blind experiments. One approach devised in clinical research to attempt to control the effect of expectations on the part of service providers and subjects of the experiment them-selves is known as the double-blind random clinical trial. In such a study a group of people to be included in an experiment—for exam-ple, on a new drug—would be divided equally into an experimental group and a control group. The experimental group would receive the drug under test, while the control group would receive a placebo, a drug that appeared the same as the experimental drug but was known to have no effect. Subsequently the two groups would be observed by an evaluator to assess their status on the condition that the drug was expected to affect. The important characteristic of the double-blind test in this case is that neither the physician administer-ing the drug, nor the subjects receiving the drug or placebo, nor the evaluators are aware of which specific individuals received the drug and which received the placebo.

This experimental approach is quite powerful for establishing the true effects of a treatment such as a drug. Cochrane (1972) sees it as the only true test of drug efficacy. It should be clear, however, that such a test cannot reasonably be applied to all medical procedures. For example, it would be quite difficult to do a double-blind test on the efficacy of tonsillectomies or the value of acupuncture in control-ling pain during surgery. It would be even more difficult to design a double-blind experiment that could assess the effectiveness of some type of complex program in producing results in some problem area. In a program setting it would be highly unlikely that a placebo for the program could be conceived of or provided in any reasonable man-ner. It would be extremely difficult to conceal from persons involved as members of either the control or the experimental group, and it is highly unlikely that any external evaluators could not know where the program was being operated or who was being influenced by it. So despite the value of the double-blind approach in clinical experi-ments, it is probably not possible to apply it effectively in any pro-gram evaluation setting. This limitation will affect, in part, all the experimental approaches that might be taken to program evaluation.

Multiple group pretest-posttest design

$$
\begin{array}{cccc}
 & t_1 & & t_2 \\
E_1 & O_{E11} & X_1 & O_{E12} \\
E_2 & O_{E21} & X_2 & O_{E22} \\
E_3 & O_{E31} & X_3 & O_{E32} \\
\cdot & \cdot & \cdot & \cdot \\
\cdot & \cdot & \cdot & \cdot \\
\cdot & \cdot & \cdot & \cdot \\
\end{array}
$$

$$
\begin{array}{cccc}
E_n & O_{En1} & X_n & O_{En2} \\
C_1 & O_{C11} & & O_{C12} \\
\cdot & \cdot & & \cdot \\
\cdot & \cdot & & \cdot \\
\cdot & \cdot & & \cdot \\
C_m & O_{Cm1} & & O_{Cm2}
\end{array}
$$

In this design there are multiple experimental groups, each with an observation at time 1, an experimental variable introduced between time 1 and time 2, and an observation at time 2. Control groups may or may not be used in this design, depending on circumstances and purpose. If used, they act as a control against any experimental effects. The major interest, however, is often in comparing the various experiments, or various programs, or various ways programs are structured, rather than comparing a program to no program.

Illustration: An education campaign as cancer control (Workman et al. 1988)

Misconceptions about cancer are widespread within various communities. The purpose of this study was to evaluate an education intervention specifically designed to refute these misconceptions and to prepare the community for further cancer control activities. To address these misconceptions a two-level, school-based strategy was developed. The first level of the strategy was to reach adults—particularly women between the ages of 25 and 45, to capitalize on their primary role in influencing the health of their families and overseeing care of their husbands, children, and frequently of their parents. The intervention consisted of two components. The first was a slide-and-tape program entitled "Beat the Odds," which was developed as a means of addressing women directly. Modeled on the format of a television quiz show, the first part of the slide/tape program included a series of questions asking participants to agree or disagree with specific statements about the etiology and treatment of cancer. This served as a pretest of knowledge and attitudes about cancer. The second section of the slide/tape program was designed to educate the audience. In this section a physician discussed various aspects of cancer and identified and refuted misconceptions.

The second component of the strategy was developed for children in grades one through eight to reinforce the message presented in the "Beat the Odds" slide/tape show. In this intervention, the message was adapted from the American Cancer Society's "My Body, My Health," "Health Network," and "Health Myself" series, which provide a general message about health habits such as smoking and some of the underlying misconceptions about cancer.

The research design attempted to assess the effectiveness of the components independently and in combination. Two experimental groups and one control group were established to test the efficacy of the interventions. Three of seven geographic subareas within the target community, each comparable in number of residents, population characteristics, and number of schools, were selected for study. Each selected geographic area, designated A, B, and C, included three schools.

Area A was designated a full intervention experimental area. In area A parents were shown the "Beat the Odds" program at parent-teacher association meetings, and children received the classroom intervention addressed to the misconceptions about cancer. In area B, a partial intervention area, parents were shown the "Beat the Odds" program, but children received a different classroom intervention concerned with cigarette smoking. In area C, only the classroom cigarette-smoking program was presented. Pre- and postintervention knowledge and attitude information with regard to cancer was collected in all three areas.

The study design permitted the analysis of three questions vis-à-vis the effectiveness of the program:

1. Were either or both interventions effective in altering the misconceptions about cancer?
2. Which of the programs proved more effective: the combination of classroom and adult programs or the adult intervention alone?
3. Which misconceptions were influenced by the intervention?

Analysis revealed that the area in which both components of the intervention were conducted had the greatest improvement in knowledge and attitudes about cancer. Minimal improvement was noted in the area receiving the single intervention component, while no improvement was observed in the control area. Moreover, it appeared that the component designed to reinforce messages through the classroom had a greater effect than the part of the program designed to influence adults directly.

Illustration: Evaluating intensive care in major medical centers (Knaus et al. 1986)

What are the effects of coordination among personnel of intensive care units on clinical outcomes of these units? To answer this question, 5,030 patients in intensive care units at 13 tertiary care hospitals were studied prospectively. Patients were stratified within each hospital by their individual risk of death using diagnosis, indication for treatment, and the Acute Physiological and Chronic Health Evaluation (APACHE) II score. Each hospital was compared vis-à-vis actual and predicted death rates in order to identify those hospitals that did significantly better or worse than expected, controlling for severity of patients. Differences occurred within specific diagnostic categories, for medical patients alone, and for medical and surgical patients combined. Moreover, these differences were related to the extent of interaction and coordination of each hospital's intensive care unit staff, providing support to the underlying hypothesis that involvement and interaction of critical care personnel can directly influence outcome from intensive care.

Data were obtained from a review of medical records. Organizational data were obtained from a questionnaire on the nature and practice of the intensive care unit completed by the unit's medical or nursing director. Visits to each of the units confirmed the validity of the responses.

In this case, the experimental variable—structure and process of the intensive care unit—varied along a number of dimensions including staffing, organization, policies, procedures, and the extent of critical care personnel's participation in patient care. Because there was no random assignment of units, but an ex post facto classification of the unit's structure and coordination practices, the critical factor was to assure that the comparison groups were equivalent on other independent variables such as severity of illness. This was done through the APACHE II system. Moreover, the selection of hospitals was also controlled; all 13 facilities had similar technical capabilities, and thus any variation was a function of their organizational structures and processes rather than their actual ability to provide treatment. Yet, potential confounding variables remain, including severity of illness and therapy used either before or after treatment within the intensive care unit, as well as important institutional differences that may affect patient selection and volume.

Design problems

The characteristics of this design, in terms of its ability to control for effects of other factors, regression, and sensitization by observation or treatment and expectations of the people involved, are all quite similar to those of the single experimental group and control group design. The multiple experimental group design, however, has the additional advantage of being able to assess from the standpoints of effectiveness and impact, and particularly from the standpoint of efficient alternative strategies by which a program can be conducted or by which an experimental variable is introduced.

Posttest only design

$$
\begin{array}{ccc}
 & t_1 & t_2 \\
E & - \quad X & O_{E1} \\
C & - & O_{C1}
\end{array}
$$

As this design indicates, no observation is made at time 1. An experimental variable, such as a program, is introduced and observations on both the experimental and control group are made at time 2.

Illustration: Birth centers (Rooks et al. 1989)

The emergence of birth centers as nonhospital facilities organized to provide family-centered maternity care for women judged to be at low risk of obstetrical complications represents a programmatic innovation worthy of evaluation. The critical issue is the safety of this type of facility. The purpose of this study was to provide a nationwide prospective descriptive evaluation of the care provided in freestanding birth centers. Analysis involved the labor, delivery, follow-up care, and outcomes of 11,814 women who were admitted in labor to 84 birth centers from mid-1985 through 1987. The women in the sample were at lower-than-average risk of a poor outcome of pregnancy on a variety of demographic and behavioral risk factors. Although the study did not have access to a control group, it did compare its findings with five outcome studies of low-risk hospital births. Comparisons reveal that birth centers offer a safe and acceptable alternative to hospital confinement for selected pregnant women, particularly those who have previously had children. Among the women involved, 70.7 percent had only minor complications or none; 7.9 percent had serious emergency complications during labor and delivery or soon thereafter, and one in six (15.8 percent) were transferred to a hospital; 2.4 percent had emergency transfers. The overall intrapartum and neonatal mortality rate was 1.3 per 1,000 births—similar to scores reported in larger studies of low-risk hospital births.

Design problems

A critical element in this design is the ability to assign individuals randomly to either experimental or control groups or the ability to control statistically for equivalency between the control and experimental groups. Obviously, random assignment is an extremely powerful tool for eliminating the effect of simultaneously occurring events, regression, and sensitization by prior measures. It may reduce the importance of the expectations of the observer by reducing the number of observations made and by expanding the number of experimental categories that can be used to assess alternative strategies. Unfortunately, randomization is often difficult to achieve in field situations. In the posttest only design, it is possible when there are sufficient subjects to control statistically for equivalence between groups.

Additional experimental designs have been detailed and discussed by other authors. For the most part, these designs are too complex for health program evaluation of reasonable type or magnitude. In fact, it should be relatively clear at this point that even the preceding designs would be difficult to apply in many program evaluation situations. The next section considers the question of when a program setting is appropriate for an experimental evaluation and what these specific settings may be.

Appropriate Settings for Experimental Design

Experimental design is appropriately applied to evaluation when the major concern is either the effectiveness of the program or the efficiency of alternative programs. Properly designed experimental studies, even in the realm of program evaluation, can provide a substantial amount of information on effectiveness and efficiency.

In general, an experimental approach is not appropriate for assessing program relevance and progress. It is probable that the evaluator conducting an experimental evaluation of a program will be primarily external to the program itself and will not be concerned with its daily, weekly, or monthly internal working. From an experimental point of view progress is irrelevant if the program can be shown either to reduce a problem or to modify a situation in the long run.

On the other hand, in assessing the results of an evaluation experiment, it may be quite useful to have information about progress—particularly if a program is designed and put in place on an experimental basis. It is one thing to design a program on paper, to plan for its implementation, to budget and allocate resources, hire staff, find quarters, and begin the program. It is something else to say that the program operated as it was expected to operate—that the resources were available in the right places at the right times, that the staff was in place, that people received the services to be provided, and so on. Such questions of progress are best answered by a monitoring approach. When it cannot be shown that a program is more effective or more efficient than some other program through an experimental design, it is extremely important to know whether the program was operating as it was expected to operate if it were to affect the state of the system. If such information is not available in an experimental evaluation of a program that appeared to have no effect, it will be impossible to separate the program as ideally operated from the program as actually operated. If information is available on progress and it indicates that the program was not implemented and carried out as projected, this fact will not, of course, mean that the program would have been effective in producing the desired results had it progressed as planned. Nevertheless, it will show that the lack of expected results cannot simply be attributed to the program strategy itself but may also be a function of poor management at any one of many different levels.

Superficially it would seem that an experimental evaluation should be appropriate to an assessment or evaluation of program impact—the long-term consequences of providing a particular program. For decision-making purposes, however, issues of impact will probably be resolved too late to affect program strategy or tactics. Experimental evaluations may be relatively expensive. Decisions about continuing with the experiment or the program that the experiment aims to test are not likely to be ones that can be put off long enough to assess the actual impact of a program on the health characteristics of a population.

Evaluation is concerned primarily with effectiveness or efficiency in the experimental or quasi-experimental setting. This concern should also be a real one for the effect of the program and should not be a political issue. Many evaluations, particularly quasi experiments, are undertaken with the expressed purpose of assessing a particular type of program or programs, when their true purpose (the hidden agenda) may be primarily political or become part of a larger political process.

In 1986, for example, the results of a six-year $5.9 million analysis to provide reliable estimates of the effects of participation in the Special Supplemental Fund Program for Women, Infants, and Children (WIC) program on nutrition and health during pregnancy and early childhood were released. The WIC program was begun in 1972 and is a $1.9 billion effort to provide food supplements and nutrition education to low-income pregnant and breast-feeding mothers and children up to five years old. It enrolls approximately 3.9 million people. The evaluation results clearly reported that WIC improves the diet of pregnant women and children, adds to maternal weight gain, increases the use of prenatal care, and reduces preterm delivery. However, when the report was reviewed within the Department of Agriculture as the sponsoring agency of the evaluation, departmental reviewers replaced original chapters and executive summaries, believing that the results as presented portrayed the program more favorably than supported by the data. Subsequent reviews by the Government Accounting Office (GAO) concluded that the replacement material contained errors, provided misleading statements, and deleted the overall conclusions of the evaluation (*New York Times,* January 19, 1990).

Despite the difficulties of trying to evaluate within a politically sensitive environment, it must be recognized that it is unlikely that any organization or political body is willing to support the cost of an experiment that does not involve an issue of substantial concern to them. If the issues to be resolved do not have major financial or political ramifications, organizations will be unwilling to expend the resources necessary to undertake a realistic experiment. In such cases, it will always be difficult to separate the political overtones from a concern for the true results of the experiment. Nevertheless, such a separation must be attempted and, to the extent possible, ensured if useful results are desired.

Short-term versus long-term designs

Experiments or experimental programs as evaluation efforts, especially evaluations involving either complex programs or several alternative ways of providing or generating the same types of services through a given program, will probably have the most reasonable chance of success if the programs are of a type that will provide an evaluation result relatively quickly. In the best case, initiation of a program on an experimental basis in any area is likely to be costly in terms of resources required, including planning and implementation expertise. Program managers and health service providers are likely to be unwilling to wait for results that may be a long time off before making critical decisions about program strategies and modifications. For example, if an experimental program does not seem to be producing expected results in a fairly short period of time, managers or health providers may terminate or modify the program in ways that would essentially invalidate the results of the evaluation. On the oth-

er hand, if an experimental program appears to be producing desired results in a relatively short time, policymakers (who are always
under pressure to provide at least a semblance of equity) may be
tempted to expand the program to a much wider population before
it has been adequately shown to be useful. Clearly the best way to
avoid both possibilities, either of which could result in tremendous
wastes of resources in the long run, would be to limit the types of
evaluation questions that experiments confront to settings in which
definitive information can be gained fairly quickly, in perhaps six
months to a year.

A second problem is that the resolution of evaluation issues
takes considerable time through the experimental approach. Actually, this problem is common to all evaluation formats but may be
most acute in the experimental setting because of the relatively high
cost of implementing and maintaining a well-designed experimental
program evaluation. It stems basically from the fact that questions
that can be resolved only in the long run through experimental evaluation may—by the time they have been resolved—be no longer
current or interesting issues.

A final problem associated with long-term designs is in maintaining an adequate population base. Over time individuals initially
involved in a program on which impact or effectiveness is measured
may selectively drop out, reducing the size of the population on
which change is to be measured. Because the dropouts are not likely
to be random, there is a high probability that they will influence
study results in consistent but unexpected ways. The problem of
dropout is known as attrition and limits the validity of the evaluation.

Evaluation versus political rationality

Because of the weakness of the pretest-posttest design with no control as an experimental approach, an experimental strategy for program evaluation should probably be avoided in a setting where no
opportunity exists to have or identify reasonable control groups or
areas or, at the very least, multiple or alternative experimental
groups or areas. Many major federal and private initiatives could
have, on the basis of evaluation rationality, been implemented and
their effects evaluated by comparing program and control areas.
Such programs include the major efforts of the JCAHO's "Agenda
for Change," HCFA's hospital and physician mortality listing program, and the NCI's Physician Data Query (PDQ) as obvious examples. But evaluation rationality is not always the same as political
rationality. From a politically rational standpoint it would have made

little sense—and may have been impossible—to implement such programs on a basis that called for extensive experimental efforts in certain areas of the country (the experimental areas) but not in others. One major reason for the difficulty, politically, of designating experimental areas would be the simple fact that all four programs have clear implications for the number of federal dollars that flow into areas where they are located. Under such circumstances a well-designed experiment would be difficult to carry out.

Randomization

Closely related to the problem of ensuring reasonable control groups or areas—or at least multiple or alternative experimental groups or areas—is making certain that assignment to the experimental or control group is based on purely experimental or evaluation factors rather than political or other considerations. For an experimental design to be useful in program assessment, the results of the evaluation or experiment must not be confounded with any factors whose effect cannot be assessed within the experiment. One clear factor, the consequences of which could not be assessed within a program or experimental program setting, would be the outcome of assigning a new program to be evaluated to certain groups or areas because their problems, which the experimental program is to alleviate or reduce, are the most acute.

Assigning an experiment program to such areas subjects the ultimate evaluation to several problems and criticisms. First, when programs are implemented in areas where certain problems are more acute than elsewhere, it is reasonable to expect a reduction in the level of the problems simply by virtue of the regression to the mean phenomenon. Second, when experimental programs are assigned to acute problem areas, improvements may be misinterpreted even if regression is not a realistic possibility. The results may be misinterpreted because it may be considerably easier for a program to produce desired results in an extreme or acute problem area than to produce even modest results in an area where the problem is less obvious.

Even if an experimental program is assigned to a particular area on the basis of other factors—such as the political importance of local citizenry, the program's ability to serve as a showcase in a particular locality or set of institutions, or for any other reason not basically dictated by the experimental design—problems may still arise in interpretation. It is naive and perhaps misleading to assume that such areas are sufficiently similar to other areas or institutions so that they would provide reasonable controls for the experiment or evaluation.

Appropriate Data for Experimental Design

The data necessary to evaluate experimental programs can be seen as more limited than those necessary for evaluations under almost any other strategy. Essentially a realistic experimental evaluation could be based on only a single indicator of program effectiveness. A program to reduce infant mortality within a given area, for example, may require no more information for a useful evaluation when based on an appropriate experimental design than the infant mortality level in the experimental area after the program has run for a predetermined period and the level in the control area for comparison.

In addition to data on effects, monitoring information to assess program progress relative to expectations can be quite useful. It is particularly important in a setting where the experimental program cannot be shown significantly more effective or useful than no program—that is, where the experimental group turns out to be no different from a control group. But monitoring-type information can be equally important in a situation where there is clear evidence of a program effect when compared to a control group. It can be determined whether the results might have been improved had more attention been paid to ensuring that the program progressed as expected. Quite possibly the effectiveness of a program in producing changes in important population characteristics might be substantially enhanced if efforts were made to ensure that it was on schedule, received the resources expected, and had, in general, the type of management necessary for a successful program.

Whether progress data are maintained for monitoring purposes or not, basically two types of information should be obtained to measure the results of the experiment or the program as an experiment itself. The first is, of course, measures of impact to assess effectiveness. Regardless of whether the experimental program is a single program design to be compared to a control group or whether it is represented by a whole series of different program strategies all compared to one another or to a control group, the absolute minimum data requirement is a relatively objective measure to assess program impact.

If the program is designed to improve the effectiveness of a local health department, some objective measure of the effectiveness of the health department must be available. It may be a composite measure of a number of different aspects of health department operation, a number of individual measures of health department effectiveness in several different areas, or a single measure that taps only one aspect of health department functioning. It is clearly necessary in any experimental evaluation to have some objective measure to be assessed as part of the evaluation. In a family planning program, for example, the objective criterion might be number of births. If the program is for malaria eradication or control, the objective criterion might be prevalence of mosquito larvae. The objective criterion in a program to reduce traffic accidents might be number of accidents per thousand miles driven.

Whatever the objective criterion to be assessed as part of the experiment, it must be measured for both the experimental and control groups and both before and after the introduction of the program. The only exception would be a situation with enough potential experimental and control units that a control in the study for possible differences between the experimental and control group at the outset of the study can be handled through random assignment. In such a case, it would be necessary to measure the objective criterion only after the study or program had been introduced and a sufficient time had elapsed for an effect to take place.

The second type of information for assessing programs via the experimental approach is maintained if the assessment is primarily one of alternative strategies for reaching the same goals—an evaluation of efficiency. If measuring efficiency is a major aspect of an evaluation experiment, it is necessary to have a good measure of the differences between programs being assessed and, through some monitoring device, to ensure that the differences exist not only at the outset of the program but also continue throughout the course of the experiment.

This matter is not as simple as it may seem. Various programs may be designed as alternative ways of reaching the same goals, and these alternative programs may be set in motion under the assumption that the design differences will be maintained through the course of the programs. Through various management and administrative decisions and minor oversights, it is quite possible that actual program operations in the different alternatives may become similar. Just as in the case of comparing an experimental group to a control group, where it is important to have good monitoring and progress information to evaluate the extent to which the program actually worked as designed, so, too, in the case of several alternative programs, such information is critical to ensure that they maintained their differences throughout the course of the evaluation.

A final point on data for experiments should be made again in regard to information about controls. In many instances, experimental controls are often assumed to be areas or all other groups of people who do not receive a program introduced on an experimental basis in one particular area or group. Within a state, for example, several counties may be designated as experimental counties and a program, such as primary care or family planning services provided through a health department, may be introduced into these counties. Those charged with the conduct of the experimental programs and those concerned with their evaluation will, in general, be likely to maintain good records of the operation of the programs over the course of the evaluation. Because the control counties or areas may often be taken for granted, evaluators may be less likely to remember to take the necessary steps to maintain similar data for them. But without such data it will be impossible to make a reasonable comparison between the experimental and control counties. In general, the same information collected about the experimental program(s) must be collected and maintained for areas with no program that are being treated as controls.

Data for Experimental Design from Two Different Programs

Consider again the CCOP and primary care programs. Using an experimental design, what data are required to evaluate experimentally the effort of CCOP to affect physician practice patterns in local communities? And what data are required to evaluate the implementation of a primary health care program for a rural county?

Illustration: Community Clinical Oncology Program (CCOP)

The evaluation of CCOP implementation and impact is, in fact, an experimental study—or more accurately of quasi-experimental design. The ultimate objective is to determine whether this particular organizational mechanism is able to facilitate the transfer of state-of-the-art technology to local physicians and make a difference in physician practice patterns.

Defining the community clinical oncology program as an intervention, the evaluation challenge is to determine whether any change in physician practice patterns is a function of the program or simply a function of larger secular trends. It is not possible to randomly assign CCOPs to communities, nor is it considered feasible to establish a series of matched control CCOPs. It is possible, however, to assess practice patterns for the identical disease sites in non-CCOP communities participating in the Surveillance, Epidemiology, and End

Results Program of the NCI. Identical data will be collected from this secondary data source and compared with the practice pattern data collected within the 20 CCOP communities.

It is also possible to have a set of "natural" experiments to examine comparisons for selected measures of implementation and impact among groups of CCOP categorized by predefined environmental structure and process variables aggregated across CCOPs. These comparisons will use both cross-sectional and longitudinal data for CCOP-specific data collected at baseline and at follow-up. For example, it may be postulated that a strong leadership style is essential for the success of the CCOP. Suppose there are 10 CCOPs with strong leaders as defined in some accepted way, and 15 CCOPs without persons characterized as strong leaders. The natural experiment would be to compare the two sets of CCOPs on some measure of program impact, such as accrual of patients to treatment or control regimens.

It is proposed that four or five important and appropriate hypotheses such as the one above can be identified and explored using CCOP natural experiments. It will be important to identify the hypotheses and the framework of the natural experiment prior to data analysis and post hoc searching of the data. The natural experiments represent the best available comparisons to be made without the use of control programs or communities. They can isolate a CCOP effect by selecting conditions in the environments that vary, such as location (rural versus urban) and resources (high and low competition for cancer patients in the community), and by comparing the performance of CCOP physicians and non-CCOP physicians in their treatment of nonprotocol patients. The accrual levels of the CCOPs will also be entered into analyses of practice patterns to determine if there is an "exposure" effect based on the activity of the CCOPs. Proposed a priori comparison categories using all 52 CCOPs might include

1. high versus low competition
2. group practice dominated versus hospital dominated
3. centralized leadership style versus other patterns
4. old versus new CCOP
5. centralized versus decentralized

Illustration: Primary care program

The first requirement for an experimental evaluation of a primary health care program is to establish an objective measure that can be used to assess its effect. The measure selected will have significant consequences for the conclusion drawn from the experiment. If the indicator is not sensitive to the changes in health status that the program is attempting to affect or is not sensitive over the relative short run, it will probably be of little use in assessing the experiment's value. Moreover, the consequences of a primary health care program may be many and varied, and thus various health status indicators might be used to evaluate the program's effect. As discussed in Chapter 10, these include measures of nutritional status, such as birth weight, weight for age, and weight for height; infant, child, and maternal mortality rates; and life expectancy at given ages.

Although there may be no totally adequate output measures to assess a primary health care program, for managerial decision making, infant, child, and maternal mortality data may be sufficient, and certainly may be the only feasible, indicators to assess the impact of primary health care.

If infant, child, and maternal mortality is accepted as a legitimate output measure for the evaluation of primary health care programs, it will be necessary in a reasonable experimental evaluation to have such information both for an experimental and a control group. It is, of course, quite likely that a community implementing a primary health care program will provide services to the entire community. In such a case, the only reasonable assessment of the effects of the primary health care program would be a pretest-posttest assessment, as discussed earlier. Then it would be most useful to consider the assessment as a time series analysis and to try to obtain time series data rather than before-and-after data.

If, on the other hand, it is feasible to implement primary health care programs sequentially or on a selected basis within jurisdictional areas such as counties, then an experimental design of a more complex and effective nature could be set up. Such an experimental evaluation might perhaps involve the implementation of primary health care in five, ten, or twenty local jurisdictional areas, using the remainder of the state as controls or only an equal number of areas as controls.

If the experimental areas have as their control comparisons the rest of the state, then they may be selected randomly from the whole state or in a controlled random way so that certain types of counties or local jurisdictional areas are to be included. If the controls are limited to an equal number of local jurisdictional areas as experimental areas, it is probably best to select matched areas at the outset, at least to pick sets of two counties each with similar characteristics and then to assign one of them on a random basis to the experimental group and one to the control group. However, the experimentals and controls are determined, it will be necessary to maintain for the control groups precisely the same type of information maintained for the experimental groups if a reasonable experimental evaluation is to take place.

Data to be used for evaluation must be routinely available at the beginning of the evaluation. If, for example, infant, child, and maternal mortality rates are not available by local jurisdictional areas, then it is probably important to select an experimental design that ensures that the experimental and control counties will be selected on a random basis from matched pairs. Then it will be necessary only to maintain data on infant, child, and maternal mortality for the local jurisdictional areas during the evaluation. Characteristics on which counties might be grouped for random assignment would include geographic area, population density, urban-rural characteristics, ethnic makeup or, if such information is available, language group makeup, and other similar information.

The ultimate payoff in an experimental evaluation is the demonstration of a difference between the experimental and control groups in terms of an objective output measure of the program under evaluation. To provide a basis for interpreting performance differences, however, it is useful to have other types of information—types that may be considered primarily monitoring data—to assess the extent to which a program has been executed in a manner consistent with implementation plans. Of particular interest to the evaluation of a primary health care program would be the difference in service provision between the experimental and control groups—particularly the ability to monitor the extent to which the experimental group received the health care services the program is designed to provide.

Physical accessibility to a health service may be a prime concern in the provision of primary health care and an important aspect of care to be measured. Of course, any particular community would need to define accessibility in its own terms, but it would probably be in terms of travel time to the target population. In any case, it will be important to keep some record of the average distance to a health facility from any part of a local jurisdictional area.

Information may also be obtained on the economic accessibility of care. Comparisons between the cost of care in nonprimary care areas and primary care areas give important information on which to judge the overall efficiency and effectiveness of services. This latter type of information is critical to decision making by program managers.

A major area of concern in monitoring primary care will be use of services. The actual number of people who use services can be rather easily obtained through a well-designed recording system. The extent to which services reach populations at risk—for example, the proportion of children immunized, or pregnant women who receive antenatal care or have delivery supervised by trained attendants—is a more difficult, but more important, measure to obtain. It will, of course, require information about the populations at risk.

Additional monitoring data useful in assessing the extent to which a primary health care program is reaching its goals could include information about the dissemination of health education, including the promotion of good nutrition, the proper use of safe water and sanitation devices, and immunizations. Further monitoring information could include the level of endemic diseases, treatments for common diseases and injuries, provision of drugs, coverage by a referral system, and, of course, information about various categories and types of health personnel and personnel availability.

The indication of clear differences between experimental and control areas on the basis of monitoring information will not necessarily result in differences in the output measures, but it is certain that differences in output measures are not likely to occur if differences in the input measures do not exist. Differences in output measures will especially not occur if the monitoring of input measures indicates that the program is not progressing according to some reasonable program plan.

Application to Decision Making and Types of Evaluation

When properly planned and executed, the experimental or quasi-experimental design approach is the most powerful evaluation technique available for assessing the actual effectiveness or impact of a given program. No other evaluation approach, with the possible exception of time series analysis, can give such a clear and definitive assessment of the true value of the efficiency, effectiveness, and impact of a program.

One important decision that can be made on the basis of experimental design evaluation data is whether a program has produced more in terms of a desired output than the absence of such a program or, alternatively, that one program strategy has performed better in regard to the desired output than some other strategy. From this standpoint the clear decision derived from experimental design evaluations is the decision to continue or discontinue a program. If this decision is to be based on the demonstrated effectiveness of the program, experimental design is the evaluation of choice.

A second type of data that can be derived directly from the experimental approach is specific information about the comparative efficiency of one program over another or of comparative efficiency among a number of alternative program strategies. Here the decision to be made would be whether to adopt the program approach that produced the most output for the least amount of input—the most efficient program.

The application of this approach to decision making is not without risk to the people most affected. Because of the disclosure that a control group of persons with syphilis in public health hospitals had never been provided penicillin treatment despite its obvious effectiveness, it has been almost impossible to withhold program benefits—or hypothesized program benefits—from groups of people who would be considered to be helped by such a program.

In fact, standard operating procedures now require that any evaluation closely monitor interventions and terminate it if it appears that the experimental treatment is clearly superior to that provided to the control group. However, given the increasing demand for the results of many evaluations in a variety of treatment and prevention areas, there is always an uneasy balance between the need to maintain the rigors of the evaluation and yet make the program available at the earliest possible time.

Discussion Questions

1. Why is experimental or quasi-experimental design usually considered the ultimate evaluation strategy and yet its actual field application is quite limited?
2. Discuss the relative advantages and disadvantages of the following designs: pretest-posttest design, pretest-posttest with control group design, multiple pretest-posttest (with control group) design, and posttest design.
3. What is the function of control groups in an experimental design? List the various problems associated with the use of controls and the methods used to ensure comparability.

13

Experimental Analysis Techniques and Interpretation

The basis of data analysis for an experimental evaluation of a program is a comparison output or outcome measures between a setting in which a program is not present and one in which it is. In a before-and-after study with no control, the comparison is between the pretest and the posttest. With a pretest-posttest design involving a control group, the comparison is between the change between the pretest and the posttest for the experimental group compared to the change for the control group. For a posttest-only design, the comparison is simply between the posttest measures.

Change or difference must be in the direction expected, but showing that a difference exists is not sufficient in itself to indicate that a program has been effective in producing a true difference in results. Even assuming that no factors except the experimental program can reasonably be expected to affect the results, the identification of a simple difference in the direction expected may not be adequate to indicate a program effect. It is also necessary to show that the difference is large enough that it might not be expected to appear by chance alone. Our objective in this chapter is to present various analysis techniques to determine whether the differences found in various settings could be assumed to be consequences of an experimental program.

The three basic study designs discussed in the last chapter—the pretest-posttest with no control, the pretest-posttest with a control, and the random posttest-only design with a control—can be examined through the analysis of difference scores, using relatively straightforward t-tests. The first part of the chapter discusses specific tests for each of the designs mentioned. A more general framework for experimental data analysis is the class of techniques known as analysis of variance; we will discuss analysis of variance and its application to the general designs mentioned in Chapter 12. Finally, a generalized statement of analysis of variance for more complex experimental designs concludes the chapter.

Analysis of Pretest-Posttest Data (no Control Group)

Although we have described in some detail the hazards inherent in relying on a pretest-posttest design with no control group for attempting to assess program effects, such a design may frequently be the only one available to an evaluator. Despite the number of possibilities that arise in the pretest-posttest design without a control group for inferring a program effect where none exists, it is still useful to understand how such an effect might be assessed statistically. To examine this situation, consider a hypothetical program to improve the public's knowledge of actions to be taken in emergency or first aid situations until competent medical attention can be obtained. The basic assumption of such a program would be that a better understanding of emergency procedures may lead to fewer deaths or more favorable prognosis from situations involving medical emergencies.

Illustration

Suppose that the program itself is a simple ten-minute film presentation of several aspects of emergency or first aid medical treatment, perceived to be important life-saving or medical-crisis—averting procedures. Obviously the ultimate evaluation of the film strip would be to determine whether people who had viewed it would at some later time be able to take control of a medical emergency in a way that would avert death or improve the prognosis following the situation. A more measurable, and certainly more proximate, output at the level of effectiveness of the film strip would be a measure of the amount of knowledge that people who saw it had about activities to be performed or avoided in a medical emergency. Of course, knowledge possessed by the viewers must be compared with some alternative setting if any statement about the effect of the film strip is to be made. The alternative setting in the case of a pretest-posttest with no control group design would be knowledge of the subject possessed by people before they viewed the film strip.

Assume that ten people are selected to view the film strip as a means of assessing its effectiveness in imparting knowledge about emergency medical procedures. Before the viewing, each of the ten is tested on his or her knowledge about emergency medical procedures; they may score from 0 to 20 points. After viewing the film strip, they are retested, and again the possibility is a score from 0 to 20 points. The effectiveness of the program for imparting knowledge can be assessed by using a simple *t*-test of the difference between means for correlated data.

Table 13-1 shows an example of constructed data that might be used to test the effectiveness of the film strip in imparting knowledge about emergency medical procedures. The data are shown for only ten persons; in general, most evaluations of a film strip of this type would involve more people. A reasonable minimum number to include in such an evaluation would be thirty people, although it is possible to use fewer, as we will show.

Table 13-1 has five columns: the first is the person identification numbers; the second represents the scores received on the 20-point test prior to seeing the film strip; the third represents the scores received on the same test by the same persons after seeing the film strip. The assumption is that these two testings will have occurred relatively close in time, since the film strip lasts 20 minutes. Both

Table 13-1 Example of a Test of the Effectiveness of a Film Strip on Emergency Medical Procedures: Pretest-Posttest, No Control

Person	Score 1	Score 2	d	d²
1	2	9	7	49
2	9	8	−1	1
3	8	15	7	49
4	5	19	14	196
5	10	18	8	64
6	17	19	2	4
7	6	17	11	121
8	11	19	8	64
9	5	10	5	25
10	12	12	0	0

$$\bar{d} = \Sigma\, d/n = 6.1$$

$$s_{\bar{d}} = \sqrt{\left[\Sigma\, d^2 - \frac{(\Sigma\, d)^2}{n}\right]\left[\frac{1}{n(n-1)}\right]} = 1.49$$

administrations of the test and viewing the film strip might involve no more than a total of one hour. The fourth column is the difference between the first and second scores, and the fifth column is the square of that difference. With this information, the mean difference, designated $\bar{d}$, and the standard error of the mean difference, designated $s_{\bar{d}}$, can be calculated as shown at the bottom of Table 13-1.

Significance tests

On the basis of these data, a test of the significance of the difference between the first and second observation is a t-test:

$$t = \bar{d}/s_{\bar{d}} = 6.10/1.49 = 4.09 \qquad (13\text{-}1)$$

With a t-test of this type, a value exceeding 2.23 (with an n of 10) would be assumed to occur less than 5 times out of 100. Thus a value of 4.09 could be said to be significant at the .05 level. The probability distribution of t is generally given as an appendix to most statistical texts.

Interpretation and limitations

Based on this example, it can be said there is a statistically significant difference between the scores of the first and second testing. The implication, of course, is that the film strip has made the viewers more knowledgeable about emergency medical procedures. It should be remembered, however, that this conclusion is based on a pretest-posttest with no control group experiment and is subject to several types of errors or threats to validity, including

1. sensitization to the test itself.

2. measurement decay.

3. history, in terms of other things occurring at the same time the film strip was being viewed (for example, the viewers may discuss the film strip or emergency medical procedures in general, increasing the overall level of knowledge available to the group).

4. time lapse; the short period of time between the test and retest decreases the possibility that other factors will have accounted for or produced the change in the scores, but it increases the possibility that instrument decay (or simply the ability to improve on the second testing by virtue of having seen or taken the test the first time) will have produced the improvements in scores.

The pretest-posttest with no control group format does not allow us, in general, to rule out the effects of other factors that may be occurring at the same time the program is in operation and that may reasonably account for changes observed between the first and second testing. With regard to the simple example of viewing the film strip, it may be reasonable to assume that few other important causal forces are operating at the same time. If the program were an experimental family planning effort, introduced nationwide in a developing country, that ran for three years, the incidence of births occurring as a measure of program effectiveness before and after the program is in operation may be substantially influenced by factors other than the program itself.

Analysis of Pretest-Posttest Data (with Control Group)

A design useful in assessing or, alternatively, in controlling for external factors is the pretest-posttest with a control group. To demonstrate the calculation of the appropriate statistics for this design, we will again use the data on measuring the effectiveness of a film strip.

Illustration

Table 13-2 contains constructed data to assess the effectiveness of the film strip. In this case, we will use exactly the same data as Table 13-1 shows for ten persons who viewed the film strip, but Table 13-2 also shows constructed data for ten others who did not see the film strip. The data are constructed to have the same mean score and variance on the first test but a different mean score with the same variance on the second test.

Analysis of variance for an experiment with repeated measures on one variable and two groups could be used to obtain a great deal of information about the differences in scores for the two groups on the first and second test. The primary question of concern, however, is whether the difference in the before-and-after scores for the experimental group is greater, on the average, than the difference of the before-and-after scores for the control group (Winer 1962). This question can be answered by a simple t-test of the difference between two means. The computations needed for this test are the average difference for the experimental group, the average difference for the control group, and the pooled standard error for these two means. The formulas for the calculation of these values are shown at the

Table 13-2   Example of a Test of the Effectiveness of a Film Strip on Emergency Medical Procedures: Pretest-Posttest, Control

Person	Score 1	Score 2	d	d^2
Experimental				
1	2	9	7	49
2	9	8	−1	1
3	8	15	7	49
4	5	19	14	196
5	10	18	8	64
6	17	19	2	4
7	6	17	11	121
8	11	19	8	64
9	5	10	5	25
10	12	12	0	0
Control				
11	9	11	2	4
12	5	14	9	81
13	6	9	3	9
14	11	6	−5	25
15	12	12	0	0
16	5	8	3	9
17	17	14	−3	9
18	10	16	6	36
19	2	4	2	4
20	8	2	−6	36

$$\bar{d}_E = \Sigma\, d_E/n = 6.1$$
$$\bar{d}_C = \Sigma\, d_C/n = 1.1$$

$$s_{\bar{d}\text{pooled}} =$$

$$\sqrt{\left[\Sigma\, d_E^2 - \frac{(\Sigma\, d_E)^2}{n_E} + \Sigma\, d_C^2 - \frac{(\Sigma\, d_C)^2}{n_C}\right]\left(\frac{1}{n_E + n_C - 2}\right)\left(\frac{1}{n_E} + \frac{1}{n_C}\right)} = 2.03$$

bottom of Table 13-2. It might be noted that the experimental and control groups need not necessarily be the same size for this t-test to be acceptable. There is a general assumption, however, that the variance for the two groups being compared is essentially the same. An F-test is available to determine whether the variance of the two sets of difference scores can be considered comparable, which is essentially

$$F = \frac{s_1^2}{s_2^2} \tag{13-2}$$

where s_1^2 is the larger variance and s_2^2 is the smaller variance. The degrees of freedom of this F-test are equal to the number of cases less 1 for both numerator and denominator. In the case of the data in Table 13-2, for example, the degrees of freedom for that F-test would be 9 and 9. The variance for either the control or the experimental group is calculated, of course, according to the standard variance formula:

$$s_d^2 = \frac{\Sigma\, d^2 - [(\Sigma\, d)^2/n]}{n - 1} \qquad (13\text{-}3)$$

For the data shown in Table 13-2, the variance for both the control and the experimental groups is the same, approximately 22.3. Consequently, it is reasonable to pool the variance for the purposes of a test of the effectiveness of the film strip. The t-test used in this case is

$$t = (\bar{d}_E - \bar{d}_C/s_{\bar{d}}\text{ pooled} = (6.1 - 1.1)/2.11 = 2.37 \qquad (13\text{-}4)$$

The total degrees of freedom for this t-test are equal to the number of cases in the experimental group plus the number in the control group minus 2, or 18 degrees of freedom. A standard statistical table giving distributions of t-probability for 18 degrees of freedom would show that a t of 2.1 or larger would occur by chance only 5 times in 100. Therefore a t-value of 2.37 would be considered evidence of a difference between the experimental and the control groups in the before-and-after scores. This would essentially be interpreted as indicating that the film strip has been effective in improving knowledge of emergency first aid procedures for the experimental group.

Analysis of Multiple Group Pretest-Posttest Data (with Control Group)

The same type of analysis procedure demonstrated for one experimental and one control group can be extended to multiple experimental and control groups in the same format. It can be extended to a number of different groups that may be considered experimental in the sense that some type of program is introduced for the group, but that program is different for each of the groups. A family planning effort, for example, might involve one program to induce people to accept sterilization, another program to induce people to use contraceptive devices, and another simply to educate people in the various family planning strategies. Analysis of variance can be used to make a direct single test of the difference or differences that may lie within any of these categories. A simple *t*-test of the difference between different scores, however, can be used to compare any two groups in a multiple category or multiple intervention evaluation, just as in the example for the data in Table 13-2.

Illustration

The data shown in Table 13-2 can also be treated in an analysis of covariance format. Instead of calculating a difference score between the first and second testings for the experimental group and two testings for the control group and then testing the difference between these different scores, the analysis of covariance approach can be used directly to test the effect of the program. It can be done by treating the score received on the second testing as a dependent variable and regressing it on the score received on the first testing, plus a dummy variable coded 1 if the observation is for a person in the experimental group and 0 for a person in the control group. If such an analysis is carried out, the format would be as shown in Equation 13-5, where $\hat{S}_2$ is the estimate of the score in the second testing, S_1 is the actual first testing score, and D represents the experimental-control dummy. The result of an analysis of covariance of this type is precisely the same as the result of the differences in means test as shown in Equation 13-4. The coefficients from the analysis are shown in Equation 13-6. A test of the coefficient on the dummy variable in Equation 13-6 is essentially the same as the test of the difference in mean differences shown in Equation 13-4 and produces precisely the same conclusion.

$$\hat{S}_2 = b_1 S_1 + b_2 D + b_0 \tag{13-5}$$

$$\hat{S}_2 = 0.453 S_1 + 5.000 D + 5.746$$
$$\phantom{\hat{S}_2 =} (1.962) \quad\;\; (1.886) \quad\; (2.374) \tag{13-6}$$

In fact, the evaluator could select either strategy for the analysis. The probability level for the coefficient on the dummy variable is almost .01 ($t = 12.6$ with 17 degrees of freedom).

Assuming that the experimental and control groups are basically subjected to the same external stimuli over the course of the program period, the pretest-posttest control group design will be effective for controlling such extraneous sources of variation or external threats to validity as history, maturation, and other items occurring at the same time of the study. What this design will not control for is the effect of having been sensitized to the posttest questions by having been initially subjected to these questions in the pretest. In the case of a pretest-posttest control group design, both the experimental and the control subjects (as the data in Table 13-2 show) were administered a test on their knowledge of first aid procedures. It is possible that the administration of this test in itself sensitized the experimental group to the important questions so that, as they viewed the film strip, they recognized and formulated answers to them. Thus, it was not the film strip per se that was the cause of an improvement in their scores but rather the combination of prior knowledge of the questions to be asked and the film strip.

Analysis of Posttest Data

A design that can solve essentially all the problems presented by the pretest-posttest control group design but that avoids the difficulty of an interaction effect between the first stage of testing and the subsequent program itself is the posttest-only control group design. Again, consider efforts to evaluate the effectiveness of a film strip.

Illustration

Table 13-3 shows constructed data for a posttest-only control group experiment. Again, the data are the same as those under score 2 in Table 13-2 for the experimental and control groups. An important and necessary assumption of this design is that the 20 people under study were randomly assigned at the outset to either the experimental or the control group. In the case of the showing of the film strip, for example, 20 people might be selected to come to a meeting on a particular evening. Once they have arrived, these 20 people could be assigned on a random basis to either the experimental or the control group. It could be done, for example, by writing a 1 on ten slips of paper and a 2 on ten other slips of paper, mixing all these slips of paper in a container, and allowing each person to draw out one. This would be an acceptable method of randomly dividing the group for the purpose of having an experimental and a control group. The equations necessary for calculating a t-test for the significance of the difference between the experimental and control groups are shown at the bottom of Table 13-3. It should be noted that the formulas for $\overline{X}_E$, $\overline{X}_C$, and $s_{\overline{X}\text{pooled}}$ are the same formulas used in Table 13-2 to test the difference between the differences, the only change being the designation of X as the score for the posttest rather than d for the

Table 13-3 Example of a Test of the Effectiveness of a Film Strip on Emergency First Aid Procedures: Posttest-Only Control

Program Group		Control Group	
Person	*Score*	*Person*	*Score*
1	9	11	11
2	8	12	14
3	15	13	9
4	19	14	6
5	18	15	12
6	19	16	8
7	17	17	14
8	19	18	16
9	10	19	4
10	12	20	2

$\overline{X}_E = \Sigma X_E/n_E = 14.6$

$\overline{X}_C = \Sigma X_C/n_C = 9.6$

$s_{\overline{X} \text{pooled}} =$

$$\sqrt{\left[\Sigma X_1^2 - \frac{(\Sigma X_E)^2}{n_E} + \Sigma X_C^2 - \frac{(\Sigma X_C)^2}{n_C} \right] \left(\frac{1}{n_E + n_C - 2} \right) \left(\frac{1}{n_E} + \frac{1}{n_C} \right)} = 2.03$$

difference between the pretest and posttest. A *t*-test for the significance of the difference between the scores is

$$t = (\overline{X}_E - \overline{X}_C)/s_{\overline{X} \text{pooled}} = (14.6 - 9.6)/2.03 = 2.46 \qquad (13\text{-}7)$$

Again, it is the same formula as given for the *t*-test for the difference between means of the two groups. A *t* of 2.46 is significant at the .05 level. The conclusion that would be drawn from these data is that, on the assumption of random assignment at the outset, the film strip was effective in producing a higher score, on the average, for the people who viewed it.

Application in Field Situations

The designs and data analysis presented above are quite simple compared to the number of complex experimental designs available. Moreover, the analysis of data from these designs has been given strictly in terms of tests of differences between means, or *t*-tests. Although this is the first level of analysis of variance, the data have not been subjected to true analysis of variance—even though they could be—because of the relatively straightforward and simple nature of the results sought.

Experimental designs can be, and often are, much more complicated than those shown here. It seems unnecessary to present more complicated designs, however, because few evaluators are likely to find themselves in a position in a real-life situation to institute any experiment much more complicated than those presented here. In fact, many program evaluators are likely to be in the situation where they must evaluate an entire program on the basis of a single output measure rather than having data for a large number of people relative to the results of the program. Such a problem may preclude the use of any statistical analysis.

Illustration

Suppose that a person wishing to evaluate the effectiveness of the film strip received, after the pretest or posttest, not an individual score for each of ten people but a total score for all ten people in the experimental group and all ten in a control group. With no more information than this, it would be impossible to determine whether the difference between the two groups was a significant one in any statistical sense. The evaluator would only be able to make such statements as that the difference between the two groups is large or small or important for substantive reasons.

To illustrate further, from an evaluation standpoint, consider again the data shown in Table 13-3. If no more were known about these data than the program group's score of a total of 146 points and the control group's total of 96 points, no statistical test of the difference between the two groups could be made. The ability to determine whether the groups are actually different from a statistical standpoint depends on knowledge of their variation.

Consider further the data in Table 13-4. In example 1 the program and control groups show the maximum amount of variation possible in a test where the scores may range from 0 to 20. Among those in the program group, seven scored a 20, one person a 6, and two each 0. In the control group, four people scored 20, one scored 16, and five scored 0. The difference between the means of the two groups is still 5. (The program group has a total score of 146 and the control group a total score of 96.) The pooled standard error for the two groups is 4.45, calculated by the formula at the bottom of Table 13-3. The *t*-statistic for the comparison is 1.12. Such a *t*-value is not

Table 13-4 Two Possible Data Strings for an Average Individual Difference of 5

	Example 1				Example 2		
Program		Control		Program		Control	
Person	Score	Person	Score	Person	Score	Person	Score
1	20	11	20	1	15	11	10
2	20	12	20	2	15	12	10
3	20	13	20	3	15	13	10
4	20	14	20	4	15	14	10
5	20	15	16	5	15	15	10
6	20	16	0	6	15	16	10
7	20	17	0	7	14	17	9
8	6	18	0	8	14	18	9
9	0	19	0	9	14	19	9
10	0	20	0	10	14	20	9

statistically significant so that the conclusion is that there is no difference between the program and control groups on the basis of the statistical analysis.

The data in example 2 of Table 13-4 show just the opposite picture. In this case, the minimum possible variance exists, for a total score of 146 for the program group and a total of 96 for the control group. Again, the difference between the means remains 5, but the pooled variance, as calculated by using the formula at the bottom of Table 13-3, is 0.23. This gives a t-statistic of 21.65, which is significant at any level. Clearly it is necessary to know something about the variation in the group or groups to be compared if any statement about statistical significance is to be made.

If the evaluator had only the information that the total score for all persons in the program group was 146 and the total for all in the control group was 96, there would be no way to assess the statistical significance of this result. It, however, is not an uncommon position for the evaluator to be in. Suppose, for example, that a family planning program is to be implemented in one province of a country and a second province is to be used as a control. Then postprogram data indicating that the fertility rate in the program province was 32 per thousand whereas the rate in the nonprogram province was 45 per thousand may be of some substantive value in the evaluator's conclusion that the program may have a useful effect. But it would be impossible—on the basis of this information alone—to determine whether the difference would be expected by chance alone or would be statistically significant.

Analysis of Variance

Although the examples discussed here may be as complex as most evaluators will see in program evaluation settings and evaluations of this degree of complexity can be adequately analyzed by using *t*-tests to assess the significance of the differences between means, it is useful to introduce briefly analysis of variance as a technique for assessing both the relatively simple experiments described in these two chapters and any of a wide range of more complex experimental designs that could be used in evaluation settings.

The *t*-test for the difference between means is essentially a test of whether there is so little overlap between the distribution of two groups of data that their means can be considered different. Analysis of variance is actually no different from a *t*-test, but at the simplest level it is an alternative approach to the same issue. Rather than a test of whether two means can be considered different, however, an analysis of variance is a test or an assessment of whether two distributions in total can be considered different from one another. The analysis of variance approach can be used in much more complex experimental settings than the *t*-test of differences of means.

Let us examine briefly the nature and characteristics of analysis of variance. Consider the simplest experimental design discussed in this chapter, the posttest design with a control group. The *t*-test for this design, shown in Equation 13-7 for the data in Table 13-3, is the mean of the experimental group minus the mean of the control group divided by the pooled variance. Analysis of variance, which will produce the same conclusion about the difference between the two groups, actually approaches the assessment as a comparison of the variance between groups versus the variance within groups.

From the analysis of variance standpoint any set of data, such as the scores for the 20 persons involved in the film strip example, has a total variance or total sums of squares. (The concept of total sums of squares comes from the notion that the variance is the squared difference between each value and the mean of all values.) This total sums of squares can be partitioned into a number of different categories. Two clear categories in the analysis of a posttest-only experiment with a control group would be the *between-group* (that is, between the experimental and the control group) sums of squares and the *within-group* sums of squares.

The definition of *sums of squares* is simply the squared difference between each observation (in this case, there are 20 observations) and the mean of all observations, indicated by $\overline{\overline{X}}$. Written in the form of an equation, the total sums of squares is

$$SS_{total} = \sum_{i=1}^{n} \sum_{j=1}^{k} (X_{ij} - \overline{\overline{X}})^2 = \sum_{i=1}^{n} \sum_{j=1}^{k} X_{ij}^2 - \frac{\left(\sum_{i=1}^{n} \sum_{j=1}^{k} X_{ij}\right)^2}{nk} \qquad (13\text{-}8)$$

where a single score for a single person is designated X_{ij} and the double summation sign represents the fact that the X_{ij} are summed simultaneously over all values of n and all values of k (n refers to the number of individual observations within each group and k to the number of groups, two). The between-group sums of squares, essentially a measure of the extent to which the groups are different from one another, is

$$SS_{between\ groups} =$$

$$n \sum_{j=1}^{k} (\overline{X}_j - \overline{\overline{X}})^2 = n \sum_{j=1}^{k} \left[\sum_{i=1}^{n} \left(\frac{X_{ij}}{n}\right)^2 - \frac{\left(\sum_{i-1}^{n} \sum_{j=1}^{k} X_{ij}\right)^2}{nk} \right] \qquad (13\text{-}9)$$

And, finally, the sums of squares within groups is

$$SS_{within\ groups} =$$

$$\sum_{j=1}^{k} \left[\sum_{i=1}^{n} (X_{ij} - \overline{X}_j)^2 \right] = \sum_{j=1}^{k} \left[\sum_{i=1}^{n} X_{ij}^2 - \frac{\sum_{i=1}^{n} (X_{ij}/n)^2}{n} \right] \qquad (13\text{-}10)$$

On the basis of these three formulas, the total sums of squares, sums of squares between groups, and sums of squares within groups are shown in Table 13-5 for the data in Table 13-3. There are $nk - 1$ total degrees of freedom, which for the data in Table 13-3 is 19. There are $k - 1$ between-group degrees of freedom (because there are two groups for the data in Table 13-3, this is 1 degree of freedom). There are $k(n - 1)$ degrees of freedom within groups, or 18. Dividing

Table 13-5   Analysis of Variance Table for
Posttest-Only, Control Group Design

Source	SS	df	MS	F
Total	495.80	19		
Between groups	125.00	1	125.00	6.07
Within groups	370.80	18	20.60	

Note: From data in Table 13-3.

the total sums of squares by the degrees of freedom for the sums of squares produces the average sums of squares, or as generally designated in analysis of variance, *mean square*. The between-groups mean square is assumed to be caused by the experimental variable itself. The within-groups mean square is essentially due to error. Division of the between-groups mean square by the within-groups mean square produces an F of 6.07, as shown in Table 13-5. This F-statistic has 1 degree of freedom in the numerator and 18 in the denominator. It is significant beyond the .05 level.

It also may be interesting to note that the F-test represents the square of the t-test. The t-test for the differences between the two groups, as shown for the data in Table 13-3, is 2.46—precisely the square root of 6.07.

Equations 13-8 to 13-10 appear on the surface to be fairly complicated. Winer (1962) provides a substantially simplified treatment of the analysis of variance calculation for a comparison between an experimental and a control group. Table 13-6 shows Winer's method. Instead of speaking of a control and an experimental group, the groups are designated as treatment groups, so that the experimental group could be considered treatment 1 and the control group treatment 2 or, in general, treatment k, for example.

The experimental designs involving one group with a pretest and a posttest and one involving both an experimental and a control group with a pretest and a posttest can be cast in the same analysis of variance form as Table 13-6 shows. Table 13-7 shows the one-group pretest-posttest with no control, and Table 13-8 the pretest-posttest with a control group.

The model in Table 13-7 can be used to assess the difference between measures at several time periods (although it can be used for only two time periods). The test of interest is the comparison of the mean square for time to the mean square residual; the F-test for this

Table 13-6   General Analysis of Variance Layout and
Computation for a Comparison between k Groups,
Some of which Represent Experimental Groups and
Some Control Groups

Notation

Treatment 1	...	Treatment k	
X_{11}		X_{1k}	
X_{21}		X_{2k}	
.		.	
.		.	
X_{n1}		X_{nk}	

$T_1 = \Sigma X_1$	...	$T_k = \Sigma X_k$	$G = \Sigma T$

$$SS_{treatment} = \frac{\Sigma T^2}{n} - \frac{G^2}{kn} \qquad\qquad df_{treatment} = k - 1$$

$$SS_{error} = \Sigma\Sigma X^2 - \frac{\Sigma T^2}{n} \qquad\qquad df_{error} = kn - k$$

$$SS_{total} = \Sigma\Sigma X^2 - \frac{G^2}{kn} \qquad\qquad df_{total} = kn - 1$$

General Form of Summary Data

Source	SS	df	MS	F
Treatment	$SS_{treatment}$	$k - 1$	$MS_{treatment}$	$\dfrac{MS_{treatment}}{MS_{error}}$
Error	SS_{error}	$kn - k$	MS_{error}	
Total	SS_{total}	$kn - 1$		

Source: Winer (1962).

comparison is mean square for time divided by the mean square
residual. The significant F for this comparison would represent a
significant change over time in the criterion measure.

Table 13-8 shows a substantially more complex analysis of several groups (in the simplest case, an experimental group and a control
group) for which several different measurements may be taken (in
the simplest case, a before-and-after measure). The general form of
the summary data shows the division of the sums of squares into
logical components. In this analysis there are three different tests of
interest. There is a test to determine whether the groups chosen are
different, on the average, both before and after treatment. This factor is, of course, not of major interest in the overall question of the

Table 13-7 General Analysis of Variance Layout and Computation for a One-Group Pretest-Posttest Design

Notation

Time 1	. . .	*Time* k	
X_{11}		X_{1k}	$P_1 = \Sigma X_1$
X_{21}		X_{21}	$P_2 = \Sigma X_2$
.		.	.
.		.	.
X_{n1}		X_{nk}	$P_n = \Sigma X_n$
$T_1 = \Sigma X_1$	. . .	$T_k = \Sigma X_k$	$G = \Sigma T$

$$SS_{\text{between subjects}} = \frac{\Sigma P^2}{k} - \frac{G^2}{kn} \qquad df_{\text{between subjects}} = n - 1$$

$$SS_{\text{within subjects}} = \Sigma \Sigma X^2 - \frac{\Sigma P^2}{k} \qquad df_{\text{within subjects}} = n(k - 1)$$

$$SS_{\text{time}} = \frac{\Sigma T^2}{n} - \frac{G^2}{kn} \qquad df_{\text{treatment}} = k - 1$$

$$SS_{\text{residual}} = \Sigma \Sigma X^2 - \frac{\Sigma T^2}{n} \qquad df_{\text{residual}} = (n - 1)(k - 1)$$

$$- \frac{\Sigma P^2}{k} + \frac{G^2}{kn}$$

$$SS_{\text{total}} = \Sigma \Sigma X^2 - \frac{G^2}{kn} \qquad df_{\text{total}} = kn - 1$$

General Form of Summary Data

Source/SS	*df*	*MS*	*F*
Between subjects	$n - 1$		
Within subjects	$n(k - 1)$		
Time	$k - 1$	MS_{time}	$\dfrac{MS_{\text{time}}}{MS_{\text{residual}}}$
Residual	$(n - 1)(k - 1)$	MS_{residual}	
Total	$kn - 1$		

Source: Winer (1962).

effect of the intervention but simply provides a way of separating out the effect of differences in groups from differences in the experimental variable. In general, this test will not be important to the evaluation. The two tests that are important to the evaluation are tests of treatments and of the interaction of the treatments and groups. If the test of treatments is significant but the test of treatments by group interaction is not, the conclusion would need to be

Table 13-8 General Analysis of Variance Layout and Computation for a Comparison between Groups on Before-and-After Measures

Notation	Treatment 1	...	Treatment k		
Group 1	X_{111}		X_{1k1}	$P_{11} = \Sigma X_{11}$	
	$X_{112}TA_{11} = \Sigma X_{11}$		$X_{1k2}TA_{1k} = \Sigma X_{1k}$	$P_{12} = \Sigma X_{12}$	
	...		...	...	
	X_{11n}		X_{1kn}	$P_{1n} = \Sigma X_{1n}$	$A_1 = \Sigma P_{1n}$
Group p	X_{p11}		X_{pk1}	$P_{p1} = \Sigma X_{p1}$	
	$X_{p12}TA_{p1} = \Sigma X_{p1}$		$X_{pk2}TA_{pk} = \Sigma X_{pk}$	$P_{p2} = \Sigma X_{p2}$	
	...		...	...	
	X_{p1n}		X_{pkn}	$P_{pn} = \Sigma X_{pn}$	$A_p = \Sigma P_{pn}$
	$T_1 = \Sigma X_1$	...	$T_k = \Sigma X_k$	$G = \Sigma T$	

$$SS_{\text{between subjects}} = \frac{\Sigma P^2}{k} - \frac{G^2}{npk} \qquad df_{\text{between subjects}} = pk - 1$$

$$SS_{\text{groups}} = \frac{\Sigma A^2}{np} - \frac{G^2}{npk} \qquad df_{\text{groups}} = p - 1$$

$$SS_{\text{subjects within groups}} = \frac{\sum P^2}{k} - \frac{\sum A^2}{np} \qquad df_{\text{subjects within groups}} = p(n-1)$$

$$SS_{\text{within subjects}} = \sum X^2 - \frac{\sum P^2}{k} \qquad df_{\text{within subjects}} = np(k-1)$$

$$SS_{\text{treatment}} = \frac{\sum T^2}{np} - \frac{G^2}{npk} \qquad df_{\text{treatments}} = k-1$$

$$SS_{\text{treatment} \times \text{groups}} = \frac{\sum TA^2}{n} - \frac{\sum A^2}{nk} - \frac{\sum T^2}{np} + \frac{G^2}{npk} \qquad df_{\text{treatment} \times \text{groups}} = (p-1)(k-1)$$

$$SS_{\text{treatment} \times \text{subjects within groups}} = \sum X^2 - \frac{\sum TA^2}{n} - \frac{\sum P^2}{k} + \frac{\sum A^2}{nk} \qquad df_{\text{treatment} \times \text{subjects within groups}} = p(n-1)(k-1)$$

General Form of Summary Data

Source/SS	df	MS	F
Between subjects	$pk-1$		
Groups	$p-1$	Group	$\dfrac{\text{Group}}{\text{Subjects within groups}}$
Subjects within groups	$p(n-1)$	Subjects within groups	
Within subjects	$np(k-1)$		
Treatment	$k-1$	Treatment	$\dfrac{\text{Treatment}}{\text{Treatment} \times \text{subjects within groups}}$
Treatment × group	$(p-1)(k-1)$	Treatment × group	$\dfrac{\text{Treatment} \times \text{groups}}{\text{Treatment} \times \text{subjects within groups}}$
Treatment × subjects within groups	$p(n-1)(k-1)$	Treatment × subjects within groups	

Source: Winer (1962).

that there is a difference between the pre- and postmeasure but that it is not due to the experimental intervention. If the treatment by group interaction is significant, whether in the presence or absence of a significant main effect of treatments, and if the results are in the direction expected, then the conclusion is that the intervention produced a significant change in the criterion measure.

Analysis of variance techniques are actually more complicated than necessary for analyzing the relatively simple experimental designs presented in this chapter. They are extremely powerful techniques for analyzing more complex experiments, particularly when a number of factors must be controlled or assessed in the experimental situation. Most program evaluators will not need to produce research designs to which analysis of variance would be logically applied as opposed to simple tests of differences and means. If they did, however, it would be well to refer specifically to a book on experimental design, such as Winer (1962).

Discussion Questions

1. What are the necessary and sufficient conditions to show program effect? Why are these conditions difficult to achieve in field situations?
2. What are the similarities and differences between a *t*-test and analysis of variance? Under what conditions is each the preferred technique?
3. Describe the difference between total sums of squares, sums of squares between groups, and sums of squares within groups.

Part VII

Basic Methods

14

Measurement

Our ability to evaluate depends on our ability to measure accurately those items that are to be assessed—regardless of the particular type of evaluation strategy involved. In a monitoring strategy, for example, the evaluator is attempting to compare existing progress between the initiation and the implementation of a program with some planned or projected criteria. The ability to measure accurately the extent to which progress toward these criteria is being achieved is precisely the problem in an evaluation of progress.

Similarly, a survey research effort to describe a problem or an analytical evaluation of the effect of different program strategies will succeed or fail on the basis of the ability to measure accurately those things that are to be assessed as part of the evaluation. If time series analysis or trend analysis is being used as the evaluation strategy, the ability to measure changes in important variables under assessment as time changes is again critical to the evaluation effort. If the measurement device used in such a situation is insensitive to changes over time, the evaluation cannot succeed.

In the experimental setting any evaluation will be only as useful as the evaluator's ability to measure accurately program effects that may occur. If these effects cannot be measured, the evaluation will not indicate any program success. Even in the case study approach to evaluation, measurement remains an important component of the process. Our objective in this chapter is to examine the subject of measurement and describe procedures used to develop measures of variables important to program evaluation.

What Is Measurement?

Measurement is the assignment of one set of entities—generally numerical values—to another set of entities—generally some empirical fact or phenomenon. In any measurement effort there is a set of rules by which the numerical values are assigned to the empirical entities. Measurement is the process of assigning the numerical values according to the established set of rules. Different sets of rules or methods for the assignment process have certain advantages or disadvantages. Consider something as simple as measuring the size of an organization.

Illustration: The case of organizational size (Kaluzny and Veney 1980)

Suppose that an evaluation requires determining the relationship between organizational size and a measure of organizational design or performance. Focusing only on size, some organizations are clearly larger than others. But the notion of larger is an abstract concept that the evaluator must translate into concrete terms. The total dollar value of the organization may be used as a measure for translating size from the abstract to the concrete, for instance. If that is the operational measure of size, the evaluator may be able to obtain the data from the records of the organization or from some regulatory agency. On the other hand, the operational definition of size may be the total area of the physical plant. Such data may be available from organization records.

Perhaps the most common definition of size used in organizational research is the number of employees. Assume that the evaluator has decided to put into operation the abstract notion of size as the number of employees in each organization. The question then becomes, What method does the researcher use to assign a numerical value to each organization to represent the empirical reality of the total number of organizational employees? At the most basic level the evaluator will probably decide to treat each employee in each organization as adding equally to the organization's score for size and simply sum up the number of individuals who work for each organization. An equally basic question, however, is how the evaluator will determine the number of workers in each organization.

Assume that the evaluator decides to apply the following method for assigning a score for each organization: The evaluator will stand outside the organization at quitting time and, as the people who work there come out, each one will be counted. On the basis of this process or this set of rules, the evaluator can assign a score to each organization, representing its size as determined by number of employees.

A consultant to the evaluator, however, might legitimately point out that this measurement tool (i.e., this set of rules for assigning a score for organizational size) has some inherent problems. All individuals employed in a given organization may not leave at the standard quitting time, for instance, and the people seen leaving the organization may not all be employees. Some of the employees may be ill or on vacation that day. If the organization has more than one exit, it would be difficult to count all the people coming out. The problems of measurement using this technique would be multiplied further if the organization happened to be in a major office building in a large city where employees from many organizations might leave work at the same time.

Based on these concerns, the evaluator might decide to employ a different measurement technique. The vice president for operations might be interviewed and then asked for the total number of employees in the organization. The answer will serve as the evaluator's measure of size. Again, the consultant may criticize the evaluator's choice of a measurement device, saying, for example, that the vice president for operations may not really know how many employees the organization has, or that the vice president may know but may have rounded the answer off so that the answer is 120 when the actual number of employees is 117. It is possible that an organization that has fewer employees may receive a score larger than another organization with more employees.

Finally, the consultant may suggest to the evaluator that the latter go to the personnel office and interview the personnel manager. There the personnel manager would be asked if the evaluator could go through the files to determine how many active employees there are in the organization. This approach, although cumbersome, may provide the most nearly correct indication of the organization's size, as indicated by number of employees. There are problems inherent even in this approach. It is possible that on a particular day some personnel records—for example, of individuals recently hired—may not yet be in the files.

In this example three methods are suggested for assigning a number to organization size: counting people as they leave work, interviewing the vice president for operations, and reviewing personnel records. Each measurement tool provides a way of assigning a number to an organization. But each rule has limitations relative to the others. Selecting a given measurement device is always a trade-off between the ease with which the rule can be applied and several important characteristics of any measurement.

Characteristics of Measurement

Several characteristics are important in measurement: quantification, scale, unidimensionality, reliability, validity, sensitivity, reproducibility, and transferability.

Quantification

The most important characteristic of measurement is its ability to quantify some phenomena of interest. Certain phenomena are relatively easy to quantify. Others are much more difficult. What might be subject to measurement as part of an evaluation could be classified as (1) physical states and occurrences; (2) performance, behavior, or practices; and (3) attitudes, beliefs, perceptions, and knowledge. Of these three categories, those factors that can be considered physical states or occurrences are probably most easily measured and quantified. Occurrences, such as births and deaths, accidents, the completion of a building, or the purchase of a quantity of drugs, are all relatively easily measured and quantified. Physical states, such as the existence of disease, numbers of facilities available, or mosquitoes in a given area, are also relatively easily measured and quantified.

Less easily quantified than physical states or occurrences are performances, behaviors, or practices—such items as the amount of money budgeted and spent, numbers of houses sprayed for mosquitoes, the extent of the use of a particular type of contraceptive, or disease averted by some practice or activity.

Perhaps the most difficult phenomena to quantify are attitudes, beliefs, knowledge, and perceptions. Attitudes, beliefs, knowledge, or perceptions toward birth control, the use of primary care clinics, physician assistants, or toward any type of program that might be of interest will always be the most difficult phenomena actually to put a quantitative value on. Much of the literature on measurement is devoted to quantification of such factors as attitudes, beliefs, knowledge, and perceptions.

Scale of measurement

Measurement can occur along four basic dimensions or scales. In terms of quantification it is useful to discuss briefly the nature of these scales. The simplest scale of measurement—the nominal scale—does not, in fact, represent quantification at all; it simply classifies. In a *nominal scale* only a distinction between similar or dissimilar items is made. Nominal scales provide such information as A equals B or A is not equal to B (Miller 1977). Nominal scales might include sex and racial classification, job title, marital status, hospital control, type of organization, or any of a number of other types of measures that simply name the members.

The first of the four scales actually to represent quantification is the *ordinal scale*. In the ordinal scale not only is the information A equals B or A does not equal B available, but also the information that A is greater than B or A is less than B. In the category of ordinal scales we might measure physical states or occurrences, such as disease exists or does not exist, birth has taken place or has not taken place, an accident has occurred or has not occurred, a facility exists or does not exist. These are all ordinal categories in the sense that the occurrence of an accident or the existence of a facility shows more or less program success than would the opposite. If the categories were irrelevant relative to program success, a measurement like disease exists or does not exist could be considered a nominal scale only; but if disease status has some consequence for the program, it must be considered an ordinal measurement. "No disease" is better than "disease." In terms of performance, acts, and practices, ordinal categories may, for example, be used to classify users or nonusers of contraceptives, people who accept the spraying of houses versus people who do not, or budgeted money expended versus budgeted money unexpended.

A common measure of attitudes, beliefs, or perceptions is the five- or seven-point scale. Persons for whom measures of attitudes, for instance, are desired will be asked whether they strongly disagree with a given statement, disagree with it, are undecided about it, agree with it, or strongly agree with the statement. This is an ordinal scale. Strongly disagreeing is not only different from but also in some sense less than (or greater than) disagreeing, which is less than being undecided, and so on.

With an *interval scale*, not only is there an order to the possible positions that a scale can take—strongly disagree, disagree, undecided, and so on—but these positions are equidistant from one another as well. In other words, if four consecutive points on the scale were denoted A, B, C, and D, then A to B is equal to B to C is equal to C to D.

The fourth and most sophisticated type of scale is the *ratio scale*. On a ratio scale, the points are ordered and spaced at equidistant intervals, and if A and B are two points on a scale and A times B equals C, then C divided by B equals A. In other words, a ratio scale is one on which multiplication and division, as well as all other mathematical operations, can be performed. This situation assumes a real zero point in the scale.

In general, it is better to quantify a measurement on a ratio scale than on an interval scale. Quantifying a measurement on an interval scale is better than on an ordinal scale, and an ordinal scale is generally preferred over a nominal scale. Not only is a ratio scale or interval scale more precise than an ordinal scale in the ability to indicate the extent to which a quantified measure is greater or less than some other quantified measure, but the mathematical operations of addition and subtraction also have a real meaning with both interval and ratio scales, and multiplication and division have a real meaning with quantification on a ratio scale.

Looking again at the three types of attributes that might be measured—physical states or occurrences; performance, behavior, and practices; or attitudes, beliefs, knowledge, and perceptions—as part of a program evaluation effort, certain aspects of these three categories may be measured on ratio scales, some on interval scales, and some on ordinal scales. Many occurrences of interest in program evaluation, for example, can be quite readily quantified on a true ratio scale.

If we are interested in evaluating a program in different areas, number of births, deaths, accidents occurring, facilities available, or persons with a specific disease state are all measures easily quantified on a ratio scale. In the area of performances, acts, and practices, it is also relatively easy to quantify activities on a ratio scale. Numbers of dollars budgeted or spent, houses sprayed for mosquitoes, contraceptives dispensed or numbers of women using birth control pills, and cases of cholera identified are all items that can be quantified on a ratio scale.

In the area of attitudes, beliefs, and perceptions, it is less clear that ratio scales can be successfully developed. The common approach to measuring attitudes is a five-point scale or continuum ranging from strongly agree to strongly disagree. This scale or continuum is nearly always translated to a numerical scale by scoring 1 for strongly disagree, 2 for disagree, and so on to 5 for strongly agree. In most practical applications the five-point scale is considered ratio, or at least interval, in measurement, but in reality such a scale is probably only ordinal. The perceptual or attitudinal difference between strongly disagree and disagree is not likely to be the same as the perceptual or attitudinal difference between disagree and undecided.

Several strategies are available for attempting to raise the level of sophistication of five-point attitude scales from ordinal to interval. The most common approach is to combine a number of similar attitude statements or perceptual statements into a single composite score, using factor analysis. It can be claimed with some credibility that scores derived from the combination of a number of attitude or perceptual items, using a factor analysis approach, will result in an interval scale. We will discuss the use of factor analysis for measurement in evaluation later in the chapter. In general, it is not possible to raise the quantification of attitude or perceptual items to the ratio level of measurement.

Unidimensionality

The characteristic of unidimensionality essentially assures that a numerical value assigned to any particular phenomenon to represent a point on a measurement scale will be assigned to one and only one real world state. Consider two statements that might be used to evaluate a particular service program:

1. The resources of this program have been used in an efficient manner.

2. This program has been effective in reaching its goals.

Persons involved in the program could be asked to respond to these two questions on a five-point scale from strongly agree to strongly disagree. Each of these measures could be used individually as an ordinal scale of perceptions about the program. Usually, however, evaluators might wish to treat both responses in a single composite score. A simple, straightforward way of producing such a composite score would be to add together the responses of each person on each of these two questions. The resulting scale would range from two, which indicates a strongly disagree response on both questions, to ten, indicating a strongly agree response to both questions.

Problems of multidimensionality do not arise for those persons who answer both questions in the same way. The person who believes that the program has been both inefficient and ineffective, for instance, can respond with a strongly disagree or disagree to both statements. If someone is undecided about both questions, that person may respond with an undecided for both, or those people who agree with both statements can respond accordingly. At this level there are no problems of multidimensionality. The scores for all people of this type will be basically unidimensional because the responses represent essentially the same perception by each person on both questions.

Problems of multidimensionality would arise, however, if a respondent believes that the program has been efficient in using resources in the best manner possible but has been ineffective in producing the results expected. On the other hand, a similar type of problem could arise if the respondent felt the program had been effective but had used its resources inefficiently. In either case, a respondent might answer strongly disagree to one of the statements and strongly agree to the other, for a total summed score of six. A score of six represents any of five substantially different response patterns: a strongly disagree to the statement on efficiency and a strongly agree to the one on effectiveness; an agree on efficiency and a disagree on effectiveness; the reverse of either of these first two; or no opinion on either. In short, scores in the midrange of the scale have little discriminating value.

Such problems of multidimensionality can be controlled to a great extent through the use of techniques like item-to-scale correlation or factor analysis when a number of measures are brought together in a summed or cumulative scale. The application of such techniques to measurement is presented in a later section.

It should be realized that it is not simply attitudes, beliefs, knowledge, or perceptions that might produce logically multidimensional scales. Many health programs have as their ultimate aim the improvement of health status. Measurement of health status is difficult because it is, in itself, a multidimensional concept. The best-known definition of health is that of the World Health Organization (WHO): Health is not merely the absence of disease but rather a state of complete physical, mental, and social well-being. If a composite measure were devised that attempted to quantify health according to physical, mental, and social well-being simultaneously, many persons would probably be at substantially different points on the three different continua and in the midranges of the composite (where a number of different mixes of physical, mental, and social well-being would produce the same numerical result), and the scale would be clearly multidimensional.

A similar type of problem of multidimensionality can occur from an entirely different source. Such a seemingly straightforward measure as number of accidents occurring in an area or within a period of time is, for some purposes (such as gross enumeration), unidimensional. But that unidimensional scale carries within itself a completely different and quite multidimensional set of attributes related to the type and severity of the accidents. An occurrence that might be considered an accident for the purpose of accumulating gross numbers might be much less consequential in terms of disability, disablement, handicap, or death than some other occurrence that would also be considered an accident for the purpose of gross numbers. But the consequence of this difference for behavior, perceptions, activities, and particularly for program evaluation may be quite important.

The same type of statement can be made about the existence of disease: Certain types of diseases are more life threatening, more debilitating, or more handicapping than other types and yet may be counted together in a single measure of the incidence or prevalence of disease. A measure that shows only the number of facilities available may carry within it an inherent measure of their quality. A measure that indicates the number of women accepting a contraceptive practice may carry within it an inherent multidimensionality of the extent to which the women adhere to the appropriate contraceptive practices. Qualifications of this sort in regard to the unidimensionality of measurement can be seen in almost any area of measurement. Although impossible, even under the best circumstances, to specify precisely what is being measured in every instance, it is important to be aware of these types of multidimensionality problems in any evaluation effort.

Validity and reliability

Validity refers to the extent to which the measurement device being used actually taps or represents reality. *Reliability* is the extent to which the measurement tool will produce the same result when used more than once to measure precisely the same item.

Even though validity and reliability are always discussed together, they are quite different concepts. A measuring device may produce a result that is highly reliable in that every time it is used to measure the same thing it produces precisely the same result. But this fact does not guarantee that a measure is valid, that it actually taps reality, or, from a different perspective, that differences assigned to different observations on the measurement scale actually reflect true differences along the dimension the measuring scale is assumed to gauge. The extent to which a measure is either valid or reliable is not easily assessed. Certain guidelines and suggestions for the assessment of validity and reliability can be made, however.

Validity

Basically, validity can be evaluated on two grounds (Kerlinger 1973): content validity (sometimes called face validity) and criterion validity. A third type of validity assessment, usually termed construct validity, is sometimes considered. But *construct validity* is simply a combination of content and criterion validity, so we will only discuss the characteristics of the two pure types.

Content validity, or *face validity*, is an assessment of whether the measure being used to describe some real-world phenomenon seems to be describing that phenomenon. A physical examination, including an electrocardiogram, would be a more valid measure of the clinical existence of heart disease than the self-report of the same person before the examination. The report of a woman about her use of oral contraceptives is likely to have greater validity than the report of her husband. The report of a patient about his or her attitude toward services received in a cancer clinic is likely to have more validity than the report of some third party.

Content validity actually has two aspects. The first is that the measuring device is directed toward the item to be measured—in a sense, a relatively simple and straightforward problem. It would be easy to agree that a measure of the incidence or prevalence of cardiovascular disease is a valid component of a measure of health status. We might also consider a measure of the incidence or prevalence of cardiovascular disease as a valid component of a measure of quality of life.

Content or face validity is an assessment not only of the extent to which the measurement device actually assesses the real-life phenomenon being measured but also of the extent to which it assesses the entire content area of that phenomenon. If, for example, we are measuring health status and we perceive it to be a multidimensional phenomenon, the prevalence or incidence of cardiovascular disease is only one single and perhaps relatively minor component of the phenomenon. We would require ways of assessing a much broader range of physical states and occurrences before we could claim that we had a measure of health status that had content or face validity.

Despite the difficulty of ensuring that a measure being applied to a particular real-world phenomenon as complex as health status has content validity, the content validity remains an important criterion for assessing the validity of various types of measurements. A measure of health that contains no assessment of disease processes will be immediately questioned on the basis of content validity, for example. A measure of the use of contraceptives based on a series of questions about attitudes or beliefs about contraceptives would be equally questionable from the standpoint of content validity. Content validity assessments should undoubtedly be made about any measure that is devised.

Criterion validity tackles the question of whether the current measure of the phenomenon produces results that are closely related to other independent measures of the same phenomenon. It is less concerned with whether the measuring device is logically a measure of the real-world phenomenon being described or whether the entire content of that phenomenon is assessed. The World Health Organization, recognizing that the health status of a person, community, or country is a difficult trait to measure with a great deal of content validity, for instance, has suggested that a useful measure of health status for communities or nations could be a combination of infant and child mortality, maternal mortality, and age-specific mortality. Clearly if health is not simply the absence of disease but also the complete physical, mental, and social well-being that WHO suggests, several categories of mortality are not going to be valid measures of health when content validity is the criterion. On the other hand, these measures will be closely associated with what WHO perceives to be health from a broad, systems standpoint and hence show criterion validity.

Criterion validity is generally assessed by using such techniques as correlation to determine the extent to which a measure that could be used for assessing some group of phenomenon is correlated or related to some other measure. The validity of a measure of health status based on a self-report of perceived health level on a ten-point scale, for instance, could be assessed by drawing a small sample of those people who responded to the self-assessment and giving them an extensive physical examination. The physician's assessment of health after the examination could be compared to and correlated with the initial self-assessment to determine the extent to which the two assessments correlate. If the two were highly correlated, the self-assessment could serve as an inexpensive measure of health that had stood the test of criterion validity.

Reliability

Reliability refers to the extent to which a measuring device produces the same results on multiple applications to the same phenomenon. If, for example, we want to measure the number of health facilities available in a number of different areas, the measuring device should include some definition of what a facility is. If this definition is loose enough or limited enough so that the person counting the facilities has substantial freedom in determining what is a health facility and what is not, different people trying to count the number of facilities in the same area may come up with widely different results. This example is not unrealistic. In the late 1960s, after the passage of Medicare, at least three different organizations actively maintained records of hospitals in the United States: the American Hospital Association, the Blue Cross Association, and the federal government. The American Hospital Association had an active list of about 6,000 hospitals. Because of a slight difference in how hospitals were defined, the Blue Cross Association maintained a list of about 7,000, but the federal government, because of still different definitional criteria, maintained a list of about 12,000 hospitals. It would be easy to see that if several individuals were told simply to count the hospitals in the United States, they might produce widely different results, based on how they decided to determine whether a particular facility was a hospital.

Determining reliability. An obvious way to assess the reliability of a measuring tool would be to take several measures of the same item and compare the results. In certain evaluation efforts this step would not be difficult. A death would be counted as a death no matter how many times it is counted. Total dollars budgeted would probably be counted the same every time. (Dollars expended in specific categories, however, might change, depending on the accounting system used.) Numbers of certain types of facilities in an area might be the same every time they were counted, assuming that the definition of a facility were relatively precise. On the other hand, a woman's self-report on her use of contraceptives might change from time to time because she failed to remember the original report or for other reasons. In the area of attitudes, beliefs, and perceptions, answers to the same questions may differ as a result of the respondent's mood, state of mind, or relative interest in participating in the survey, even though underlying perceptions had not, in fact, changed.

There are problems in measuring the same item on more than one occasion. On the one hand, if we measure something that is not likely to change, such as death or birth, multiple measures are not necessary. Reliability would seem evident. On the other hand, if the reliability of the measuring instrument is a question, particularly in regard to responses to questionnaire items, an effort to measure the phenomenon more than once in the same manner could lead to an overestimation of reliability when people remember their previous answers and without thought provide them again, or an underestimation of reliability if people became exasperated with the questions, or other possible combinations of these situations.

The use of multiple tests of the same thing has led to the idea of a reliability test known as *split halves*. In this case, a number of questions all generally describing the same area would be asked and scores calculated on half the questions would be correlated with or compared to scores calculated on the other half.

A logical extension of the split-half technique is the multiple correlation between a number of items purporting to measure the same thing. If, for example, a cancer clinic is being evaluated and one area of concern is the attitude of clients, there might be a series of eight to ten questions all focused on the overall attitude toward clinic services. A measure of the reliability of this group of questions or items would be the multiple correlation between all the items. For a detailed discussion of this approach to the measurement of reliability, see Kaluzny and Veney (1980).

Increasing reliability. Validity and reliability have the interesting property that increasing one generally leads to decreasing the other. It is particularly true that in order to increase the reliability of a test or measuring device, additional items can be added to the measuring tool. If, for example, the measure of reliability consisted of five statements on perceptions about the cancer clinic program, reliability can be increased through the correlation technique by adding more items. At the same time, however, if the original five items are perceived to be relatively valid measures of attitude toward the clinic, the addition of five new items will decrease the overall validity of the total test because they will tap additional dimensions of people's attitude toward the clinic. These conclusions can be shown mathematically but are beyond the scope of our discussion.

Sensitivity

Sensitivity refers to the ability of a measure to reflect changes in the state of the real-world phenomenon under evaluation. If the measures being employed in an evaluation are not relatively sensitive to changes in the real-world states, a particular program effort that has a true effect on the real-world state may be seen as ineffective. This situation could occur only because the measurement tool is not sensitive to changes in the real world.

To illustrate, the World Health Organization has, as noted, suggested as measures to evaluate the impact of primary health care efforts several categories of mortality—infant and child, maternal, and age-specific. A major problem with mortality, whether age- and sex-specific or simply mortality in general, is that it tends to be highly insensitive to changes in health status other than the gross change of death itself. If health is a function of mental, physical, and social well-being, many changes can take place in these levels of well-being that are never reflected in mortality data. A program like primary health care designed to affect and influence a wide range of health concerns or a wide spectrum of the health concept may have profound consequences for mental and social well-being and for certain aspects of physical well-being and not be reflected at all in changes in mortality.

But sensitivity is not simply a problem that can be identified as associated with such gross and fairly obvious differences as the difference between health per se and mortality. Measures may be closely related to real-world phenomena and perhaps appear to measure these phenomena and yet still have the problem of sensitivity, particularly measurements or attempts at measurement of attitudes, beliefs, or perceptions. A scale might be constructed of six or eight items related to how a person feels about a particular mental health clinic, for example. The items in the scale may be statements about the clinic to which people can respond on a five-point scale, strongly disagree to strongly agree. People, however, are often unwilling to select extreme points on a scale as answers even though these extreme points might best reflect their perception. If these questions were directed to a number of people who had used a particular mental health center, they might simply, because of the way people are inclined to respond to such scale items, provide responses that differed very little as their perceptions of the clinic changed when, in fact, their real feelings toward the clinic might be quite different. In many situations where measures are not sensitive to changes in real-world phenomena, the result will underestimate the result of the program effort.

Reproducibility and transferability

Both reproducibility and transferability are critical in measurement techniques whose purpose is discovering "scientific knowledge" but may be less important in evaluation. Nevertheless, it is appropriate to include a brief mention of them under the general subject of measurement.

Each is a component of reliability. *Reproducibility* refers specifically to the extent to which a given researcher or evaluator can reproduce measures used in one setting to apply to the same phenomenon in other settings. For example, an index of perception about medical services developed in the United States for application to U.S.

citizens may be of little value if a similar program is to be evaluated in a different setting, such as within a developing nation. The extent to which an evaluator can take a measure that has been developed to provide an assessment in one setting and reproduce similar results in another setting is a result of the reproducibility of the measure.

Transferability might be considered a similar characteristic. The distinction between reproducibility and transferability centers on the uses of the measuring device. The issue for reproducibility is whether a given evaluator can use the same measuring tools, whereas in transferability the issue is whether other evaluators can use the measuring tool and use it in similar settings or in other settings.

In general, transferability from one researcher to another or one evaluator to another is a characteristic often assumed to exist in measurement, and in many cases, this assumption is accurate. The major categories of physical states or occurrences, performance, behavior, and practices particularly provide for a high degree of both reproducibility and transferability.

It is in the area of attitudes, beliefs, and perceptions that reproducibility and transferability present difficulty. A classic example of the lack of transferability would be the Rorschach test of personality characteristics. The interpretation of a Rorschach test is, by its very nature, subjective, and the test itself is not highly transferable from one researcher or one evaluator to another.

The Rationale for Measurement

Measurement provides a means for learning something about a program that can be used for evaluation purposes. Two specific points should be made about measurement and its relationship to program activities, however.

Comparisons

Measures are taken for the purpose of comparison. A great deal of information may be collected about any given program—the number of dollars budgeted for the program, dollars spent, personnel involved, visits made by clientele, or the number of drugs dispensed by the program. The items measured may be endless.

All this measurement, however, is meaningless for evaluation purposes unless it involves some comparison. The comparison may be between the measure produced by the program—for example, number of clients served—and some ideal measure as specified or set up prior to the implementation of the program. In this case, the comparison is between actual productivity or progress and some ideal or established norm. The comparison can be between different programs providing basically the same types of services—for example, the cost of providing them through one program as opposed to providing the same services through another program. A comparison might be between different areas served by the same or similar programs, so that the numbers of immunizations given might be compared from one county to another. Comparison can be over time, such as comparing the proportion of dollars budgeted to dollars spent by a program in each of five succeeding years or comparing the number of outpatient visits per month from one month to the next.

All are legitimate comparisons that can be made in a program evaluation context and certainly do not exhaust the number of such possible comparisons. Nevertheless, comparison between units over time or between performance in a standard or norm is critical to program evaluation and is an underlying assumption of the whole measurement effort. If no comparison is anticipated on the basis of measurements taken, then such measurements are relatively meaningless.

Variation

If comparisons between some standard or some norm and performance are to be carried out, if comparison between units of observation is to be successful, or if comparison over time is to have any meaning, then a basic assumption of measurement or, perhaps more specifically, of measurement goals, is that they should provide evidence of variation. A measure that shows no variation across a range of observations is useless.

It is possible that a particular measure to assess certain characteristics of a program will not show substantial variation over time or from one unit of analysis to another or between performance and a standard. On one level this situation may be all right in the sense that if the standard is being met, or if all units of analysis are performing equally, or if there is no change over time, then no variation should be evident. In many circumstances, however, the lack of variation in a measure is not so much a consequence of the absence of true differences, divergence from a standard, differences between units of analysis, or changes over time as of sensitivity of the measure. The measure is not adequately sensitive to reflect the variation that exists. If a measure is so insensitive that it does not reflect true changes or differences in units of analysis, it is worthless as a measure for evaluation purposes.

It is also possible that certain aspects of program evaluation or program assessment may involve attempts to assign certain types or levels of performance, outputs, outcomes, effectiveness, and so on to certain levels of input. It is possible, for instance, that in several programs operating in basically the same way a range of results is observed in terms of the outputs. A program of immunization that operates in several different geographic or political areas may have widely differing results in terms of numbers of persons immunized. An evaluation of these programs that would attempt to explain this difference in numbers of persons immunized might include some relation between numbers of persons immunized and, say, number of dollars per capita available to each of the separate programs. If every program has the same number of dollars per capita for the program in each area, however, the measure is basically worthless as an explanatory measure in regard to the number of people immunized. It is a basic fact of scientific procedure that variation from one measure of interest cannot be accounted for by another measure that is essentially a constant or shows no variation. Stated another way, if the number of dollars per capita expended on each of several programs providing immunizations was constant, it could not account for a difference in the number of people immunized.

Types of Measures

The only limits on the types of measures used in program evaluation are those imposed by the creativeness and imagination of the evaluators. Nevertheless, we can discuss specifically several different types of measures that can be used in evaluation, some of their characteristics, certain settings in which they may be more or less appropriate, and how they might be constructed. Five types of measures are considered: (1) numbers, (2) rates, (3) attributes, (4) perception measures, and (5) composite measures.

Any type of measure used is a means of assessing some attribute of a specific unit of analysis. The unit of analysis might be a person, a program, or a program in a given year. It might be a geographic location or a community (political entity). It might be an organization, such as a hospital. All the measures to be discussed could be applied to some extent to any of these units of analysis. But several types of measures seem to adapt more readily to certain types of units of analysis than others. For example, rates are more useful in discussing geographic areas or programs than individuals. Perception measures are often more useful when the individual is the unit of analysis. Nevertheless, all these measures could be used in a setting where any unit of analysis is assumed. In discussing these measures in general, we will assume the unit of analysis to which the measure is most likely to be applied. Where it is clear that substantial adjustments in the use of the measures would be required for other units of analysis, we will make that point.

Numbers as measures

Numbers are certainly the simplest form of measures that might be applied to program evaluation. If a certain type of health services or social services program is operating in a given geographic area, its characteristics and those of the area in which it operates can be described in terms of numbers—for example, the size of the population (number of people living in the area); numbers of births, deaths, hospital beds, or clinics available in the area; dollars budgeted to or expended by the program; or number of people served by the program. Numbers are appropriate in characterizing programs or the areas within which they are operating. It is quite common, for instance, to compare program areas or operations or population served or dollars budgeted to indicate the relative size of a program. Numbers can also be applied to measures of characteristics of people being served by programs—height and weight, age, or expectation of life at birth all are numbers that can be readily applied to individuals who may be the clients or recipients of service from a particular program.

Basically, as with any type of measure, three different comparisons might be made. One comparison is between the actual number and some ideal number for the same measure. A second is between units of analysis (whether people, programs, geographic areas, etc.). The third is among the values of the measure on a specific unit of analysis at different times. In monitoring program progress, the number of dollars expended on services at the end of any given fiscal period could be compared to the number of dollars expected to be expended on services. If these two numbers coincide, then an evaluation of progress would indicate that, at least for this measure, the program was on track. A measure representing the actual number of persons provided services through some type of program could be compared at the end of some appropriate period of time to the number of persons who should have received services based on some program plan. It, again, would serve as a valid measure of progress and, to a certain extent, of effectiveness.

Comparisons across units of analysis are also possible. The number of services provided by each of several programs operating under the same basic circumstances could provide information about their relative effectiveness. Alternatively, the number of services provided by a single program in each of several successive time periods, such as months or years, could be used as a means of assessing or evaluating program progress over time or, alternatively, program effectiveness or impact over time.

Numbers are useful as measures of program progress or effectiveness and are easily obtained for purposes of program evaluation. There is a major difficulty with numbers as such, however—the problem of relative scale. Two programs providing different numbers of services may do so because they are comparatively more or less effective. Or they may do so because they are serving different-sized populations and thus have different numbers of potential clients to draw from or because they have different numbers of program personnel, and hence more personnel to provide services, or because they have differing budgets with greater or fewer resources with which to provide the services. These problems lead to the use of rates as measures.

Rates as measures

A rate is essentially a ratio of two measures. The ratio of the total number of physicians in an area to the total number of people living in that same area is a rate. It may be expressed as physicians per capita (in the United States, approximately .0018). It might be expressed as the percentage of persons who are physicians (in the United States, approximately 0.183 percent of the population), or it might be expressed as physicians per 1,000 or 1 million population (approximately 1.829 physicians per 1,000 population in the United States). In any case, whether the ratio or rate is expressed on a per capita basis, a percentage basis, or a per 1,000 or per 100,000 basis, the result is the same. A rate provides a means of standardizing some number measure of interest, such as number of clients served, by some measure of the size of the unit of analysis assumed important in determining number of clients served. For example, the number of clients served per 1,000 dollars budgeted (the number of clients served divided by the total number of dollars available and multiplied by 1,000) is a rate or ratio measure that can be used in comparing organizations or programs. Because rates are standardized measures that take into account important scale aspects of programs or areas served by programs, they become measures not only of program effectiveness but also of program efficiency. The number of clients seen per program employee or the number of immunizations given per 1,000 dollars of program expenditures allows direct comparisons of the effectiveness and efficiency of one program with other programs of greater or smaller size.

Rates can be based on almost any measure that has conceptual meaning—numbers of services, physicians, dollars expended, or clinics per person or per 100,000 persons represent useful rates based on numbers of people served. Alternatively, the base could be numbers of dollars expended or budgeted or time, such as services provided per month or dollars expended per day. In many cases, it may be reasonable to deal with what might be considered double rates, such as visits per clinic per day, visits per physician per day, or budgeted dollars available to a program per capita per service area.

Rates are particularly useful for making comparisons across a number of similar programs of substantially different size. Rates can provide a standardized means of evaluating not only progress but also efficiency, effectiveness, and, in certain instances, impact.

When rates are used to describe disease or morbidity states, a distinction is made between occurrence or onset and persistence, particularly between acute and chronic diseases. Acute diseases are defined as having relatively rapid onset and short duration, whereas chronic diseases are those of perhaps less rapid onset but certainly a longer duration.

To recognize this distinction, disease rates are frequently expressed in terms of prevalence versus incidence. *Prevalence* refers to the number of persons at any time (scaled to some relevant base, such as percentage or per 100,000) who actually show evidence of a disease. *Incidence* refers to the number of persons (again scaled to an appropriate base) who succumb to the condition or disease within a given time range. Certain diseases may have frequent onset and long duration; they have both high incidence rates and high prevalence rates. Diseases like colds, flu, measles, and mumps may have high incidence (although most childhood infectious diseases are declining markedly) but relatively low prevalence. They are of short duration, and the persons who have them rapidly recover. Other diseases that may have relatively low incidence—such as diabetes or arthritis—because they are long-term chronic conditions, have a much higher prevalence than incidence. New persons are added to the ranks of those with the condition, but relatively few leave these ranks except through death. In assessing or evaluating the effect of any type of health-related program, particularly as that program is expected to reduce the rate of disease, it is important to consider whether the rate reduction concerns incidence, prevalence, or both.

Attributes as measures

Attribute measures generally refer to those taken on a strictly nominal scale—that is, a scale that serves to differentiate, but not to order, categories. In general, attributes cannot be used as objective criteria by which programs are assessed or evaluated. Instead attribute measures serve as a means of clarifying the nature of the program or ensuring that expected target populations are being reached. Attribute measures of importance in program evaluation might include such variables as sex, race, ethnicity of the country or region, and profit versus nonprofit status. The purpose of a particular program may be to provide services to a mixed community of native-born Americans and recent Spanish-speaking immigrants. An important aspect of program evaluation, then, might be to ensure that the proportion of persons receiving services from the clinic would be approximately the same as the proportion distribution in the population between native-born Americans and Spanish or Spanish-surnamed immigrants. In such a case, the attribute variable, ethnicity or place of birth, would be an important attribute for defining categories within which the program is assessed. Similarly, a program directed toward the control of hospital costs might have as one of its important aspects the control of hospital costs in both for-profit and not-for-profit hospitals. Here the nominal or attribute variable profit versus not-for-profit status would be important as a component measure for evaluation purposes.

Perception measures

Perception measures represent a broad category of measures that are generally defined along ordinal or interval scales—or, in certain instances, along ratio scales—and that can be useful in many aspects of program evaluation. Perception measures refer to a broad range of attitudes, beliefs, knowledge, and even consensual agreement that can be used in program evaluation. It is an area that has received extensive attention from psychologists, social psychologists, and sociologists.

Historically, numerous and different types of efforts have been made to measure attitudes, beliefs, or perceptions in more or less consistent and scientific ways. These include the use of such techniques as Thurston scaling, the semantic differential, Guttman scales, and Likert scales. We will not attempt to discuss all these types of perception-measuring devices, but several are presented because of their relevance to evaluation. For a detailed discussion of perception measures see Kerlinger (1973) and Miller (1977).

Likert scale

In recent years the most common technique for measuring attitudes, perceptions, beliefs, and, to a certain extent, knowledge and consensus has been the Likert scale. It has the advantage over many other attitude or perception measurement techniques of being fairly simple, straightforward, and, for the most part, easy for people to respond to.

A *Likert scale* refers to a statement or series of statements made in either a positive or negative manner. Respondents are asked to check one category from among several categories of answers that best represents their feeling about or belief in the statement. In general, each statement has five response categories, which may be labeled strongly disagree, disagree, undecided, agree, and strongly agree. In rare instances, Likert scales are constructed with three categories—that is, simply disagree, undecided, and agree—or seven categories providing a finer differentiation along the continuum from strongly disagree to strongly agree.

Exhibit 14-1 shows a set of questions used to evaluate the perceptions of health department personnel about a primary care program funded by a state department of health services but delivered through local health departments. Each of the nine statements in Exhibit 14-1 represents a separate attitude or perception about a Division of Health Services–funded primary care program provided through a local health department. The possible responses to these statements range from strongly disagree through strongly agree. Two points might be made in regard to these nine statements. First, they cover a fairly diverse set of perceptions about primary care programs in health departments. Question 2, for example, relates to people's perception about the impact of a primary care program on their personal position, question 6 relates to the perception that primary care programs will force small health departments to merge into larger ones, and question 7 relates to some perception about the quality of the health department as a consequence of having a pri-

Exhibit 14-1 Example of Likert Scale Items: Questions Designed to Evaluate the Perceptions of Health Department Personnel about a Primary Care Program

Listed below are a series of statements that have been made about the DHS-funded primary care program in local health departments. Please indicate how closely these statements reflect your feelings about the program.

	Strongly Disagree	Disagree	Uncertain	Agree	Strongly Agree
1. DHS-funded primary care programs were helpful in motivating county funding sources to provide resources for adding and improving similar programs.	1	2	3	4	5
2. The DHS-funded primary care program has had a substantial impact on the way I do my job.	1	2	3	4	5
3. The DHS-funded primary care program has made my job substantially more difficult.	1	2	3	4	5
4. The DHS-funded primary care program has been difficult for many local health departments to implement.	1	2	3	4	5
5. A DHS-funded primary care program was unnecessary since most local health departments are already providing these services through other programs.	1	2	3	4	5
6. In order to implement a primary care program along the lines suggested by DHS, smaller county health departments have been forced to merge into larger ones.	1	2	3	4	5
7. DHS-funded primary care programs have improved the quality of local health department activity.	1	2	3	4	5
8. DHS-funded primary care programs have improved the appropriateness of local health department activities.	1	2	3	4	5
9. The DHS-funded primary care program has not yet had any impact on my health department.	1	2	3	4	5

mary care program. Clearly it would be possible for respondents to these nine questions to have different views about the individual items. Readers interested in recent progress in utility measures should see Drummond et al. (1987) and Torrance and Feeny (1989).

Although the individual items indicated in the first set of perceptions represent a diverse set of characteristics of primary care programs, they may not include everything that an evaluator may wish to know about the perceptions that a group of people hold about such programs. In any effort of this type to generate statements that can be used to assess attitudes, perceptions, or beliefs about a program or some aspect of it, it is important that these statements cover all aspects of the program to be assessed.

With attitude or perception measures constructed by using the scale or item statements shown in Exhibit 14-1, the basic value of the statements lies in comparisons between programs, between areas in which a program is operating, or over time within a given program. Gross values of the results are relatively useless for evaluating a program except to the extent that it would be important to hope that the respondents would be more inclined to answer at the end of the continuum that reflects more favorably on the program; but, in general, when many people respond to a given item, the tendency will be for the mean for all people to be relatively close to the midpoint, and no absolute statement of agreement or disagreement may be possible. Furthermore, sometimes there may be no standard by which to judge whether the response meets some norm for the program.

Trade-off or utility measures

A utility measure has been used in management science to account for decision making under risk situations. In regard to program evaluation, the notion of utility or trade-offs derived from utility may be successfully used to construct unidimensional measures of such factors as perceived health status for the purpose of evaluating changes in health status or other concepts similarly difficult to measure. Torrance (1972) describes one application of the utility–trade-off approach to measuring health status.

The approach begins with an extensive list of different types of mental, physical, or social ailments that might be considered health problems. These problems are then presented to a group of respondents who are asked to select the worst possible condition. To illustrate, let us consider an abbreviated list of such conditions, including good health, asthma, diabetes, end-stage uremia, and quadriplegia.

Time is an important consideration in this measurement. The amount of time that a person might be expected to spend in a given state will be closely related to that person's perception of how relatively good or bad the state is. So a comparison, for example, between asthma and diabetes would include the respondent's additional knowledge of the length of time in either of the two states. For simplicity, we will assume that the time in each state would be equal and would be one year. The first step is to select the state in which the judges or respondents would least prefer to be for a year's time. Assume that the respondents have selected quadriplegia as the worst state. Given that quadriplegia has been selected as the worst possible state, the next step is to assign a score to that state on a range from zero to one. Zero would be considered death or the worst possible health state.

The score of the worst state (quadriplegia) would be assigned on the basis of the Von Morganstern Standard Gamble. Respondents are asked to choose between two alternatives. The first alternative is that the respondents would be in good health for, say, one year, then would assume the worst state, quadriplegia, for one year, and finally would die. The alternative is that the respondents would be in good health for one year, at the end of which they would take a drug that would have a probability p of keeping them completely asymptomatic for one year, after which time they would die, or a probability of $1 - p$ of the drug's causing immediate death. The score assigned to quadriplegia on the scale of zero to one is the value of p for which people would be indifferent as to whether they accepted quadriplegia or elected to take the drug. For the assignment of a value to any health state other than the worst, the process is somewhat different. In these cases, the alternatives are a period of time (such as one year) in a given state, followed by good health, or the taking of a pill, which has a probability p of producing total good health for the time period and $1 - p$ of putting the person in a worse state (such as quadriplegia) for the same time period, followed by good health. The utility for such a state would be p for that state plus $1 - p$ times the utility for the worse state.

If we wished to calculate the utility for diabetes relative to quadriplegia, for example, the alternatives would be diabetes for one year, followed by good health; or taking a pill, which would produce immediate good health for the year with a probability p, or quadriplegia for the same time period with a probability of $1 - p$. The utility of diabetes, then, is the value of p selected by the judges for the alternative plus $1 - p$ multiplied by the utility for quadriplegia. If p was chosen as .8 for diabetes and the utility for quadriplegia was .1, then the utility for diabetes would be .8 + .1(.2) or .82. This is shown in Figure 14-1.

Several important points must be mentioned about this type of scaling technique for measuring health. First, the issue of time is critical. The scores that we derived for diabetes and quadriplegia are based on one year of time (of course, this is simply a hypothetical example). It may be that either state would take on different values if maintained for different periods of time. Consequently, it is necessary in constructing a scale of this type to specify clearly the time period involved and to include a varying set of time periods for each condition.

A second concern is the difficulty of construction. Such a scale assumes that a very large, perhaps comprehensive, list of conditions will be judged in terms of their relative desirability for the construction of an overall scale. This would clearly be a major effort. Moreover, the scale is a perishable commodity since many conditions, because of advances in medicine, might become less undesirable over time. This problem is not fatal to the use of the technique, however, because it can be applied to selected specific types of conditions for the purpose of cost-benefit analysis in comparing the benefits of different programs of treatment or prevention that affect different types of conditions. If the approach were to be used to derive a general measure of health status, however, it would be costly, time consuming, and difficult.

A third point is the problem of determining what state people are actually in. If a trade-off measure is used to assess changes in

Figure 14-1 Example of Health Status Measurement Based on Utility Theory

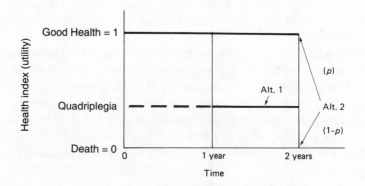

overall health status for a community as a consequence of some type of health services program, the cost of collecting information about the state of health that people in the community actually enjoyed would be quite great. This would be true even if it were done on a sample basis, although the sample would certainly provide a more workable approach.

Composite measures

Composite measures may involve attributes, numbers, rates, perception measures, or combinations of these categories. A composite measure is basically derived by putting together several other measures in some combination to produce one single measure from the composite.

Weighted and unweighted sums

The most common approach to generating composite measures is to produce the weighted sum of a given set of measures about some attribute of a program under evaluation. The composite measure would be essentially of the form

$$C_i = \sum_{j=1}^{m} w_j Z_{ij} \qquad (14\text{-}1)$$

where C_i represents the composite score, w_j the weight for the jth variable, and Z_{ij} the standardized score for the jth variable for person i, and the summation is over all m variables. It is important, of course, that the variables to be made a composite or summed are transformed to standard score form—that is, Z score—before the summation is done. If, for example, average family income were to be made a composite with the portion of families below the poverty level as some measure of economic health, family income—which has a mean of perhaps \$14,000 or \$16,000—would completely overwhelm the proportion of families below the poverty level, which is perhaps .20 or .25.

The simplest type of composite score is a score in which the weights w_j are all equal. If the weights are all equal, usually it is reasonable to assume that they would be simply one; then the composite score is the sum of the Z scores.

A more complex scaling system or system for putting together a composite score would be one in which the weights w_j differ from variable to variable. Consider a constructed score for each Standard Metropolitan Statistical Area (SMSA) in the United States, which represents a quality of health and education component of an overall quality of life score (Lieu 1979). Seven rates were used to make up the health portion of the health and education score—infant mortality per 1,000 live births, death rate per 1,000 population, dentists per 100,000 population, hospital beds per 100,000 population, hospital occupancy rates, number of physicians per 100,000 population, and per capita local government expenditures on health. In addition, sex education factors provide a score for the education portion of the health and education component.

In the composite score, equal weights were assigned to the health and the education portions. Moreover, equal weights were assigned to infant mortality and the death rate. Table 14-1 shows the specific variables included in the measure of health and education for each community. The numbers in parentheses on the left side of the table represent the weights w_j for each of the thirteen variables.

It is clear from Table 14-1 that the total composite score will be weighted most heavily by the two death variables and the two educational attainment variables, all four of which receive weights of .125. The medical care availability and accessibility variables each receive a score of .05, which means that taken together they are all equal to the health (or death) measure. If the subject of an evaluation was a program or series of programs to improve health and education in a number of geographical areas, this composite score could serve for evaluation purposes as a measure of the extent to which the programs were successful.

The logic of Lieu's (1979) weighting factors in constructing a health and education component score is fairly straightforward. Equal weights were given to individual and community conditions within the health and the education portions. Beyond this logic, however, the weighting may be quite arbitrary. In certain situations, logic may dictate the assignments of weight. For the health and education component, there seems to be some clear logic to the assignment of a one-fourth weight to each of the four separate categories. In other instances, differential weighting might be less easy to justify. As Lieu points out, one strategy for differential weighting, however, could be a survey of persons assumed to be knowledgeable about the importance of various factors in determining some aspects of program performance or, in this specific instance, community life.

Guttman scales

The Guttman scaling technique is based on the assumption that dichotomous attributes can be ordered in such a way that, for the least common attribute to exist or have a positive value for a given respon-

Table 14-1   Factors in Health and Education Component

Factor Effect and Weight	*Factors*
Individual Conditions	
Health	
− (.125)	1. Infant mortality rate per 1,000 live births
− (.125)	2. Death rate per 1,000 population
Education	
+ (.063)	1. Median school year completed by persons 25 years old and over
+ (.063)	2. Percentage of persons 25 years and over who completed four years of high school or more
− (.063)	3. Percentage of males ages 16 to 21 who are not high school graduates
+ (.063)	4. Percentage of population ages 3 to 34 enrolled in schools
Community Conditions	
Medical Care Availability and Accessibility	
+ (.05)	1. Number of dentists per 100,000 population
+ (.05)	2. Number of hospital beds per 100,000 population
+ (.05)	3. Hospital occupancy rates
+ (.05)	4. Number of physicians per 100,000 population
+ (.05)	5. Per capita local government expenditures on health
Educational Attainment	
+ (.125)	1. Per capita local government expenditures on education
+ (.125)	2. Percentage of persons 25 years old and over who completed four years of college or more

dent or organization, all other attributes will also exist or be positive responses for the same respondent or organization. For the next least common attribute to exist, all attributes except the least common are assumed to exist and so on through the second least common attribute, the third, and so forth. Any organization having only one attribute will have the most common one. If such is the case, and a respondent or organization receives a particular score on the scale, it indicates immediately the position of the organization or respondent relative to the items that make up the scale.

Illustration. To provide a simple illustration of the Guttman scaling technique, assume a set of responses from ten hospitals to the question of whether the hospital provides each of five services: rehabilitation, mental health, medical social work, family planning, and home care. Table 14-2 shows the constructed data for the responses of the ten hospitals about whether they provide any one of the services. If the service is provided, a 1 appears in the column.

As the table shows, seven of the ten hospitals provide rehabilitation services. Five provide mental health services, five have medical social work services, three have family planning services, and two provide home care services. The programs are ordered by the number of hospitals providing the service.

If a scale is to exist in the data, there should be a distinct pattern in which the hospitals not providing rehabilitation services (hospitals H, I, and J) will also, in general, not provide any other services. This is, in fact, the case. Furthermore, those hospitals not providing mental health services (hospitals F, G, H, I, and J) should also not provide medical social work, family planning, or home care. Only hospital F violates this requirement. Of the hospitals not providing medical social work services, only hospital E provides family planning or home care; and of those not providing family planning services, only hospital C provides home care. Despite these "errors," it is possible to test whether the data demonstrate the characteristics of a Guttman scale.

Table 14-2   Example of Guttman Scale Using Constructed Data for Ten Hospitals

Hospital	Rehabilitation Services	Mental Health Services	Medical Social Work Services	Family Planning Services	Home Care Services	Maximum Marginal	Scale Score
A	1	1	1	1	1	5	5
B	1	1	1	1	0	4	4
C	1	1	1	0	1	4	3
D	1	1	1	0	0	3	3
E	1	1	0	1	0	3	2
F	1	0	1	0	0	3	1
G	1	0	0	0	0	4	1
H	0	0	0	0	0	5	0
I	0	0	0	0	0	5	0
J	0	0	0	0	0	5	0
Total	7	5	5	3	2	41	

The criteria for the existence of a Guttman scale are actually a combination of three separate calculations. The first criterion is the *coefficient of reproducibility* (CR)

$$CR = 1 - \frac{E}{nm} = 1 - \frac{3}{50} = .94 \qquad (14\text{-}2)$$

where E is the number of errors. An error is counted for each entry (1 or 0 in the table) that must be changed for each hospital to be a scale type; n represents the number of observations (hospitals) and m the number of items (programs). The second criterion is known as the *minimum marginal reproducibility* (MMR), defined in Equation 14-3 as the sum of the most frequent response for each organization

$$MMR = \frac{MM}{nm} = \frac{41}{50} = .82 \qquad (14\text{-}3)$$

where MM is the maximum of ones or zeros for each organization (the maximum marginal). The third criterion is the *coefficient of scalability* (CS)

$$CS = \frac{CR - MMR}{1 - MMR} = \frac{.94 - .82}{.18} = .67 \qquad (14\text{-}4)$$

In order for a Guttman scale to be present, it is commonly accepted that the coefficient of reproducibility should be greater than .9. The minimum marginal reproducibility must be less than .9, and the coefficient of scalability should be greater than .6. These levels are rather arbitrary but have the weight of usage on their side. If these criteria are accepted, it is clear that the constructed example for the ten hospitals forms a Guttman scale. The coefficient of reproducibility is .94, the minimum marginal reproducibility is .82, and the coefficient of scalability is .67. Furthermore, it can be seen in the table that hospitals A, B, D, G, H, I, and J are all pure scale types. That is, they fit the perception of the underlying scale perfectly. Hospitals C, E, and F are nonscale types. They contain one error each.

A scale score of 5 can be assigned to A, 4 to B, and so on for the pure scale types with confidence that the result will be clear and unambiguous. A score of 3 for a pure scale type means that the hospital provides rehabilitation services, mental health services, and medical social work services. A decision must be made in order to assign a scale score to hospitals that contain errors. Hospital C, for example, has an error either in the negative response to family planning or the positive response to home care. If it is decided that the positive response to home care outweighs the negative response to family planning, the hospital would be assigned a score of 5. If the reverse is decided, the hospital would be assigned a score of 3. Although this decision will not have a major influence on overall relationships between the Guttman scale variables and other variables, it is likely to have consequences for the interpretation of results for hospital C and is always a difficult decision to make. Nevertheless, some such decision must be made for every organization that includes an error (hospitals C, E, and F). If it is decided that the affirmative answers will be treated as errors, the figures shown in the scale score column in Table 14-2 would be assigned to the ten hospitals. Scales could then be used as independent or dependent variables for further analysis of the data.

Factor analysis

A technique for finding composite weights involves a certain empirical logic for determining the weights and at the same time ensuring that the resulting scores will not be such that midpoint values are ambiguous. The technique, which has widespread use for this type of application, is known as *factor analysis*. For a more detailed discussion of factor analysis, see Nie et al. (1975); and for its application to health services, see Kaluzny and Veney (1980).

Illustration. To see how factor analysis works and to examine some of its results, let us consider some select data for counties in North Carolina that correspond relatively closely to the measures included in Lieu's health section of the health and education score. These measures are the infant mortality rate for each county measured in terms of deaths per 1,000 live births; the death rate for each county measured in terms of total deaths per 100,000 population; and the number of active physicians, dentists, and hospital beds per 100,000 population. Hospital occupancy rates and per capita local government expenditures on health, two variables that Lieu uses, are not included in this set of data.

Factor analysis begins with a matrix of correlations among the variables to be scaled. Table 14-3 shows the correlation matrix between the five variables taken from the North Carolina data for which we would like to produce a factor analysis result. In any set of data, such as that shown in the correlation matrix in Table 14-3, there is some variance shared with other variables in the data set and some variance unique to each independent variable. To a certain extent, the intercorrelations represent this shared variance. A correlation of

Table 14-3   Correlation Matrix for Data from North Carolina Counties

	Infant Mortality	Death Rate	Physicians/ 100,000	Dentists/ 100,000	Hospital Beds/ 100,000
Infant mortality	1.00000	0.17841	−0.12941	−0.17621	0.00045
Death rate	0.17841	1.00000	−0.14085	−0.17094	0.02646
Physicians/100,000	−0.12941	−0.14085	1.00000	0.89886	0.24655
Dentists/100,000	−0.17621	−0.17094	0.89886	1.00000	0.19337
Hospital beds/100,000	0.00045	0.02646	0.24655	0.19337	1.00000

Source: Data taken from North Carolina Health Statistics Pocket Guide, Public Health Statistics Branch, Division of Health Services, Department of Human Resources, Raleigh, North Carolina.

0.90 shown for the two variables physicians and dentists per 100,000 population indicates that there is more variance shared between those two variables than between, for example, physicians per 100,000 population and the infant mortality rate with a correlation of −0.13.

One purpose of factor analysis in determining whether variables should be summed together and in determining the best empirical weights is to find a transformation of the original correlation matrix that will account for as much variance in the original correlation matrix on the basis of a single vector. The vector that best reproduces the original correlation matrix is called the *first principal component factor;* its values are referred to as *factor loadings.* Table 14-4 shows the first principal component factor for the correlation matrix given in Table 14-3.

The factor loadings shown in factor 1 are the actual correlations between the five variables included in the factor and the factor itself. As Table 14-4 shows, physicians and dentists per 100,000 population are most highly correlated (at approximately 0.92) with the first principal component factor. What this means is that factor 1 is basically a measure of the physicians and dentists per capita or per 100,000 population. The low correlation between the variables infant mortality, death rate, and hospital beds per 100,000 population indicates that these variables are not closely associated with the underlying factor.

To understand further what a factor analysis means in this situation, consider the notions of *communality* and *uniqueness.* In any data set, such as is represented by the preceding five variables, there is the assumption that a certain variation in the data is common to

Table 14-4   Factor Loadings and Communality:
One Factor Solution of Data in
Table 14-3

	Factor 1	*Communality*
Infant mortality	−0.17767	0.031567
Death rate	−0.17730	0.031435
Physicians/100,000	0.92471	0.855089
Dentists/100,000	0.92515	0.855903
Hospital beds/100,000	0.22873	0.052317

several variables in the data set and that a certain variation in the data is unique to each single variable. Looking at the factor loadings in Table 14-4, it is possible to determine what portion of the variance in each of the five variables is common (communality) and which part is unique. The square of each of the factor loadings represents the communality for each variable, shown in the communality column in Table 14-4. Communality is, in fact, the square of the factor loading.

As the communality column indicates, only about 3 percent of the variance in birth rate, death rate, or hospital beds per 1,000 population is shared with any of the other variables in the data set; so 95 percent or more of the variance in those three variables is unique to each variable independently. It can be seen to a certain extent in the correlation matrix in Table 14-3, but it is much more apparent from the result of the factor analysis. The clear result of this information is that a summed score made up of all five variables weighted equally is likely to produce a result in which intermediate range values are multidimensional or at least confused in pattern and meaning. If a summed score is to be created from these five variables, it should be done on the basis of weighting that reflects the correlations shown as factor loadings in Table 14-4.

Most factor analysis programs will produce the factor scores resulting from a factor analysis of the data, weighting each of the variables proportionally to the factor loadings. When the result is as clear as in Table 14-3, where physicians and dentists per 100,000 population are the only two variables that share a large proportion of the variance in common, it would be quite reasonable simply to ignore the infant mortality, death, and hospital bed rates and produce a measure of physician and dentist services available, which would be the simple sum of the standardized scores for physicians and dentists for each of the counties under consideration.

Discussion Questions

1. Distinguish between a nominal, ordinal, interval, and ratio scale. Consider a primary care program and designate measures of impact that illustrate each type of scale.
2. What is the difference between content validity, criteria validity, and construct validity? Why is validity more difficult to deal with, methodologically, than reliability?
3. Discuss the advantages and disadvantages of using composite scores. In

what ways does Guttman scaling and factor analysis resolve the problem of assigning weights when using composite measures?

4. Are the following response categories considered a unidimensional or multidimensional scale? Why?

Not done in my organization	Done in organization but I am not responsible or involved	I am not responsible but I intend to influence	I have made policy	I supervise	I perform
1	2	3	4	5	6

15

Sampling

Sampling has two main functions: (1) describing a total population on the basis of an examination of only a small part of it and (2) being certain that results obtained from an experiment reflect its true effect. Our objective in this chapter is to apply the principles of sampling to program evaluation. We distinguish between descriptive sampling and sampling for more analytic evaluation. Various types of sampling designs are considered, together with external-internal validity, bias, and precision. We conclude by selecting a sample of health departments to illustrate basic sampling procedures.

Descriptive versus Analytic Sampling

Sampling for descriptive purposes involves populations of interest already defined. Such a population may be all the persons served by a health services program, all the people within a geographic area where a new planning program has been instituted, or all the hospitals in a state. It may be too costly or physically impossible to obtain information about all members of a population of interest. Thus, a sample may be drawn on the basis of some known and agreed-on criteria to be used as the basis for estimating the characteristics of the total population.

Sampling for analytic purposes is a means to ensure that differences found between an experimental group and a control group can actually be attributed to the experimental intervention and are not a function of other external or unmeasured factors. Sampling, or in this case, random assignment of units under study to experimental or control groups, represents an effective control for factors to be excluded as possible causes of observed differences in outcome measures for the experimental and control groups. In every instance, the units to be included in the sample, or the decision about whether a particular unit is in an experimental or control group, must be the result of a random process or chance. A sample drawn on a random basis or chance is generally referred to as a *random sample,* or frequently as a *probability sample.* In this chapter we refer to random sample or probability samples more or less interchangeably. The design of a sample involves a number of basic terms and concepts: the mean, variance, standard deviation, and the standard error of the means. The *mean* refers to the average value of the variable of interest and is calculated as

$$\mu = \frac{\Sigma X}{N} \tag{15-1}$$

where X is the value of the variable of interest and N is the number of observations.

The *variance* is a measure of dispersion—that is, the extent to which the number of observations differ from one another for some variable of interest. It is calculated as

$$\text{Variance} = \sigma^2 = \frac{\Sigma (X - \mu)^2}{N} \tag{15-2}$$

The square root of the variance is the *standard deviation:*

$$\text{Standard deviation} = \sigma = \sqrt{\sigma^2} \tag{15-3}$$

The *standard error of the mean* (also known as the *standard deviation of the sample mean*) is the average squared difference between the mean for each sample and the true population value μ:

$$\sigma_{\overline{X}} = \text{SE}_{\overline{X}} = \sqrt{\frac{\Sigma (\overline{X} - \mu)^2}{N_{\overline{X}}}} \tag{15-4}$$

The use of these concepts and terms is described later in the chapter.

Issues of Sample Design

Validity

When a sample is selected for the purpose of evaluating a program, the evaluator must be concerned about two types of validity: internal and external.

External validity

External validity deals with the question of whether what is observed from the sample is true of the whole population. If, for example, the evaluator finds that the greater proportion of sample program recipients favor the program, is it possible to conclude that the greater proportion of all service recipients are favorable toward it? If the selection of a sample to be used for evaluation is done on a random or probability basis, sampling statistics or sampling theory provides a means by which to determine the validity of findings from the standpoint of inferences from the sample to the population and, in the case of experimental studies, the internal validity of the results on a sample itself. But the critical factor is whether the sample has been selected on a random or probability basis. If it has not, if the sample is a haphazard one, a sample of convenience, or a purposeful sample, there is no theoretical basis on which to assess the validity of the results either internally or externally.

Because randomization or the notion of a probability sample is so critical to sampling and to the internal and external validity of results obtained from evaluations that involve sampling, some discussion of randomization and its characteristics is needed. Consider first the question of extrapolating from a sample to the total population—external validity.

Illustration. In drawing a sample to provide data that describe the total population, the evaluator is attempting to estimate, on the basis of the sample, certain important population values or characteristics. Suppose that the evaluator is trying to estimate the level of need in the population for primary health care services. The evaluator has available a scale that has been used to measure need in other populations. This scale, which physicians agree is valid, is based on physician examinations and questionnaires directed to the respondents that are capable of classifying people on an interval scale from 10 to 1, which represents high (need) to low (no need) for personal health services. The evaluator will draw one sample of 100 persons from the population. These individuals will complete questionnaires and have physical examinations from the physicians. On the basis of this information, the evaluator will make an estimate of the probable level of need in the population.

Assume that in the population of 10,000 people for whom an estimate of need is being determined, 1,000 people would actually be recorded by the assessment instrument as being in each of the ten levels. One thousand would be ranked 1, one thousand would be ranked 2, and so on. In this case, the true mean level of need in the population would be 5.5. If every one of the very large number of possible samples of 100 was drawn from this population of 10,000— the total number of samples of 100 that can be drawn from a popula- tion of 10,000 without replacement is 10,000! (factorial) divided by 100! times the quantity 10,000 minus 100!—the distribution of mean values (average assessment of need) for all these samples would be approximately normal with its midpoint at 5.5. This distribution would have a standard deviation or standard error of the mean of 0.29. The population variance for a set of data consisting of an equal number of values 1 through 10 is approximately 8.24 (Equation 15-2). The standard error of the sampling distribution of the mean can be calculated as

$$SE_{\bar{X}} = \sqrt{\frac{\sigma^2}{n} \cdot \frac{N-n}{N}} = \sqrt{\frac{8.25}{100} \cdot \frac{9900}{10,000}} \qquad (15-5)$$

In a normal distribution the standard error of the mean has the interesting property that approximately 95 percent of the means of all the many samples of 100 that can be drawn from a population of 10,000 will be within two standard errors of the population mean. Or, in terms of the present distribution, 95 percent of all possible sample results will show a mean between 4.93 and 6.07. Using another per- spective, because a normal distribution is symmetrical, only 2.5 per- cent of the samples will have mean values smaller than 4.93 (a sample, for example, in which of the 100 cases selected, all 100 were values of 1), and only 2.5 percent will have mean values greater than 6.07.

What has been described here are population values. The mean of 5.5 is a population value—that is, a value that pertains to the entire 10,000 cases. The standard error of 0.29 is again a value that applies to the entire set of samples that can be taken from these 10,000 cases, and the confidence limits of 4.93 to 6.07 represent population-based confidence limits. The important point, however, for estimating characteristics of a population is that data from a sample will work in almost precisely the same way. If a single sample of 100 cases is selected on a random basis, a standard error of the mean can be calculated by using the variance from the sample as an estimate of the true population variance. An estimate of the standard error of the mean can be calculated from the estimate of the variance, and confi- dence limits can be established about the estimated means of the population in exactly the same way. Assume, for example, that the actual sample of 100 produced a mean value of 5.2 as the point estimate of the level of need, and a standard error for that mean of 3.33 as the estimate of the true standard error of the mean. We could then be 95 percent certain that the true need level of the population lay somewhere between 4.54 and 5.86. What this means is that if we were able to select every sample of the many samples that could be drawn from a population of 10,000, sampling 100 at a time, 95 out of every 100 of those samples would produce a confidence limit of two standard deviations on either side of the estimated mean, which would include the true mean value of 5.5.

This type of statement can be made if sampling is random. If sampling is nonrandom, there is no statistical means to determine the accuracy of the estimate. Random selection ensures external validity—that is, ensures that an assessment of the validity of the estimate can be made. Nonrandom sampling does not provide external validity.

Internal validity

Internal validity is concerned with the question of whether the evaluator's observations or conclusions about relationships within the sample drawn actually exist for that sample. Suppose, for instance, that an evaluator draws a sample of persons who have access to a particular health services clinic and from this sample determines that over half the people sampled are satisfied with the services. Here internal validity would be concerned with the extent to which that statement about the members of the sample is true. In this case, internal validity primarily involves how the determination is made as to whether people favor or do not favor the program. In other cases, the question of internal validity may be a sampling problem, particularly with regard to experiments.

Internal validity is similar to external validity in that it may depend on random sampling, but it is more specifically directed toward the issue of whether what has been observed within the sample is, in fact, true for that sample rather than true for some population. The issue of internal validity as it pertains to sampling arises specifically when the evaluation takes an experimental format. In the experimental setting some type of program is provided to one or more "experimental" groups of recipients while an alternative program or no program at all is provided to some other group or groups of persons, or other areas that are considered the controls. (This ignores, of course, the essentially nonexperimental before-after study with no control group, whether a panel study or a longitudinal time series analysis.)

Illustration. Assume again that the subject of interest is the level of need for primary health care services within a population of 10,000 people. It is assumed that the provision of a certain level of primary health care services will reduce this need as evaluated by the instrument described in the preceding discussion. A hundred persons in the population will be selected to receive these primary health care services for a specified period of time. A hundred other persons in the population will be selected as controls; these individuals will not receive any special treatment, although they are free to obtain services in any way that they might have obtained them prior to the study. If every possible sample of 100 persons were drawn from this population of 10,000 and compared to every other sample of 100 persons in the complete absence of any program, this comparison (or the absolute value of the mean of the first sample minus the mean of the second sample) would produce a distribution with its minimum value at 0 (where both samples of 100 persons had exactly the same mean score) and its maximum value at 9 (where everyone in one of the samples had a score of 10 and everyone in the other sample had a score of 1). The distribution would look something like that shown in Figure 15-1.

If the difference between the mean in each of the many alternative samples being compared is now divided by the average standard error of the two samples,* a *t*-test of the difference between the means can be performed. Because the best estimate of the variance for any sample is the population variance of 8.25, the best estimate of the pooled standard error for two samples (from the footnoted formula) is 0.071. If the difference between each possible pair of samples is divided by the pooled standard error, the result will be essentially a one-sided *t*-distribution. What this means is that 95 percent of all the sample pairs will produce *t*-values of less than 2 (actually less than 1.96). There is less than a 5 percent chance of getting a value of

---

*The *average standard error* is generally called the *pooled standard error* in a comparison between means. It is calculated as

$$SE_{pooled} = \sqrt{\frac{n_1\sigma_1^2 + n_2\sigma_2^2}{n_1 + n_2}\left(\frac{1}{n_1} + \frac{1}{n_2}\right)}$$

where n_1 refers to the size of the first sample, n_2 to the size of the second sample, σ_1^2 is the variance of the first sample, and σ_2^2 the variance of the second sample.

Figure 15-1   Distribution of Difference between Means of Two
Samples of 100 (Hypothetical)

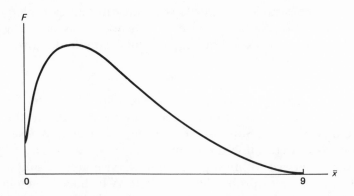

a difference between two means divided by the pooled standard error that will be greater than 2.

Returning to the original idea of a single experimental sample
and a single control sample, if they are randomly selected, then the
probability is .95 that they will have at the outset mean values that,
when divided by the pooled standard error of the two groups, will
produce a *t* less than 2. Next, if after the experimental group has
received personal health services for a period of time the difference
between the groups divided by their pooled standard error is greater
than 2, the researcher would conclude that there is a very small
probability (.05 or less) that the two samples differed before the onset
of the experiment and so would accept the alternative hypothesis that
the experiment made a difference in the level of need. This conclusion could be drawn even in the absence of any measurement of need
before the beginning of the experiment. If such an experimental
setting uses random selection to assign persons to the two comparison groups, the experiment will have internal validity. If random
selection is not used for group assignments, there is no way of assessing the probability that people's status beforehand will not be reflected in the measure of level of need after the experiment and,
consequently, no way of assessing its internal validity.

Bias, accuracy, and precision

Bias, accuracy, and precision are three important characteristics of
any sample design. The terms actually refer to the estimates made

from a particular sample. In general, these terms are applied to samples drawn for the purpose of making estimates about populations. In that sense, they would refer to samples taken from the survey research strategy or perhaps monitoring or case study approaches. It is also possible, however, to talk about bias, accuracy, and precision of estimates based on experimental sample designs.

Bias

In the case of descriptive samples, *bias* refers specifically to whether the expected value of an estimator being used is the same as the true value being estimated. Suppose, for instance, that the purpose of an evaluation is to determine the extent of need for a specific type of medical care service within a geographic service area. Using a random or other type of probability sample for which each member of the population has a known and nonzero probability of being selected and using a nonratio estimator to determine the level of need in the population will give an unbiased result. It will be unbiased because every possible sample of an equal size from the population has a known nonzero probability of selection and the mean value of all these estimates would be the true population value. The selection of any single sample by this strategy would result in an unbiased estimate.

If, on the other hand, the sample did not provide some possibility that every member of the population would have a known and nonzero chance of selection, the resulting estimate would be biased. The expected value or mean of all possible samples drawn in a manner in which every member of the population does not have a chance for inclusion would produce a biased estimate. The most common way in which biased estimates occur is when there is a difference between the target population (the one about which some statement is to be made) and the sampled population (the one actually available for selection).

In an attempt to estimate the need for a certain type of primary health care service in a geographic service area, bias could be introduced into the estimate in a number of ways. It is possible, for example, that the population actually sampled to determine need is those persons who come to a clinic for services. If only the people who come to the clinic for services of some type are possible selections for a sample to estimate need for the entire service area, the sample will be heavily biased by the fact that people who do not use clinic services have no possibility of being selected. Other sampling strategies can produce similar problems of bias. Suppose that a city is the service area for a health care provider in question; then the sample of persons in that service area might be drawn by using the telephone directory or tax listing for the community. Either approach, although better than a sample taken from persons coming to the clinic, is still likely to produce a biased result. Not every family has a telephone. Persons with unlisted telephones or new arrivals in the community will not be listed. Not everyone is included on the tax rolls, and it is often difficult to gain access to these rolls. So bias can be introduced in estimations when either approach is used as the sampling frame.

Similar types of phenomena can occur in experimental work when persons or other units of observation, such as organizations, are selected from a larger group to be included either in a control or an experimental group that will ultimately be compared to determine the effect of some program. If a sampling strategy is used for selecting the experimental and the control groups that will result in all possible pairs of samples being selected for comparison to one another, the result of this selection strategy will be an unbiased estimate of the effect of the experiment, at least as far as sampling is concerned. If, on the other hand, the sampling strategies used make it likely that only certain persons or organizations are selected for the experimental group, while other persons or organizations are selected for the control group, the result of the experiment in terms of sampling will be biased. It is as important in experimental work as in surveys or case studies to avoid bias if possible. In particular, if two strategies for sampling are available, each of which is essentially identical in cost, the one that produces the least bias should always be preferred.

Accuracy

Accuracy refers only to the extent to which the estimate of the population is close to the true population value, regardless of whether the estimating was done on a biased or unbiased sample. Accuracy is basically independent of bias. A sample may produce an accurate or inaccurate estimate and still be unbiased. Or, alternatively, a biased sample could produce a relatively accurate result. Accuracy is measured by the difference between the sample estimate of the population value and the true population value.

Precision

Precision is a measure of the degree of variation in the estimates that might be made on the basis of all possible samples drawn in a particular manner. The best measure of precision is the standard deviation of the sample. If the standard deviation of the sample is large, precision is determined to be relatively low. If the standard deviation is small, precision is assumed to be fairly high.

Clearly the desirable situation for any sample is one that is unbiased, relatively accurate, and highly precise. It is not always possible to combine all three characteristics. In certain circumstances it is possible that a biased estimate, such as one taken from a sample based on a telephone directory, may be the only estimate available or that the variation in the population is so great that a high degree of precision is impossible to obtain. Nevertheless, a basic assumption of sampling is that bias will be ruled out to the extent possible and that the sample will produce an accurate and precise estimate.

Estimating optimal sample size

In many evaluation settings the question of how large a sample should be arises. There is no easy answer in all applications. In many types of program evaluation the evaluator will be forced to accept a sample size smaller than would be ideal. If, for example, a certain type of primary care program is being implemented within a number of local governmental jurisdictions and the desire is to compare some overall measures of health between those local jurisdictions and other control jurisdictions over some period of time, the evaluator must be satisfied with this number of places as the total universe of observations. In fact, in this sense, the issue of sample size does not arise because the evaluator has the total universe.

In other applications the determination of an optimal sample size may be nearly impossible. When several variables are to be assessed at one time—for example, when the evaluation may involve something like analysis of covariance or regression—the determination of optimal sample size may be extremely difficult and probably not worth the time and effort of the evaluator. Then it is likely that the best strategy for determining sample size is simply to get as large a sample as feasible, given time and money constraints.

In one setting, however, it may be both desirable and possible to determine an adequate sample size. Suppose that a certain number of persons are to be selected for special treatment of a costly nature and some comparison is to be made afterward between a control group and the treated group to determine if there is a difference between the two groups. If the treatment is costly, it would make sense to select as small a sample as possible while still being able to detect an expected difference of a certain amount.

To put this issue in concrete terms, consider a special program to reduce hypertension. Suppose that a number of persons are coming to a hypertension clinic and are receiving certain types of traditional advice and traditional treatment, including recommendations about diet, periodic checkups, and so on. A program substantially more costly than the normal treatment but, at the same time, one expected to have a greater impact on blood pressure reduction is to be assessed to evaluate this impact. Given that it is a costly program, it would be desirable to evaluate the impact on the basis of the smallest program possible.

In order to determine a necessary sample size in either the control group (the group treated in the conventional manner) or the experimental group (the group that receives the new treatment), it is necessary to know two items. The first is how much of a difference between the two groups must be detected in order to conclude that the difference is useful in some substantive sense. The second is what the standard deviation or variation in blood pressure within groups is likely to be. On the basis of such information, it is possible to make an estimate of the sample size necessary.

In general, a diastolic blood pressure at 90 mm Hg is judged normal, and a diastolic blood pressure at 95 mm Hg would be judged hypertensive and in need of some type of treatment. With this in mind, it might be reasonable to expect that a reduction of as little as 5 mm Hg on average between groups could be considered a difference of substantive import. The second piece of information necessary is the standard deviation of diastolic blood pressures within the two groups. It is not possible to know the standard deviation of the diastolic blood pressure within the specially treated group before the study has been conducted. It may be estimated, however, if the variance or standard deviation of the diastolic blood pressure in the control group (that is, the normally treated group) is available. It might reasonably be assumed that the diastolic blood pressure for the new experimental group will be essentially equal to that for the control group. Let us say, on the basis of knowledge of the variance in the diastolic blood pressure for the control group, that the expected standard error will be 5 mm Hg. In this case, a first approximation of the sample size needed will be

$$N = \frac{2S^2}{(\frac{1}{2}D)^2} = \frac{2(25)}{\frac{1}{4}(25)} = 8 \tag{15-6}$$

where N = sample size
S = standard deviation
D = difference between groups

What this would indicate is that 8 persons are needed in both the experimental group and the control group to derive a *t*-value for the test of difference between means (discussed in the chapter on experimental design) that is at least 2. (In large sample situations, a *t* of 2 is usually considered significant at the .05 level.)

If a sample of 8 in each group is selected, however, the total *n* on which the comparison is made is 16. A *t*-test on the basis of 16 observations requires a value of approximately 2.1 to be significant at the .05 level. Therefore the actual sample size should be increased (perhaps even doubled) in order actually to be able to detect a difference as great as 5, on the assumption that the standard error is 5 in a situation where the .05 level of significance is being accepted.

A sample size as small as 16 or even 32 persons to test the effectiveness of a new treatment for blood pressure or hypertension seems very small, indeed, and should not be a major barrier in terms of cost to the conduct of such a study. The fact that the sample size is so small is a function of the relatively large difference between the two groups that will be accepted compared to the relatively small standard deviation of expected blood pressure within the two groups. In situations where smaller differences between the control and experimental group relative to the amount of variance within the two groups is expected, the sample size may be substantially increased. In any case, the final word on sample size is to select or accept as large a sample as can be afforded.

Types of Samples

For descriptive-type evaluations attempting to determine the level of need for services or results of a program on the basis of a case study or a survey, three kinds of sampling strategies might generally be considered applicable: simple random sampling, stratified sampling, and cluster sampling.

Simple random sampling

A simple random sample is one in which every member of the population, whether persons, organizations, geographic areas, or political entities, has an equal probability or possibility of being selected. As the name implies, it is the simplest type of sample. If, for example, an estimate of the level of need for primary health services within a health care service area were to be estimated and if there were a reasonably accurate list of all persons living within this area, a simple random sample could be drawn to produce an estimate of level of need if an instrument were available to assess need.

Illustration

Suppose that 20,000 persons were in the area under consideration, and the decision had been made to select 400 as a sample to whom the survey instrument would be administered and the decision about the level of need for the entire population would be based on this sample of 400. If such were the case, each person in the population would have a .02 probability of being selected for the sample.

Given that a numbered, ordered list of all people in the area is made available for sample selection, one strategy for selecting a simple random sample of approximately 400 from 20,000 people in the population would be to select one random number from a random number table to be associated with each of the 20,000 people on the list. If that random number were in the lowest 2 percent of all numbers that could be generated by the table, the person associated with the number would be included in the sample. On average, this would produce approximately 400 people for the sample. An alternative strategy that would result in exactly 400 persons being included in the sample would be to select 400 random numbers in the range 1 to 20,000 from a random number table and include in the sample the persons who corresponded to these 400 numbers from an ordered and numbered list of the population. This approach is discussed in more detail later in the chapter.

A similar sampling strategy could be employed if the evaluation were concerned with estimating, for example, the level of health services available throughout an entire county. In this case, it might be substantially easier to get a complete list of eligible sampling units—that is, a complete sampling frame. If some estimate of the primary health care services provided by local health departments within the state is to be produced, it would be quite easy to compile a list of all counties in the state. The list would not exceed 254 counties (Texas has 254 counties; next largest is Georgia with 158), and from this list a random sample of counties could be drawn.

Limitations

Although simple random sampling is conceptually straightforward, it has two major problems: precision and bias. Because in a simple random sample every possible sample has an opportunity to be included, there is some small probability that the sample selected could consist of the most extreme members of the population. In reference to the estimation of the need for primary health care services in a service area, it is conceivable that with a simple random sample the 400 persons with the least need, or the 400 with the most need, or any other sample that would yield a relatively inaccurate estimate of the population mean, although not biased, might be selected.

The second major problem of a simple random sample is the difficulty of obtaining a complete and accurate sampling frame. Even with a problem as small as sampling from an area of 20,000 people, it is clearly quite difficult to obtain an accurate list of these 20,000 people to ensure that the target population and the sample population are the same. A strategy to attempt to reduce the degree to which the result of sampling will be inaccurate is the stratified sampling approach. A strategy to reduce the possibility that the target and sampled population will not be the same is the cluster sampling approach. Both these samples can be useful alternatives to simple random sampling and are discussed below.

Stratified samples

A stratified sample is designed specifically to increase precision and hence the probable accuracy of sample results. In stratified sampling the population is divided into two or more strata that are assumed to be closely associated with the characteristic of the population to be estimated. When estimating the need for primary care services, the population might be divided into two strata consisting of those persons who had sought services in any of the health care agencies in the area during some specified period of time and those persons who had not. The assumption would be that persons who had sought services would be more likely to have a need for them. An alternative strategy would be to stratify the population on the basis of age on the assumption that perhaps the very young and very old are more likely to need primary care services than people in middle age. Other stratification variables could probably also be useful.

When a decision has been made about the stratification variable, two different approaches can be used to determine the size of the sample to be taken from each strata. Sampling can be based on drawing an equal number from each of the strata defined—generally the best approach when comparisons between strata are to be made. Or sampling can be based on the probability of selection proportional to the size of the strata. In general, when evaluating for descriptive purposes—usually the type done for the purpose of establishing the state of a system or determining the state after some intervention—overall estimates will be needed, and sampling probability proportional to strata size will be most useful. Essentially, if the group of people within an area were divided for sampling purposes into those who have visited a clinic and those who have not and, moreover, if it were known, say, that 32 percent of all area residents have visited the clinic, then 32 percent of the sample should be taken from among the clinic visitors and 68 percent of the sample from among those who are nonclinic visitors. In general, this process will give the most efficient sample for estimates of the overall need for services in the population.

Stratified sampling reduces the probability that extreme samples from the population will be selected and so increases the likely precision of the sample. Assume that the population is divided into two strata, those who have and those who have not sought services from any health care facility within the past year. It is agreed that a specified number for the sample will be drawn from each of the two strata. Let us say that 200 persons will be drawn from those who have sought services and 200 from those who have not. If we are fairly confident that people in least need of services have a low probability of being among those people who have sought services or, alternatively, that those people in most need of services have a low probability of being among those who have not sought them in the past year, then it should be clear that we will be unlikely, in using this stratification technique, to draw a sample dominated by persons in either group. Consequently, we have reduced the probability of obtaining a highly inaccurate or extreme appraisal of the need for services in the population. The extent to which we have increased precision and reduced the probability of an inaccurate result is directly related to the extent to which need for services is associated with membership in one of the two stratification groups.

Limitation

A major problem of stratified sampling is defining a sampling frame. In the example of the service area and the question of need for primary health services, stratification does simplify definition of the sampling frame for those who have visited the clinic. The frame then becomes all persons who have used clinic services. But it does not simplify the problem of getting a total list of persons who have not used clinic services but who are residents, however defined, of the area. Consequently, the problem of ensuring that the target and sampled populations are the same remains, as well as the problem of potential bias resulting from selection of a sample that does not have as its expected value the true population value.

Cluster samples

A strategy that may be used to increase the probability that the sampled population and target population are the same and that has certain advantages over either simple random or stratified sampling is the cluster sample. Cluster sampling is a technique whereby the sample is drawn in two or more stages. At the first stage the total population to be sampled is drawn and divided into several clusters on the basis of some meaningful variable. These clusters will be mutually exclusive and all inclusive. To illustrate, a sample representing all people in a state could be drawn, with the first clustering being counties, so that a sample of counties would be drawn from the state at the first stage. In the second and subsequent samples, smaller units within clusters could be drawn, representing either the specific units to be sampled—in which case, the sampling would end at this point— or some larger unit that contained the units to be drawn.

In a study of health departments in North Carolina, for example, one unit of analysis was ultimately to be health department employees. The sample was drawn in two stages. The first stage included as a sampling frame or target population all health departments in the state of North Carolina. From this population 16 health departments were drawn. Then at the second stage employees within these 16 health departments were sampled to make up a sample of health department personnel for the entire state.

The advantage of this approach is that a detailed list of health department employees need be drawn up, in general, only for the 16 health departments actually included in the sample at the first stage. No list of employees need be available for health departments excluded from the sample. This process reduces substantially the amount of work required to construct a useful list of people to be sampled.

To consider the example of an estimate of the need for primary care services in some health service area, a cluster sample can make it unnecessary to construct an accurate list of all people in the area. As an alternative, it would be possible to use logical divisions, such as census tracts or blocks, postal zones, or some other logical set of divisions, and draw a sample of clusters from them. Then it would be necessary to construct an accurate list only of those persons residing within the clusters selected. If city blocks were selected as clusters, for example, a relatively accurate list of persons to be sampled at the second stage could be constructed simply by going to one or two households on the block and asking who lived in the other households. Alternatively, a sample could be drawn by numbering all the housing in the sampled block and simply drawing a sample of them.

Cluster sampling can be carried out at more than two stages. A national sample of the United States, for example, might begin with a cluster sample of states. Within states, a cluster of counties might be selected; within counties, townships; and within townships, people.

While cluster sampling can serve to reduce the possibility of missing potential respondents and hence biasing results, it should also be clear that it can be useful in reducing such factors as the cost of actual data collection if the data will be collected by interview or by some other strategy that requires someone to contact the respondents personally. If a simple random sample of personnel within health departments were selected, say, to produce information about employees working within health departments in a given state, it is quite likely that the majority of health departments would be included so that the evaluator would be forced to visit every health department or the majority of them to obtain data. If a cluster sample is drawn, it is only necessary to visit those health departments which are included in the initial cluster.

Limitation

Cluster sampling has the disadvantage, however, that employees within health departments, for example, are likely to be more similar to one another than they are to people in other health departments in many aspects of their responses. This means that there will be relatively high variation between clusters. Although similarity of people within strata is an advantage for stratified sampling, it is a disadvantage for cluster sampling because all clusters are not represented. In consequence, most cluster sample–based estimates of population parameters are likely to be less precise than stratified sample estimates and are frequently less precise than simple random sample estimates.

Other multistage samples

Cluster sampling is one type of multistage sampling. A second type of multistage sampling similar in execution, although not necessarily in concept, is the kind in which information is desired at two or more levels. In a study of health departments, for instance, it may be important to the evaluation to have information about individual employees and their perceptions of departmental activity as well as information about aspects of the health departments themselves. Thus, the sample might be drawn on the basis of health departments as clusters at the first stage and employees as units of analysis at the second stage, but data will be collected about both the individual employees and the departments within which they operate.

With a sample of this type, estimates can be made about the population of health departments and the employees who work in them; information also becomes available across the individual health department interface. When data for evaluation purposes are desired at several different organizational levels, a relatively uncommon, but certainly fatal, mistake is the selection of samples independently at different levels.

Illustration: A five-year health plan in a developing country

This evaluation had two major aims. The first was to characterize the nature of the health system as it operated at five different levels of organization: central, district, health clinic, individual field worker, and household recipient. The second aim of the evaluation was to examine the communication, supervision, and service links among the district officers, health clinic, and field workers and the links between services and recipients of care.

In the sample design, samples were drawn independently at each of the five levels. The district sample, for example, was drawn from a sample of 20 districts out of 75 districts in the country. For health clinics, the country was again divided into districts, and the second sample of 20 districts was selected. In certain instances, the latter overlapped with the original district sampling, but the second selection resulted in a total selection of 31 separate districts from each of the two stages. Moreover, 9 districts had been selected by chance alone as representative of both district and the health clinic, and 11 were included as one or the other. The high proportion of overlapping districts in the two selections was partly the result of selection with probability proportional to the number of health clinics at the district and the clinic level. A second step in sampling at the clinic level was to select a sample of approximately 100 clinics from the 20 districts selected in the second phase. The result of this selection procedure was then to produce one sample to describe the characteristics of districts and a second to describe the characteristics of clinics.

Independently, either sample was perfectly adequate for the task at the level selected, but taken together the samples were almost entirely inadequate for any discussion of relationships between levels. One question in the evaluation, for example, was what knowledge district-level persons had of clinic-level activities in a number of specific areas. The strategy for determining the extent of knowledge was to compare the statements by district personnel with those of clinic personnel. Unfortunately, because the districts and clinics had only a chance occurrence of actually overlapping with one another, few conclusions could be safely drawn from any comparison of the statements by district and clinic personnel.

The same types of sample selection (drawn independently) were taken at the health worker level, with workers selected independently of either districts or health clinics, and at the individual household level. The result, of course, is that any comparison across levels becomes extremely tenuous.

Suppose that, say, district officers said that salaries always arrived on time, but clinic respondents said they did not. The inference for researchers to draw was either (1) district officers were not aware of happenings at the clinic level or (2) the district officers were unwilling to admit a breakdown of salary flow to the clinic level. Unfortunately, the sample design does not allow such inferences to be drawn. Given the sample design employed, the lack of correspondence between the two levels could be a function of sampling alone. Regardless of how carefully two samples are drawn, it is never possible to be certain that differences between two levels are not the result of different samples or that similarities are not equally fortuitous.

Nonrandom samples

All samples are not based on probability. Many samples in evaluation applications are what may be called haphazard samples—that is, the units observed have been selected on a basis that appears to be random but that, in fact, may not be. One type of haphazard sample is the *sample of convenience*. If something is to be known about all the people who use a particular clinic for some type of service, the sample for obtaining this information might be the first 50 people who arrive at the clinic during a period of one week; it is in no sense a random sample and should not be treated as such. Conclusions drawn from such a sample are generally applicable only to the sample itself.

Another common type of nonprobability or nonrandom sample is the *representative sample*. In such a sample, units are selected because they seem to be representative of the population as a whole. If an evaluation is to be carried out on a program that exists in all counties within a state, the representative sample might include a high-income county, a low-income county, a rural county, an urban county, and so on. Although conclusions drawn from such a sample might be more useful in the long run than conclusions drawn from a haphazard sample or a sample of convenience, they are still generalizable to the whole population only with a great deal of caution.

Sample selection: An illustration

Consider the simplest sampling situation, one in which each element (organization) in the population has an equal probability (less than one) of entering the sample. Assume that a study of county health departments is being conducted within a state that has 120 counties, each with one health department. Resources are available to draw a sample of 30 health departments from the 120. Each health department thus has 30 chances out of 120, or 1 of 4, of entering the samples.

It is possible to draw a probability sample of 30 health departments from the 120 in the population that ensures that each department has a probability of exactly one-fourth of entering the sample. One strategy is to assign a distinct number (for example, one number from the sequence 1 through 120) to each health department. Next, the investigators obtain a table of random numbers.* The researcher then selects 30 numbers in the range of 1 to 120 from the random number table. The health departments whose numbers correspond to the numbers selected will be included in the sample.

Table 15-1 represents a portion of a typical random number table. Each number is four digits. Because the sequence 1 to 120 is three digits long, only the second, third, and fourth digits in each of the random numbers in Table 15-1 would be considered in selecting the health departments. In general, it is acceptable to start at the beginning of the table or at any place within the table to begin the draw. Once a starting point is selected, the researcher can proceed in

---

*See, for example, Arkin and Colton (1963) or Kendall and Smith (1939). Many statistics books contain abridged random number tables in appendixes. Sequences of pseudorandom numbers having most of the characteristics of true random numbers can be generated with a variety of computer packages, including SAS (SAS Institute, Inc. 1988) and SPSS (Norusis 1988).

Table 15-1 Table of Random Numbers (First 2,000 of 8,000 Numbers)

First Thousand

	1–4	5–8	9–12	13–16	17–20	21–24	25–28	29–32	33–36	37–40
1	23 15	75 48	59 01	83 72	59 93	76 24	97 08	86 95	23 03	67 44
2	05 54	55 50	53 10	53 74	35 08	90 61	18 37	44 10	96 22	13 43
3	14 87	18 03	50 32	40 43	62 23	50 05	10 03	22 11	54 38	08 34
4	38 97	67 49	41 94	05 17	58 53	78 80	59 01	94 32	42 87	16 95
5	97 31	26 17	18 99	75 53	08 70	94 25	12 58	41 54	88 21	05 13
6	11 74	26 93	81 44	33 93	08 72	32 79	73 31	18 22	64 70	68 50
7	43 36	12 88	59 11	01 64	56 23	93 00	90 04	99 43	64 07	40 36
8	93 80	62 04	78 38	26 80	44 91	55 75	11 89	32 58	47 55	25 71
9	49 54	01 31	81 08	42 98	41 87	69 53	82 96	61 77	73 80	95 27
10	36 76	87 26	33 37	94 82	15 69	41 95	96 86	70 45	27 48	38 80
11	07 09	25 23	92 24	62 71	26 07	06 55	84 53	44 67	33 84	53 20
12	43 31	00 10	81 44	86 38	03 07	52 55	51 61	48 89	74 29	46 47
13	61 57	00 63	60 06	17 36	37 75	63 14	89 51	23 35	01 74	69 93
14	31 35	28 37	99 10	77 91	89 41	31 57	97 64	48 62	58 48	69 19
15	57 04	88 65	26 27	79 59	36 82	90 52	95 65	46 35	06 53	22 54
16	09 24	34 42	00 68	72 10	71 37	30 72	97 57	56 09	29 72	76 50
17	97 95	53 50	18 40	89 48	83 29	52 23	08 25	21 22	51 26	15 87
18	93 73	25 95	70 43	78 19	88 85	56 67	16 68	26 05	99 64	45 69
19	72 62	11 12	25 00	92 26	82 64	35 66	65 94	14 51	68 65	18 67
20	61 02	07 44	18 45	37 12	07 94	95 91	73 78	66 99	53 61	93 78

Continued

Table 15-1 Continued

First Thousand

	1–4	5–8	9–12	13–16	17–20	21–24	25–28	29–32	33–36	37–40
21	97 83	98 53	74 33	05 59	17 18	45 47	35 41	44 22	03 42	30 00
22	89 16	09 71	92 22	23 29	06 37	35 05	54 54	89 88	43 81	63 61
23	25 96	68 82	20 62	87 17	92 65	02 82	35 28	62 84	91 95	48 83
24	81 44	33 17	19 95	04 95	48 06	74 69	00 75	67 65	01 71	65 45
25	11 32	25 49	31 42	36 23	43 86	08 62	49 76	67 42	24 52	32 45

Second Thousand

	1–4	5–8	9–12	13–16	17–20	21–24	25–28	29–32	33–36	37–40
1	64 75	58 38	85 84	12 22	59 20	17 69	61 56	55 95	04 59	59 47
2	10 30	25 22	89 77	43 63	44 30	38 11	24 90	67 07	54 82	33 28
3	71 01	79 84	95 51	30 85	03 74	66 59	10 28	87 53	76 56	91 49
4	60 01	25 56	05 88	41 03	48 79	79 65	59 01	69 78	80 00	36 66
5	37 33	09 46	56 49	16 14	28 02	48 27	45 47	55 44	55 36	50 90
6	47 86	98 70	01 31	59 11	22 73	60 62	61 28	22 34	69 16	12 12
7	38 04	04 27	37 64	16 78	95 78	39 32	34 93	34 88	43 43	87 06
8	73 50	83 09	08 83	05 48	00 78	36 66	93 02	95 56	46 04	53 36

9	32 62	34 64	74 84	06 10	43 24	20 62	93 73	19 32	35 64	39 69
10	97 59	19 95	49 36	63 03	51 06	62 06	99 29	75 95	32 05	77 34
11	74 01	23 19	55 59	79 09	69 82	66 22	42 40	15 96	74 90	75 89
12	56 75	42 64	57 13	35 10	50 14	90 96	63 36	74 79	09 63	34 88
13	49 80	04 99	08 54	83 12	19 98	08 52	82 63	72 92	92 36	50 26
14	43 58	48 96	47 24	87 85	66 70	00 22	15 01	93 99	59 16	23 77
15	16 65	37 96	64 60	32 57	13 01	35 74	28 36	36 73	05 88	72 29
16	48 50	26 90	55 65	32 25	87 48	31 44	68 02	37 31	25 29	63 67
17	96 76	55 47	92 36	31 68	62 30	48 29	63 83	52 21	81 66	40 94
18	39 92	36 15	50 80	35 78	12 84	23 44	41 24	63 33	99 22	81 28
19	77 95	88 16	94 25	22 50	55 87	51 07	30 10	70 60	21 86	19 61
20	17 92	82 80	65 25	58 60	87 71	02 64	18 50	64 65	79 64	81 70
21	94 03	68 59	78 02	31 80	44 99	41 05	41 05	31 87	43 12	15 96
22	47 46	06 04	79 56	23 04	84 17	14 37	28 51	67 27	55 80	03 68
23	47 85	65 60	88 51	99 28	24 39	40 64	41 71	70 13	46 31	82 88
24	57 61	63 46	53 92	29 86	20 18	10 37	57 65	15 62	98 69	07 56
25	08 30	09 27	04 66	75 26	66 10	57 18	87 91	07 54	22 22	20 13

Source: Reproduced from M. G. Kendall and B. B. Smith, *Tables of Random Sampling Numbers*, Tracts for Computers XXIV (London: Cambridge University Press, 1939), p. 2, by permission of the Biometrika Trustees and the Department of Statistics, University College, London.

any consistent direction through the table, using each succeeding number.

If the selection started at the beginning of the table with the number 2,315, only the last three digits of that number, 315, would be considered. Because 315 is larger than 120, the researcher would simply skip to the next number. Similarly, 548, the next number in the list, is also larger than 120, as is 901, and so on. The first number that is actually small enough to be included in the sample is the number 061 in the second row, columns 21 to 24. Health department 061, then, would be the first health department selected for the study. The next health department to enter the study would be health department 032 in columns 9 to 12 of row 3; health departments 043, 005, and 003 would also be included in the study. Selection would continue in this manner until 30 departments had been chosen for the study. The fact that numbers larger than 120 were skipped does not affect the randomness of the sample. If the same number had come up twice (as 062 does in row 23, columns 9 to 12 of the first thousand, and row 6, columns 21 to 24 of the second thousand), the number is ignored the second time, and the researcher proceeds to the next number within the range. This strategy would also not affect the randomness of the sample. The approach will produce a sample in which each health department in the population has a one-fourth probability of being included in the study.

This example of an approach to the selection of a random sample is applicable to simple random sampling if we are assuming that the sample of 30 health departments is drawn from all 120 in the state. It would also be applicable to stratified sampling if the departments were divided into separate strata on some basis (for example, urban and rural). Selection could take place in exactly the same way within strata. The example also applies to a cluster sample selection. If, say, the health departments selected are considered not only as health departments but also as clusters of employees, then employees within the 30 health departments selected could also be selected either by taking all employees or by selecting a sample of employees with some probability.

This selection approach also applies to experimental designs. Suppose that an experimental program was to be introduced into 15 of the 30 health departments, and the other 15 health departments were to remain as controls (but from which certain types of information would be collected to use for comparisons); then the sampling approach could be exactly the same. The first 15 health departments selected could be the experimental group. The second 15 health departments selected could be the control group. Alternatively, odd-numbered health departments could be the experimental group, and even-numbered departments could be the control group. Either approach would allow a legitimate comparison between a reasonable experimental and a reasonable control group.

Sample Design and Evaluation Strategies

If it were possible in any evaluation setting to observe the entire population of interest, sampling would be a subject of little interest to program evaluation. But in many evaluation settings it is neither physically possible nor financially feasible to obtain information on or observe the entire population of entities to be evaluated. When less than the total number of units of interest can be observed or measured, sampling becomes a real concern. In many instances, it is only through the selection of a sample that a reasonable evaluation can be conducted.

As noted throughout, there are basically five different evaluation formats: monitoring, case studies, survey research, trend analysis, and experimental design. In each of these strategies the role of sampling should be considered.

Monitoring

In most monitoring formats, sampling is not likely to be a major concern. Monitoring is usually applied to a single program or a limited number of programs selected because they are one of a kind or, at most, the several programs that make up the total universe. In such programs, it is probably the management itself doing the monitoring. Or perhaps the monitors are consultants working directly with the program management. These evaluators or managers generally have access to the entire universe of information about most aspects of the program for which progress information—monitoring data— is useful or necessary. Information for monitoring purposes, for instance, might include weekly or monthly expenditures of funds or comparisons of funds expended to funds budgeted by time period. It might include information about the daily patient census or services provided each week or quarter.

Still, certain aspects of monitoring data may be available only on a sample basis. If a program is designed to deliver some type of service to clients, one possible aspect of program progress that might concern administrators is the continuing perception of the program in the eyes of its clients. If clients are generally satisfied with the services being received, management may elect to allow the program to continue providing services in more or less the same way. On the other hand, if over a period of time clients appear to be dissatisfied with the services or if their satisfaction declines, management may wish to take steps to increase client satisfaction. Specific information about client satisfaction may be available on a routine basis. Such information as appointments missed might be considered a measure of client dissatisfaction. Missed appointments may be information that is available routinely, but if a more direct measure of client satisfaction—say, answers to a direct question or set of questions on satisfaction with the program—is wanted, such information might be most easily collected on a sample basis. If the sample were to assess client satisfaction with services, one way to make certain that clients would respond to questions about satisfaction with services would be to query them at the time they received the service. A sample strategy would be needed in which a client could be identified as being in the sample at the time service was delivered and the questionnaire or set of questions could be addressed to that client.

Case studies

There are two levels at which sampling should be discussed in regard to the case study evaluation format. At one level the entire issue of sampling may seem irrelevant because the situation selected for case study purposes represents the entire universe. If the specific case is unique and is selected not for the purpose of generalizing to some larger population but for program activity evaluation within the specific example, then there is no need to sample. To illustrate, an evaluation of how a specific strategic alliance dealt with its hospitals to ensure nonduplication of facilities could be undertaken in order to gain a better understanding of the process with which the alliance pursued these objectives. The results of such an evaluation—the evaluator's conclusions—would clearly pertain to this alliance alone. But at the same time there would be a basic assumption that the results might apply reasonably well to other alliances as well. Nevertheless, the particular alliance selected would have been chosen because it had dealt with the problem of nonduplication of services in a particular way or because it was an area of interest to the evaluator on some other ground. In this sense, the alliance under study is different from all other alliances and to that extent represents the entire universe. And yet this alliance is one of many alliances, and its selection might be considered a purposeful selection from a larger population. Still, it is unlikely that selecting any program or organizational form as the subject of a case study—or choosing a particular area in which a larger program or organization is operating as a case study example—should be done on a random basis. Because case studies are exploratory, in many respects, the specific case selected for study should clearly be chosen for some reason other than randomness.

Moreover, once a specific program or organizational form, such as a strategic alliance, or a political or geographic entity, such as a county, state, or region, has been selected as the subject of a case study, it may be possible to evaluate the program or aspects of it within a given area without considering any type of sample selection. The procedure for evaluating how a particular alliance has worked with its constituent hospitals to ensure nonduplication of services might involve direct interviews with the alliance's executive officers and officers of the participating hospitals. Then it is probable, given the size of most alliances, that the evaluators would want to meet and obtain additional information from each executive officer of the alliance and all constituent hospitals. In such a case, sampling would be basically unnecessary for evaluation purposes.

On the other hand, part of the evaluation might be assessing the impact of an effort to ensure nonduplication of various hospital services on physicians who use them for their patients within this alliance area or on patients who seek them. If such an interest was included in the evaluation, it might be unreasonable to anticipate the possibility of reaching every physician in the alliance or every patient or potential patient to assess their attitudes toward the alliance's efforts.

In this situation it is not uncommon to see a sample design embedded within a case study. Here a case study is being carried out on the strategic alliance as a whole, but specific pieces of information about the alliance may be obtained from a sample of persons within the alliance on a survey basis. Such an evaluation approach, although part of a case study, is no different from survey research as the overall evaluation tool.

Survey research

Sampling is a central component of survey research. Survey research as an evaluation tool can be used to assess the state of the system—to ascertain its relevance before the program has been undertaken. Surveys can also be used after a program has been in operation to assess at certain levels effectiveness, efficiency, and impact. Survey research can also be used in certain settings to evaluate the relationship between program output and certain aspects of program input. Each situation requires a sample to select information for analysis.

Trend analysis

As an evaluation tool, trend analysis is generally concerned with data that represent the universe of all data available. Trend analysis might be applied to such data as the hospital cost per patient day before and after the passage of the Medicare bill to assess the impact of Medicare on hospital costs. Or it might be applied to highway death tolls before and after reducing speed limits to 55 mph to assess the impact of that directive on highway deaths. For such an analysis, the entire population of observations would probably be used for the evaluation of impact.

When a long time series is required for assessment of program interventions, however, it is possible that the entire universe may not be available for study. It is possible that data representing more limited geographic areas, such as states, might be readily available to someone wishing to assess the impact of the speed limit reduction so that the data set—a given state—becomes a sample of all states in the population selected because it is available to the evaluator and, as such, should, to be absolutely correct, be considered its own entire population or universe.

Experimental design

Experimental design is the most powerful evaluation format. It has been used with considerable success in evaluating the effectiveness of drug treatment, for example, through random clinical trials. Experimental designs are less applicable, as noted, to program evaluation for a number of reasons. One is the difficulty of identifying control groups to use in comparison to experimental groups or areas. Still, experimental design as a program evaluation tool should receive consideration in any evaluation context and should depend heavily on sampling or—more specifically in terms of experimental design—on random selection.

In an evaluation based on experimental design, the evaluator's concern is to determine whether the program or project as structured and carried out was the causal factor in producing some observed outcome. How this is done depends on a comparison between one or more experimental groups, programs, or program areas and one or more control groups, programs, or program areas. In such a comparison, it is imperative that the evaluator rule out any other factors that may have produced a particular observed level of outcome—that is, produced a difference between the experimental and control programs.

There are two ways to attempt to ensure that any difference between the experimental and control groups is a function of program input, and not of some other characteristic or set of characteristics. One is matching and the other is random selection.

In the matching strategy the people or organizations who are the subjects of an evaluation are matched on any characteristics assumed to be associated with outcomes that the program to be implemented may produce. Once this matching has been carried out, it is common to select an equal number of persons, groups, organizations, or areas from the matched sets for inclusion in the experimental and control categories, respectively. Depending on the unit of analysis, matching can be done on basic characteristics that might be considered associated with response to the experimental variable.

After the matching is finished, random selection is almost always used to determine the specific evaluation units to be assigned to the experimental or control group. If matching has been carried out, for example, so that every unit in the potential evaluation population has been matched with only one other unit, the decision about assigning the two units to either the experimental or control group should still be based on chance. The flip of a coin, say, could be used to determine which one of this matched pair would be a member of the experimental group. If matching is not so complete, it is even more important that units be selected randomly from the two sets of groups.

If matching is not done to control for variables that might influence the results of the evaluation, such variables can still be controlled through the technique of complete random assignment. Here all units subject to the evaluation would be assigned to the experimental category or the control category on a random basis without regard to whether their characteristics matched or not. The process of random assignment itself, if carried out properly, will provide a control for differences among the units to be examined that might be reasonably expected to affect the outcome.

Unfortunately, random assignment can never totally ensure that the possible effects of confounding factors have been controlled. Random assignment is most effective when the number of units to be compared or observed is relatively large (perhaps more than 30 observations in both the experimental and control group). It is less effective when the number of units to be compared gets small. If the evaluation is to be an assessment of the impact of a family planning program, for instance, in a limited number of different regions of a country—perhaps six to eight—random assignment is not a powerful tool in controlling for characteristics that might be related to results of the evaluation. No statistical procedure is likely to be particularly useful with such a small group. The best that the evaluator can do is probably to match the areas of the country as closely as possible and assign the matched areas to the experimental and control group, respectively.

When random assignment is used, the basic approach is simple random sampling. There is no need in an experimental setting to use more complex designs, such as stratified, cluster, or multistage sampling.

Discussion Questions

1. What is the difference between descriptive and analytic sampling? What types of evaluation questions are best answered by each type of sampling strategy?
2. Why is the appropriate sample size so important to evaluation—yet so difficult to achieve?
3. Distinguish between a simple random sampling, stratified random sampling, cluster sampling, and nonrandom sampling. What are the conditions that determine their appropriate use in evaluation activities?
4. What is the role of internal and external validity in different types of evaluation strategies, such as monitoring, case studies, survey research, trend analysis, and experimental design? Illustrate the types of evaluation questions appropriate to each type of validity for each type of evaluation strategy.

16

Operations Research Techniques and Interpretation

Evaluation techniques are used when the outputs are known but the best method or program design for achieving those outputs is unknown. Evaluation methods, as an aid to cybernetic decision making, can provide the means for continually assessing program outputs and assuring continual improvement of outputs through successively better decisions. In the cybernetic mode, there is no formula or algorithm that leads to the optimal or preferred result, only the availability of information about the result of a particular strategy that is then used to modify the strategy so as to become more effective.

This chapter will again contrast the cybernetic decision-making mode to the mechanistic decision mode and provide illustrations from an outpatient clinic. In the mechanistic decision mode, there are various operations research techniques available for making decisions that produce the best result under a defined set of circumstances in exactly the same way as the square root algorithm described in Chapter 2 produces the square root of a number. If a manager applies the technique correctly, there is no need to monitor the progress of the program or compare its outputs to outputs derived through the application of alternative decision strategies. The result will be, by the nature of the technique, the best result available under a given set of conditions.

As with other techniques described in this book, the presentation is designed to introduce the techniques and illustrate their application within a health service setting. Selected techniques are presented, including model building, linear programming, queuing theory, and inventory control.

Model Building

A first step in the application of operations research techniques to decision making is almost always the development of a mathematical model of how a given system operates. In the simplest formulation, a mathematical model is the statement in equation form of a relationship between a dependent variable, or a program or process output, and one or more independent variables, or program inputs. In general, program inputs may be divided into two groups; those over which the decision maker has some control, and those that are essentially uncontrollable.

For example, the number of clients who can be served in a clinic might be considered as determined by a minimum of three components: the number of providers associated with the clinic, the number of clients a provider can serve in a given unit of time, and total amount of time available. A mathematical formulation of this would be very simply

$$C = P \cdot ST \cdot TT$$

where C = clients served
        P = number of physicians
        ST = clients served per unit of time
        TT = total time available

Thus, if a clinic had three physicians, a physician spent 15 minutes with each patient (four patients per hour), and each physician worked for six hours a day, the clinic could serve 72 patients ($C = 3 \cdot 4 \cdot 6$) in a day.

This mathematical model is so simple as to seem almost trivial. Yet it can provide information to decision makers about types of decisions that *must* be made in operating the clinic, even if not, at this stage, the decisions that *should* be made. If an administrator was faced with an increasing demand for services, so that the ability to serve 72 patients per day was not adequate for the needs of the organization, the mathematical model provides direct information about how the problem might be solved. The administrator might consider one of three possible options to increase the number of patients served: increase the number of physicians, increase the number of patients that physicians are able to serve in a given amount of time, or increase the number of hours that physicians work.

There is, of course, a fourth option open to the decision maker. That is simply to ignore the increased demand and use the limited service availability as a rationing device. This solution has been adopted widely in the Western world as health care costs have risen. From the standpoint of either evaluation or decision making, however, this decision is based essentially in the political realm and cannot be effectively informed by evaluation or operations research techniques, at least as the issue is posed.

But assuming that the decision maker will not decide to ignore the increased demand, the three decisions available are essentially as indicated above. It may also be that the decision maker has no control over one or all of the inputs to patients served. Inputs may be divided into those that are subject to control by the administrator and those that are not subject to such control. It is also often true that which inputs are under an administrator's control and which are not may depend largely on the context.

In the example above, all three inputs are potentially controllable. But it may well be that a decision maker may have little or no control over the amount of time a physician spends with a patient. In large part, this is likely to be a matter of practice patterns. An administrator may be able to determine the number of physicians available or the number of hours they are available during a day. But in virtually all cases, this would require additional resources. A valuable aspect of operations research techniques is their ability to identify the decision that provides the greatest output for a given level of cost, or alternatively, the least-cost alternative for a fixed output.

Illustration: Clinic staffing

Using the model above, an administrator may wish to increase clinic capacity to serve patients from 72 patients per day to 90 per day. If it is assumed that time spent with a patient is fixed, then the only two decision variables are number of physicians and hours that they work per day. To add one physician would increase the capacity of the clinic to 96, which would solve the problem of capacity, but would leave an excess capacity of 6 patients. An alternative would be to increase the number of hours worked by physicians to seven and one-half per day. This would increase the capacity of the clinic to exactly 90 patients per day.

On an annual basis, perhaps a new physician may cost $120,000 for a six-hour workday. In addition, there may be a fixed cost of $50,000 per year to add another physician, for examining-room space, administrative costs, support costs, and so on. To increase the amount of time spent by physicians on a daily basis may cost an additional $90,000 at the same hourly rate of reimbursement. So, a decision to add one physician will produce the desired capacity of 90 patients for an additional $37.78 per patient with a slack of 6 patients per day, while the decision to add hours to the workday will produce the desired capacity of 90 patients for an additional $20 per patient. This is a simple example to illustrate the application of models to decision making. In this case, it is possible to arrive at the optimal solution with little effort. Operations research techniques can assist in making the same type of decisions when the alternative decisions (variable inputs in the model) and the alternative constraints (costs associated with various decisions) are much more complex.

Clinic Staffing with a Mechanistic Solution: A Linear Programming Example

Linear programming allows an administrator to arrive at an optimal solution to a management problem in an entirely mechanistic way. Once the problem is presented in the proper form, the application of an algorithm known as the *simplex method* will produce the optimal answer (that is, the best solution) without any feedback, in much the same way as the square root of a number is found according to the method shown in Chapter 2.

Illustration

A group of administrators is confronted with the need to provide as many hours of clinic care as possible to persons coming to their facility. In this sense, the problem is like the one above. But now, let us assume that not only can physicians provide needed patient care, but in addition, that the administrators have the option of hiring physician assistants to provide care as well. The administrators know from long experience that physicians, on the average, can see and treat four patients per hour. Physician assistants, on the other hand, both because they are in general less experienced and because they have been trained to spend more time with patients, will be able to treat no more than three patients per hour. The administrators have a budget that provides $1,400 per day for direct patient care salaries. They must pay physicians $70 per hour and physician assistants $35. In addition, there are three examining rooms in the clinic, each of which can practically be used for 10 hours per day. So the total hours of patient care time by either physicians or physician assistants cannot exceed 30 hours per day. Finally, the administrators know that it will be necessary to have a physician at the clinic at least 6 hours per day, both for supervision of the physician assistants, and because some of the presenting diagnoses cannot reasonably be dealt with by physician assistants.

Let us also assume that the administrators are operating in a community in which it is possible to hire either physicians or physician assistants on an hourly basis, so they are free to make the decision about how much time during a day either physicians or physician assistants work. This, of course, would be a highly artificial assumption for many administrators, but not unrealistic for others. The question, then, is what mix of physician and physician assistant time should the administrators buy in order to maximize the number of patients who can be seen at the clinic while remaining within the constraints of time and money.

It is possible to solve this problem in a cybernetic (that is, feedback) mode. Approaching the problem this way, the administrators could say that since physician assistants are cheaper than physicians, use as many hours of physician assistant time as possible. If the administrators were to buy 30 hours of physician assistant time per day, the result would be a capacity for 90 patients. But they know they must have at least 6 hours of physician time as well, and since they have only space enough for 30 hours of time in total, they can buy no more than 24 hours of physician assistant time. Calculating total patients that can be seen using 24 hours of physician assistant time and 6 hours of physician time, they see that the clinic capacity is now 96 patients per day. But they also can see that with 24 hours of physician assistant time and 6 hours of physician time, they are expending only \$1,260 per day on clinic personnel ($24 \cdot 35 + 6 \cdot 70 = 1,260$). So they realize that they can increase the number of physicians (who can see more patients than physician assistants) and still remain within their budget.

The administrators might then begin to increase the number of physician hours, for example, in two-hour intervals, to try to reach the maximum number of patients while not exceeding their daily budget. If they contract for 8 physician hours (and thus 22 physician assistant hours), total patients will increase to 98 and total cost will increase to \$1,330. They still have money to work with. If they increase physician time to 10 hours and reduce physician assistant time to 20 hours, total patients will rise to 100 per day and total cost will rise to \$1,400, which is the limit available. A little further tinkering with the figures will demonstrate to the administrators that they can do no better with their constraints of money and time (clinic space) than a combination of 10 hours of physician time and 20 hours of physician assistant time.

The administrators have solved this problem in the cybernetic mode. Even though they did not actually put into place a decision to contract for a certain number of physician hours and a certain number of physician assistant hours, they have done essentially the same thing "on the back of an envelope." But this is a problem that can be solved directly, in what we have termed a mechanistic mode, without any feedback at all, using linear programming.

To employ linear programming to solve this problem, the administrators must first be able to formulate the problem in the form of a set of mathematical equations that represent the outcomes they are seeking. The primary thing the administrators wish to do is maximize the number of patients who can be seen in a day at the clinic. They know physicians can see four patients per hour and physician assistants can see three. They can state this knowledge in terms of an equation:

$$\text{Maximize: } Z = 4X + 3Y \tag{16-1}$$

where Z = total number of patients who can be seen
X = number of hours worked by physicians
Y = number of hours worked by physician
    assistants

The administrators know also that maximizing the function shown above is subject to constraints of money to pay for daily salaries and of available examining-room space (and thus total hours during which practitioners can see patients) and the constraint that there must be at least 6 hours of physician time available during the day:

$$70X + 35Y \leq 1{,}400 \tag{16-2}$$

$$X + Y \leq 30 \tag{16-3}$$

$$X \geq 6 \tag{16-4}$$

In words, these can be read in the following way. Equation 16-2 says that the total amount of money paid for both physicians and physician assistants on a daily basis must not exceed $1,400 (must be less than or equal to $1,400). Equation 16-3 says that the total hours worked by both physicians and physician assistants must not exceed 30 hours, and Equation 16-4 says that there must be at least 6 hours of physician time each day.

Having cast the problem in this form, the administrators can use the simplex method, a mathematical algorithm, to solve directly for the optimum mix of physician and physician assistant time to maximize patients seen while remaining within the constraints of money and space. The first step in the simplex method is to rewrite the equations in the form shown in Table 16-1.

In looking at Table 16-1, it is possible to see the original set of equations with some additional information added. The headings of the table include X, the designator for physician hours, and Y, the designator for physician assistant hours. In addition, there are also S_1, S_2, and S_3, which represent "slack" in the system. In general, there will be as many slack variables as there are constraints (in this case, three). The next letter, A, designates an artificial variable that is included to allow the use of a "greater than or equal to" constraint (the third constraint) in the simplex method. This will be explained further below. The final letter, Z, represents the column in which the final solution will be found.

Line (1) in Table 16-1 represents the expression to be maximized, the objective function. It could be read as

$$4X + 3Y = 0$$

The problem, then, is to change this in some way so that

$$4X + 3Y = \text{the largest value possible}$$

The M in column A will not enter into the solution. To assure this, it is considered to be a very large negative value, such as $-10,000$. Only positive values in the objective function are considered in carrying out the simplex process.

Line (2) in Table 16-1 represents the constraint that the cost of physician hours ($70X$) plus the cost of physician assistant hours ($35Y$)

Table 16-1 Simplex Method Formulation for Maximization Problem

	X	Y	S_1	S_2	S_3	A	Z
(1)	4	3	0	0	0	M	0
(2)	70	35	-1	0	0	0	1,400
(3)	1	1	0	-1	0	0	30
(4)	1	0	0	0	-1	1	6

cannot exceed $1,400. The -1 is shown under S_1 to eliminate the "less than" aspect of this constraint, so that

$$70X + 35Y - 1S_1 = 1,400$$

Similarly, line (3) in Table 16-1 represents the constraint that the number of hours available for clinic services (because of the limitation of space) is 30. The -1 under S_2 eliminates the "less than" aspect of this constraint, so that

$$1X + 1Y - 1S_2 = 30$$

Finally, line (4) in Table 16-1 represents the constraint that there must be at least 6 hours of physician time available during the day. To remove the "greater than" aspect of this constraint, a -1 is shown under S_3 so that

$$1X - 1S_3 = 6$$

In this case, however, it is also necessary to include an artificial variable, A, in the equation shown in the line (4) to assure that any surplus represented by S_3 will be nonnegative, so that the final version of the third constraint is

$$1X - 1S_3 - 1A = 6$$

As indicated earlier, A is an entirely artificial variable that will not appear in the final solution, but which is there only to allow the simplex solution to work.

Now that the form of the simplex method is specified as shown in Table 16-1, it is possible to discuss the algorithm that will produce the maximum number of patients to be seen during any day while remaining within the constraints of time and money available.

To begin the simplex algorithm, it is necessary to identify what is known as a *pivot value*. The pivot value is found by first selecting the largest value of the objective function. In Table 16-1, the largest value of the objective function (line 1) is the 4 associated with X, the number of hours of physician time. This identifies a column, the X column, in which the pivot value will be found. The pivot value is selected from the X column by finding the entry, among the constraints (excluding line 1), that gives the smallest result when the entry in the Z column is divided by the entry in the X column. This will be the pivot value. In Table 16-1, the pivot value is the 1 in line (4), column X ($1,400/70 = 20$; $30/1 = 30$; $6/1 = 6$). The entire row in which the pivot value is located is then transformed by dividing the row by the pivot value. In this case, no change is produced in line (4) and the result is

(4)
$$
\begin{array}{ccccccc}
X & Y & S_1 & S_2 & S_3 & A & Z \\
1 & 0 & 0 & 0 & -1 & 1 & 6
\end{array}
$$

The next step in the simplex process is to subtract from each of the other three lines in Table 16-1, a multiple of the transformed line (4) that will reduce the entry in the pivot column (column X) to zero. Thus, for line (1), the objective function, each value in the transformed line (4) is multiplied by 4 and subtracted from line (1). For line (2), each value in the transformed line (4) is multiplied by 70 and subtracted from line (2). Line (3) is simply subtracted from line (4). These operations produce the result shown in Table 16-2.

The simplex process is continued by finding in Table 16-2 the largest value in the transformed objective function for the next step. This is the value 4 in column S_3. Then, in that column, the pivot value is the value in lines (2), (3), or (4) that gives the smallest result when divided into column Z, only considering positive values in column S_3. This is the 70 in line (2) (980/70 = 14; 24/1 = 24). This is the new pivot value. All values in line (2) are then divided by the pivot value, producing the following as line (2) in Table 16-3.

(2)
$$
\begin{array}{ccccccc}
X & Y & S_1 & S_2 & S_3 & A & Z \\
0 & 0.5 & -0.014 & 0 & 1 & -1 & 14
\end{array}
$$

Then, just as in the development of Table 16-2, a transformed line (2) is subtracted from each row in Table 16-2 to produce the result in Table 16-3.

Again, to continue the simplex process, the largest value in the transformed objective function in Table 16-3 is found. This is the 1 in

Table 16-2 Simplex Method: Step Two

	X	Y	S_1	S_2	S_3	A	Z
(1)	0	3	0	0	4	M	−24
(2)	0	35	−1	0	70	−70	980
(3)	0	1	0	−1	1	−1	24
(4)	1	0	0	0	1	1	6

Table 16-3 Simplex Method: Step Three

	X	Y	S_1	S_2	S_3	A	Z
(1)	0	1	0.057	0	0	M	−80
(2)	0	0.5	−0.014	0	1	−1	14
(3)	0	0.5	0.014	−1	0	0	10
(4)	1	0.5	−0.014	0	0	0	20

column Y. The same process as followed above is used to produce the result shown in Table 16-4.

The simplex process is now finished. This is determined by the fact that there are no columns in the original objective function (that included only X and Y) for which there is a positive value in line (1). The maximum number of patients who can be seen given the constraints of time and money is shown as the negative number under Z in line (1). One hundred patients per day is the maximum that can be seen. Line (4) shows the number of hours of physician time that should be used to achieve that total, 10 hours. It is possible to see that these 10 hours are associated with physician time because of the value 1 in line (4) under X. Line (3) shows the number of physician assistant hours to use, 20 hours. Again, there is a 1 in line (3) under Y. The 4 under Z in line (2) indicates that the constraint of at least 6 hours of physician time each day is exceeded by 4 hours. Thus, there are 4 hours of slack physician time in the optimal solution. Moreover, this last constraint, even though it may be very important to the administrators in their decision making to assure that the necessary skills are available in the clinic, has no effect on the optimal solution.

We have already seen that this problem can be solved through trial and error, or as we have put it many times in this book, in a cybernetic mode. In that sense, one might ask why the simplex approach is necessary. The answer is that the simplex method is a technique for solving a variety of maximization problems that may in-

Table 16-4 Simplex Method: Step Four

	X	Y	S_1	S_2	S_3	A	Z
(1)	0	0	0.028	2	0	M	−100
(2)	0	0	−0.028	1	1	−1	4
(3)	0	1	0.028	−2	0	0	20
(4)	1	0	−0.028	1	0	0	10

volve many more terms in the objective function than appear in this example, as well as many more, and more complicated, constraints. Furthermore, linear programming is just one of a whole class of mathematical programming techniques that may be used to solve a wide variety of optimization problems. The purpose of this section is not to give anyone the skills necessary to solve an optimization problem using the simplex method, but rather to introduce the method and to make the reader aware of this technique as one of the operations research tools for decision making.

Clinic Staffing from a Different View: A Queuing Solution

The administrator in the example above has satisfied himself that the clinic has been adequately staffed to serve 100 patients during a 10-hour period and that all of his space and money have been used up through the combination of 10 hours of physician time and 20 hours of physician assistant time. Unfortunately for the administrator, if patients begin to arrive unscheduled at the clinic at an average rate of 10 per hour, he will soon discover that, despite what he learned from the linear program, waiting lines ("queues") will begin to form in his clinic and to grow to amazing lengths. To see that this will be the case, the administrator can use another operations research tool known as queuing theory.

Queuing theory is a body of knowledge that is useful for examining the nature of waiting lines. It is concerned with what happens to a waiting line when people arrive at a facility on a random basis and are served at a particular rate. In the case above, the assumption is that patients are arriving at the clinic at the rate of ten per hour, or on the average, one every six minutes. But if the arrivals are essentially random, as they would be expected to be if they were unscheduled, then experience shows that arrivals would not occur exactly every six minutes, but would be likely to follow relatively closely what is known as a *Poisson distribution*. While we will not go into the characteristics of Poisson distributions here, what this means, essentially, is that during some six-minute periods there would be more than one arrival and during other six-minute periods there would be none at all.

Further, it is assumed to be the nature of treatment in a clinic facility that while it is possible for the physician to serve, on the average, four patients per hour (15 minutes per patient) and physician assistants to serve, on the average, three (20 minutes per client), it is also likely that some patients will take longer than others, so that actual treatment time will also be variable. Experience has shown that in situations such as this, treatment time, or service time, tends to follow a *negative exponential distribution.*

If it is assumed that arrivals are random and follow the Poisson distribution while amount of time required for treatment follows a negative exponential distribution, queuing theory provides a formula for determining what will happen in terms of waiting time and queue length in a given facility. To examine this, we will adopt the basic notation used by Warner et al. (1984, p. 132).

The waiting time for one client $[W(X)]$ is

$$W(X) = \cfrac{\cfrac{\rho^x}{X!(1 - \rho/x)} \cdot \cfrac{1}{\sum\limits_{j=0}^{x-1} \rho^j/j! + \cfrac{\rho^x}{X!(1 - \rho/x)}}}{\mu X - \lambda} \qquad (16\text{-}5)$$

and the expected length of the waiting line $[L(X)]$ is

$$L(X) = W(X) \cdot \lambda \qquad (16\text{-}6)$$

where λ = average number of clients arriving per hour
μ = average clients served by one provider per hour
X = number of providers
$\rho = \lambda/\mu$

On the basis of these formulae, it is possible to determine the somewhat anomalous result that in an environment where there were exactly ten persons arriving for services each hour, and where the service capacity was exactly ten per hour, other things being equal, the waiting time and waiting line would both approach infinity. In the real world, of course, this would not happen, because at some point either the providers would increase their pace or the doors would be shut and no more clients admitted. However, with three providers serving a total of ten clients each hour and somewhat fewer than ten clients arriving per hour, Table 16-5 shows the expected waiting time and length of the waiting line for several ranges of clients. It can be seen from Table 16-5, that even if arrivals average only nine per hour, there will be an expected wait of about 50 minutes and about seven people waiting at any one time.

Table 16-5 Expected Waiting Time and Length
of Waiting Line for Three Providers

Arrivals per Hour	Expected Wait (hours)	Expected Line Length
9.8	4.81	47.16
9.5	1.81	17.23
9.0	0.82	7.35

Linear Programming versus Queuing Theory

How can the results of linear programming, which indicates that ten persons can be served per hour, and queuing theory, which indicates that even nine per hour will back up the system, be so different? The difference lies in the basic assumption of linear programming that there is never a wait for the next person to be served (as there is with a real queue) and that the service time is always exactly the same (as it is not in a real service situation). Linear programming in this case provided a general notion about the optimum mix of service providers given certain limited resources. Queuing theory, on the other hand, provides a much more realistic picture of the type of burden on the system if the patient load approached the theoretical maximum of the linear programming solution.

Even queuing results will not necessarily adhere to actual events. The mathematically solved queuing solution depends on the basic assumption of a Poisson arrival pattern and a negative exponential service pattern. In real life, providers are likely to work faster as lines become longer, potential clients are likely to leave when lines become too long if they can, and doors are likely to be closed in extreme cases of service lines becoming too long. All of these factors take the solution out of the realm of classical queuing and make the results of queuing theory less than wholly applicable. Nevertheless, queuing theory provides a basic understanding of what happens in the service provision setting.

Decision Analysis: Dealing with the Problem of Long Queues

The administrator of the clinic in the above situations might decide that it is of substantial concern that the average waiting time for a patient at the clinic may be nearly 50 minutes even if the clinic actually has a client load of 90 patients per day. He may also anticipate that there could be a reasonable possibility that the patient load would increase to as much as 110 patients per day. If this latter event occurred, there would be no reasonable way for the existing staff to deal with the patient load.

The administrator knows that available clinic hours can be increased by adding hours to the time already worked. Assume that it is possible to add two additional hours to the ten hours that the three examining rooms are used, so that it would be possible to have a service provider (possibly hired on an hourly basis) available twelve hours each day in each of three examining rooms. Alternatively, the administrator knows that it would be possible to hire an additional provider if an examining room was added to the clinic. The question is: Is it better to hire additional provider time on an hourly basis or to add an examining room to the clinic and hire an additional full-time provider? And is this question answered differently if the demand remains constant at 90 clients per day or increases to 110 clients per day? Decision analysis can provide a strategy for such decisions.

Decision analysis is usually pictured in the form of a tree diagram as is shown in Figure 16-1. Figure 16-1 begins with a decision point indicated as A on the left hand side of the figure. At this point, the administrator has the option of making a decision to hire additional medical staff on a part-time hourly basis or to add an additional examining room to the clinic and essentially add an additional full-time person. In either case, the administrator expects to add only six hours of clinic time—in the first case extending the hours during which the three existing clinic rooms are used to twelve, or if an additional clinic room is opened, by cutting back the time during which the clinic is open to nine hours per day, so that the total clinic hours in either case will be 36 as opposed to 30 prior to the decision.

If the administrator chooses to add one office, the annual cost will be an additional $50,000 for the office space plus $63,000 for six additional hours of a physician assistant ($35 · 6 hours per day · 300 days per year) or $113,000. If the administrator decides to add overtime, the cost will be only $63,000 per year. Points B_1 and B_2 in Figure 16-1 indicate chance events. The administrator believes that the client demand at the clinic will remain at 90 patients per day or will increase to 110 patients per day over the coming year. He also believes that if an office is added there is a .7 likelihood that the client load will increase and a .3 likelihood that it will remain at 90. On the other hand, if only overtime is added, the administrator suspects,

Figure 16-1 Decision Analysis Tree Diagram for Dealing with the Problem of Long Queues

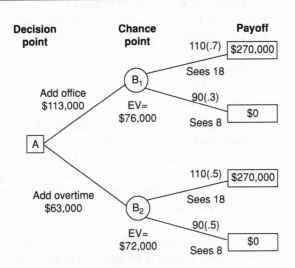

because the hours may be more inconvenient for many people, there is only a .5 likelihood that the volume will go to 110 per day and an equal likelihood that it will remain at 90.

A further necessary piece of information for decision analysis is the payoff of these different decisions and possibilities. The administrator expects that if the client load goes to 110, either by increasing office space or by adding overtime, the number of clients seen by the additional medical personnel will average 18 per day. The administrator knows that the average clinic visit returns $50 in revenue, so that the payoff from 18 patients per day would be $270,000 per year. Alternatively, if there is no increase in clients, the administrator expects that the extra medical personnel will see only 4 to 8 persons per day, essentially just taking up slack in the system and cutting the waiting times. But in this case, the payoff from the additional staff would be 0, because the expectation is that all clients would be served by existing staff.

Within the context of this reasoning, the expected value (EV) of each alternative decision, given the possibility of uncertainty in outcomes (probability of an increase in patients or a constant patient load) is found by

$$EV_i = \left\{ \sum_{j=1}^{J} PO_{ij}p_{ij} \right\} - C_i$$

where EV_i = the expected value for decision i

PO_{ij} = the payoff for decision i and chance event j

p_{ij} = the probability that chance event j will occur given

decision $i \left(\sum_{j=1}^{J} p_{ij} = 1 \right)$

C_i = the cost for decision i

Using this formulation, it can be seen that the decision to add an office leads to an expected value of $76,000, while the decision to add overtime, primarily because of the higher probability that the patient load will not increase, leads to an expected value of only $72,000. In decision analysis terms, it is better for the administrator to add an office than to increase the number of hours available with the existing offices.

Clearly, however, the conclusion reached above is highly dependent on the probabilities assigned to the two chance alternatives, as well as to the level of the two alternatives. If the probability of increased client traffic was the same for both decisions, the result would have indicated that overtime was the best choice, since it is cheapest. If there was a smaller differential in the number of clients seen in a day, the results would have also indicated that adding overtime was the best choice.

A Different Problem for the Clinic: Inventory

The clinic manager is responsible for maintaining an extensive inventory of supplies and equipment and assuring that these are always available when needed. While the clinic has a part-time pharmacist who handles the pharmaceutical supplies, the manager also feels responsible for being certain that the supplies of pharmaceuticals are always adequate for the everyday needs of the clinic. Further, the manager knows that placing orders for supplies costs money in terms of time required to decide on the size of the order, and staff time needed to fill out and mail order forms. At the same time, the manager is constantly aware that storage space at the clinic is limited, so that maintaining a quantity of supplies larger than needed actually represents a cost to the clinic in terms of other supplies that cannot be stored, and even in the necessity to rent additional storage space.

Within this relatively straightforward statement of an inventory problem, operations research techniques provide a deterministic solution that will arrive at the proper ordering quantity and ordering frequency to assure the minimization of inventory ordering and storage costs if it is assumed that the manager can determine the cost of placing an order and the cost of holding the inventory.

The basis of this example of the application of operations research techniques is what is referred to as the *economic ordering quantity* (EOQ). The EOQ makes several basic assumptions about the inventory control problem, including the following:

1. The demand for the item is constant over time.
2. The unit holding and ordering costs are independent of quantity ordered.
3. Replenishment is scheduled so that new stock arrives just at the time that the old stock is entirely exhausted.
4. Orders for different items are independent of one another.

Illustration

The clinic will see about 90 patients per day, or between 28,000 and 29,000 patients per year. Assume that each patient seen requires the physician, on the average, to use two pairs of rubber gloves. This means that the manager must assure the timely, and most cost-effective, availability of about 57,000 pairs of rubber gloves each year. Assume further that the manager has spent some time studying the cost of placing orders for various supply items and has determined that the cost of placing any order for rubber gloves is $7.00. The cost of storage space has been calculated for a box of rubber gloves (they come 100 to a box) as being $.80 per year. Given this trade-off between cost of ordering and cost of storing, and the need to assure constant availability, how often are orders for rubber gloves placed and how many are ordered each time?

The EOQ calculation is based, in general, on an annual supply cycle, although longer cycles could be assessed. We will assume here that the concern is with an annual cycle. In this formulation, then, the following parameters can be specified:

- annual demand   (*D*)   570 boxes
- ordering cost   (*K*) $7.00
- holding cost   (*H*) $ .80
- quantity ordered   (*Q*)   To be determined

Within this formulation, the following is true. Annual ordering cost (T_o) is equal to the annual demand divided by the quantity ordered at each order multiplied by the cost of ordering, or

$$T_o = \frac{D}{Q} K$$

Annual holding cost (T_h) is equal to the average inventory $(Q/2$ if demand is constant) multiplied by the cost of holding one box, or

$$T_h = H\frac{Q}{2}$$

Then total annual cost (T) is

$$T = T_o + T_h = \frac{D}{Q} K + H\frac{Q}{2}$$

Both calculus and graphic solutions to this problem will show that the minimum value of T is obtained when T_o and T_h are equal, or when

$$\frac{D}{Q} K = H\frac{Q}{2}$$

or, when

$$Q = \frac{2KD}{H}$$

With this information, the optimal ordering quantity can be seen to be

$$Q = 2 \cdot 7.00 \cdot 570/.80 = 99.87 \text{ boxes}$$

With this number of boxes of gloves, the total inventory cost of rubber gloves for one year will be

$$T = T_o + T_h = 570/99.87 \cdot 7 + .80 \cdot 99.87/2$$
$$= 39.95 + 39.95 = \$79.90 \text{ per year}$$

Of course, it is unlikely that the clinic will be able to buy 99.87 boxes of rubber gloves at one time, so if the quantity is changed to 100, the total cost per year comes out to

$$T = T_o + T_h = 39.90 + 40 = \$79.90$$

In this case, the difference in the price of the next higher number of boxes was not detectable at the level of cents.

This formulation also indicates to the manager how often gloves must be purchased. This will be simply the number of days in a year times the quantity purchased at any one time divided by the annual demand, or every 64 days.

The EOQ also provides useful information in the situation where it may not be possible to purchase supplies in exactly the most economic quantities. For example, let us assume that rubber gloves can be purchased by the clinic at a reasonable purchase price only if obtained in lots of 60 boxes (perhaps 60 boxes are packaged in a larger carton). The optimal purchase in terms of inventory costs, as seen above, is approximately 100. Will it be more efficient for the clinic to purchase gloves as one carton of 60 boxes each time it makes a purchase, or will it be more efficient to purchase two cartons of 60 boxes each, for 120 boxes at each purchase? The EOQ provides the answer. The purchase of 60 boxes at a time will give an annual cost of $66.50 for ordering and $24.00 for holding, for a total of $90.50. The purchase of 120 boxes at a time will give a total of $33.25 for ordering and $48.00 for holding, for a total of $81.25 (only $1.35 more than the optimal solution). Thus, in this case, it is better to buy the larger amount each time, rather than the smaller. This will be true because the cost of holding is small compared to the cost of ordering. If the reverse were true, a different solution would have resulted.

This is the simplest of all inventory models. The point should be made that a separate calculation must be done for each item of inventory. There are more complex models, but the purpose here is to provide an introduction to the types of decisions that can be made with operations research—in this case, inventory models—not to make the reader an expert in the technique.

Discussion Questions

1. What is the relationship of operations research techniques to the cybernetic model and decision making?
2. Under what conditions are operations research techniques the method of choice? Illustrate your answer.

17

Cost-Benefit and Cost-Effectiveness Analysis

$\mathbf{C}$ost-benefit and cost-effectiveness analysis are treated formally in this book as the last chapter in the topics covered on the subject of evaluation. In the sense that cost-benefit and cost-effectiveness analysis are not a specific type of evaluation tool per se, but rather a set of techniques that would be well applied to any evaluation, there is logic in the position of this chapter. To the extent, however, that virtually no evaluation can ignore the issues of cost and the most efficient ways in which to produce a desired result, cost-benefit and cost-effectiveness analysis must be considered an integral part of any evaluation effort. Cost-benefit and cost-effectiveness analysis address specifically the efficiency element of evaluation discussed in the first chapter of the book.

Benefit versus Effectiveness

The first issue to address in a chapter on cost-benefit and cost-effectiveness analysis is the distinction between the two. Both techniques are concerned with program costs, but cost-benefit analysis makes the explicit point of converting all desired program outputs to dollar values. Cost-effectiveness analysis, on the other hand, does not convert desired program outputs to dollar terms. The most obvious result of this difference is that cost-benefit analysis can, to the extent that desired program outputs can be valued in dollar terms, compare programs that may have entirely different outputs, even entirely different goals. Cost-effectiveness analysis, in contrast, is limited to those situations where the outputs are essentially comparable, not only in quality, but in many cases, in quantity as well.

This distinction has at least two important consequences. Cost-benefit analysis would seem to be the more desirable tool to use, because it is, in theory, able to assess a wider range of alternative programs against one another. However, it is often the case that cost-benefit analysis cannot be used, except in the most trivial sense, because some or many of the desired outputs, and often the most important ones, cannot be converted to some dollar (or rupee or shilling) value. On the other hand, cost-effectiveness analysis, which may be used to assess alternative programs against the important, nontrivial desired outputs, is limited by the difficulty of establishing a scale of measurement that can solve the problem of even slightly different outputs, either in quantity or quality.

We will return to the dilemma posed in the paragraph above later in the chapter. But before dealing with that concern, let us examine the general techniques of cost-benefit and cost-effectiveness analysis in somewhat greater detail and with some examples.

Cost-Benefit Analysis

Illustration

In the most simplistic terms, cost-benefit analysis is a comparison of the costs of a program to the benefits to be derived. If it costs $16,000 in the first year to initiate a program and an additional $1,000 per year to keep it going for four subsequent years, the total cost of the program is $20,000 for five years. If it is projected that the benefits from the program will equal $10,000 in the first year and decline at the rate of $2,000 per year over the life of the program (perhaps this is a training program where there are fewer persons trained in each year), then the total benefits derived from the program are, in dollar terms, $30,000. The net difference between the costs and the benefits (the net benefit) is a positive $10,000. Thus, it looks like a good idea to initiate the program.

But there are two reasons that it may be wise to do some further analysis before actually initiating the program. The first is that there may be other programs that will return a greater net benefit for the money invested. The second is that the above paragraph assumes there are no other opportunities lost for the use of the $20,000 invested in the program. It is necessary to deal briefly with the first of these and at more length with the second.

To consider the first issue, suppose there is a program that will cost $4,000 in each year of operation for five years. Unlike the program above, there are essentially no start-up costs (the initial year's $16,000). Let us also assume that this program returns $36,000 rather than only $30,000, but that the benefits are not realized until year 3, when they start at $8,000, followed by $10,000 in year 4 and $18,000 in year 5. If a manager had only $20,000 to invest in a new program, he might reasonably decide that the second program, which returns a net of $16,000 for the investment, is more desirable than the first, which only returns a net of $10,000. If the only consideration was the absolute difference between costs and benefits, then the second program is clearly superior.

Net present value

The fact that the value of money is not constant over time must be considered in cost-benefit analysis. In general, if I can have a dollar today, it is better (more valuable to me) than a dollar that I will acquire one year from now. Even if we disregard inflation that is certain to erode the value of the dollar that I will receive one year from now, making it worth less in buying power than a dollar today, there is also another issue. The dollar I obtain today can be invested at some rate of interest (r) to produce $1 + r$ dollars in one year. Thus, in considering the costs and benefits of any given project, or when comparing one or more projects, it is usually desirable, if not essential, to take into consideration the time value of money. The time value of money is often stated as the net present value (NPV) of a quantity of money that will be obtained at some point (T) in the future. If the interest rate (or as it is often called, the *discount rate*) is r, then the NPV of a quantity of money, P, to be received one year in the future, is

$$\text{NPV} = \frac{P}{1 + r} \qquad (17\text{-}1)$$

In particular, if the P is one dollar and r is .05, then the NPV of one dollar received in one year is $1/(1 + .05)$, or .952.

If we are interested in the benefits of a program that will be implemented and active over some period of years, t, then the NPV of the money invested in the program, costs (C), and the returns from the program, benefits (B), will be

$$\text{NPV} = \sum_{t=1}^{T} \frac{B_t - C_t}{(1 + r)^t} \qquad (17\text{-}2)$$

This equation indicates that the net present value of the program is the sum of the difference between the costs and benefits of the program over its lifetime, reduced by one plus the discount rate raised to the power of the number of years that have elapsed since program start-up.

One problem with this cost-benefit formulation, of course, is that it assumes a particular discount rate, or rate at which the value of uninvested money would be expected to decline over time. In general, the discount rate can only be estimated. In many cases the decisions reached through cost-benefit analysis may depend directly on the assumptions about the discount rate. To see this, let us examine the consequences of alternative discount rate assumptions in regard to the two projects discussed above, one that returns a net $10,000 for an investment of $20,000 and the other that returns $16,000. Table 17-1 shows a comparison of the two programs in terms of the time value of money.

Table 17-1 shows several different discount rates and the calculation of net present values for the projects in each year, 1 through 5, based on that discount rate, as well as the total NPV (the

Table 17-1   Comparison of Two Projects with Comparable Investments

		Year 1	*Year 2*	*Year 3*	*Year 4*	*Year 5*	*NPV*
Program A							
Benefits		$10,000	$8,000	$6,000	$4,000	$2,000	
Costs		16,000	1,000	1,000	1,000	1,000	
Discount	0	−6,000	7,000	5,000	3,000	1,000	$10,000
rate	.1	−5,455	5,785	3,757	2,049	621	6,757
	.2	−5,000	4,861	2,894	1,447	402	4,603
	.3	−4,615	4,142	2,276	1,050	269	3,122
Program B							
Benefits		$ 0	$ 0	$8,000	$10,000	$18,000	
Costs		4,000	4,000	4,000	4,000	4,000	
Discount	0	−4,000	−4,000	4,000	6,000	14,000	$16,000
rate	.1	−3,636	−3,306	3,005	4,098	8,693	8,854
	.2	−3,333	−2,778	2,315	2,894	5,626	4,724
	.3	−3,077	−2,367	1,821	2,101	3,771	2,248

last column). At a discount rate of 0, each project has an NPV of exactly the difference between the total investment and the total return, making program B more attractive. At a discount rate of .1 (10 percent) or .2 (20 percent), program B is still superior on the basis of the NPV. If a discount rate of .3 is projected, however, program A becomes the one with the higher NPV and remains so at all higher discount rates. A logical consequence of the fact that the two programs shift position with regard to NPV is that there is a discount rate, in this case, approximately .21, where both programs are equally attractive. If the discount rate is projected to be below that level for the next five years, then option B is preferred. If the discount rate is projected to be above that level then option A is preferred.

This comparison between programs A and B suggests at least one generalization. Programs with relatively large returns that come late in the program life will tend to be preferred over programs with more modest returns that come early in the program life when a low discount rate is projected. Programs that have early modest returns will be preferred over programs with larger later returns when a high discount rate is projected.

It should be pointed out here that it will not always be true that the desirability of one program over another will be determined by the level of the discount rate. It is easy to postulate one program that will be more attractive than another and will "dominate" the other program no matter what the discount rate. A program with the same stream of investments as that in program A in Table 17-1, but with a stream of returns that was equal to $10,000 in each of the five years of program operation, would be a clear example of such a dominant program. The decision to choose this latter program over program A would be independent of discount rate.

Internal rate of return

The NPV is generally accepted as the best measure of the value of a program, either as assessed against no program, or as assessed against alternative competing programs. The internal rate of return (IRR) is the discount rate at which the NPV of a given project is equal to zero, or the discount rate at which returns from the project will exactly equal outlays. The IRR is defined as that discount rate, r, that satisfies the equation

$$0 = \sum \frac{B_t - C_t}{(1 + r)^t} \qquad (17\text{-}3)$$

The IRR, although commonly employed as a means of comparing one program to another, has several fundamental problems. It is possible to calculate the IRR for programs A and B in Table 17-1 and determine that the IRR for program A is approximately .81, while the IRR for program B is about .47. If no other information was available, the common decision rule would be to select that program with the higher IRR, that is, program A. But we have already shown that the NPV of program B is higher than program A at values of r lower than .21.

The IRR has other problems as well. In general, the IRR applies easily and clearly only to those programs in which the first years of a program's life are characterized by an investment stream that is greater than the stream of returns, but in which returns exceed investments in later years. As defined in Equation 17-3, it can be shown mathematically that the IRR will take on as many values as there are shifts, over the life of the program, between costs exceeding benefits and benefits exceeding costs. In particular, for example, it is possible to imagine a program in which investments exceeded returns early in the life of the program, returns exceeded investments during the middle years of the program life, and then investments again exceeded returns at the end of the program (that is, two changes of the relative status of costs and benefits). Such a program would have two different values of the IRR that would be equal only by chance. On the other hand, if it was possible to implement a program that in the first year would begin to realize benefits greater than costs (for example, a five-year program that costs \$1,000 per year to initiate and that realizes benefits of \$2,000 per year from year 1), there is no IRR. The IRR would be undefined, because the relative position of benefits and costs never shifts and the sum of the benefit stream will always exceed the sum of the cost stream.

The benefit-cost ratio

The benefit-cost ratio also provides a means of assessing the value of a program. But it, too, presents difficulties when comparing programs. The benefit-cost ratio (B/C) is defined as

$$B/C = \sum \frac{B_t/(1 + r)^t}{C_t/(1 + r)^t} \tag{17-4}$$

It should be clear that any program with a B/C greater than 1 will return a net benefit to society, and any program with a B/C less than 1 will be a net loss. But the B/C, when used to compare programs, will not in general yield the same results as the NPV. In the case of programs A and B in Table 17-1, for example, the *B/C* would prefer program B even at discount rates as high as .3, when the NPV of program A is clearly higher. In most cases, it is agreed that the NPV is the measure of choice in assessing costs and benefits, in determining whether a program will be a net benefit to society, or in choosing between two or more competing programs.

Cost-Effectiveness Analysis

Cost-effectiveness analysis is a program assessment that does not convert the outputs of the program to dollar terms. In cost-effectiveness analysis the output may be measured in episodes of illness averted, deaths averted, years of life added, doses of vaccine administered, children fully immunized, persons served by a water system, or any other set of units that are relevant to the project being assessed.

In general, cost-effectiveness analysis will be concerned with comparing two or more mutually exclusive programs that provide the same benefits at different levels, or provide the same level of benefits at differing costs. For example, a cost-effectiveness analysis might be conducted to assess the relative advantage of an immunization program in a developing country that is based on centrally directed immunization campaigns compared to one based on routinely available vaccine for immunization at local health departments. Less frequently, cost-effectiveness analysis might be used to assess the marginal benefits to be derived from additional program efforts. As an example, it might be of interest to assess the cost of a second wave of vaccinations during a vaccination campaign that had already been carried out in a given community area. To better understand cost-effectiveness analysis, let us examine both examples.

Consider a comparison of centrally directed immunization campaigns to routinely available immunization at local health departments. A country wishes to provide immunization to an area in which there are 40,000 eligible children to be immunized every six months. Immunizations can be provided through centrally directed immunization campaigns that involve teams of workers who go out on a semiannual basis to immunize all eligible children in the area, or they can be provided through immunizations routinely available at local health centers.

The experience of the Ministry of Health indicates that the local availability of vaccine has resulted, in the past, in approximately

13,260 children effectively immunized over a typical six-month period at an estimated total cost of $1,486. The ministry projects that the campaign approach, carried out over a period of two weeks every six months, could result in the equivalent number of children immunized at a cost of $3,060. Table 17-2, below, compares these two approaches in terms of cost effectiveness.

This is a result typical of cost-effectiveness analysis. On the basis of this result, it appears that the campaign approach to immunization is twice as expensive as the local availability of vaccine. If the Ministry of Health was satisfied with the status quo in terms of the number of children immunized, it should accept the local availability of vaccine as the preferred approach and not consider the campaign approach.

One reservation about this conclusion, however, is that it is based on a comparison of the two approaches assuming a proportion of children immunized as would be expected from an existing program of supplying locally available vaccine. Typically, the costs of realizing a given level of effectiveness will not be linear for a particular program approach across the entire range of possible program outputs. To illustrate this point, consider Figure 17-1. Figure 17-1 shows a hypothetical graph of costs for clinic-based immunization and campaign-based immunization over the range from 0 to 100 percent of eligible children immunized.

As Figure 17-1 shows, the hypothesized cost of both immunization strategies increases at an increasing rate as the proportion of children immunized increases. This is a reasonable expectation, because as a larger proportion of the eligible children are immunized, it becomes increasingly difficult and costly to identify and locate the remaining children and to obtain agreement from their parents. Curves for both programs go off the chart before reaching 100 percent based on the not unreasonable expectation that complete

Table 17-2 Cost Effectiveness of Two Program Strategies for Immunization

	Campaign	Local Availability
Children immunized	13,260	13,260
Percent immunized	33.15	33.15
Total cost	$3,060	$1,486
Cost per immunization	$ .23	$ .11
Cost per percent	$92.31	$44.82

Figure 17-1   Comparison of Two Immunization Programs

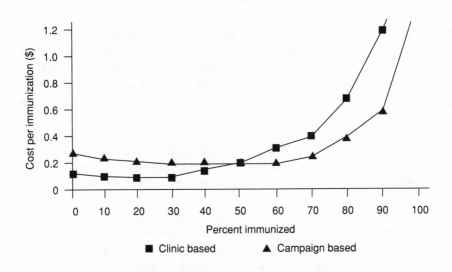

coverage in most circumstances is almost prohibitively expensive. The figure also shows the reasonable expectation that at low proportions of children immunized, there will be a higher cost—in this case, only marginally higher—that represents the fixed costs associated with any level of program activity.

But a second point that is made in this figure—and in cost-effectiveness terms, the more important point—is that the preferred program in terms of cost effectiveness may actually, and quite reasonably, depend on the level of effectiveness to be achieved. After initial start-up costs, the cost per immunization increases for either program approach. But while the cost of clinic-based immunization is less expensive than campaign-based when the level to be achieved is below 50 percent, clinic-based becomes increasingly more expensive as the proportion of children immunized exceeds 50 percent. Thus, if the Ministry of Health planned to produce immunization levels above 50 percent it would seem logical to go to a campaign-based approach.

Figure 17-1 also provides initial and somewhat approximate information for assessing the marginal benefits to be derived from additional program efforts. For example, if a campaign approach was utilized and it was carried out over a period of time necessary to immunize approximately 60 percent of eligible children (in our example of an area in which there were 40,000 such children, this would be 24,000 children), the cost would be approximately $.23 per immunization, or a total of \$5,520. If the program had set out to immunize 80 percent of the children initially, the cost per immunization would have been about \$.38 per immunization, or \$12,160. The reasons for this—difficulty in accessing the remaining eligible children and gaining permission from their parents, which translates into more time in the field—have been indicated above. The difference between the two total figures gives a good working figure for the cost of launching a second wave of immunizations to increase the proportion of children immunized to 80 percent when a first wave immunized only 60 percent. Under these circumstances it would be reasonable to estimate that each additional immunization will cost approximately \$.83. So the cost of immunizations in a second wave would be almost four times as much as the cost of immunizations in the first wave.

There is one remaining point to be made in regard to this presentation of cost effectiveness as a comparison between two different types of programs that are aimed generally at producing the same end result. The locally available vaccine approach to immunization and the campaign approach are not necessarily mutually exclusive. It is quite possible that a ministry of health could adopt both strategies, making immunization routinely available at local clinics and also undertaking periodic campaigns. In this case, the cost of each strategy would have to be reestimated. One result, however, would be almost certain. The cost of completed immunizations for the campaign-based strategy would increase. This is, again, because it would be more difficult, and hence more costly, for campaign workers to identify eligible children in the field, since many of the children they would see would have already received immunizations at local clinics.

Assessing Costs and Benefits

The preceding section discussed the basic concept behind cost-effectiveness analysis. In this analysis, benefits are not assessed in the same way that they are in cost-benefit analysis. In general, however, costs are assessed in the same way in either approach. To that extent, this section is equally applicable to either cost-benefit or cost-effectiveness analysis.

The first step in assessing costs and benefits is to understand what they are and where they may arise. To take the latter point first, consider again the simple program diagram shown as Figure 17-2.

Figure 17-2 Simple Diagram of Program Flow

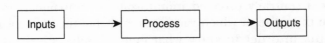

This diagram is an excellent starting point for discussing an assessment of costs and benefits. Costs of a program are to be found in the box labeled "inputs." Benefits (or effects) are to be found in the box labeled "outputs." In quite simple terms, anything that represents a program input is a cost. Anything that represents a program output is a benefit (there may actually be some unintended and undesired program outputs that represent negative benefits). A case might be made that program costs could also be identified in the process box. For example, a committee might require a period of time to reach a decision, part of the program process. But the time of the members of the committee can also be valued as an input, as can any other opportunities lost because of the time taken for the decision. Thus this discussion of costs will be limited only to the input box.

There are various ways of determining what should be included as program inputs. Bainbridge and Sapirie (1974) see the program inputs that will make up the components of the costs of a program as including salaries and expenses, transportation, space, supplies and equipment, capital equipment, consultative or contractual services, training, publication, and miscellaneous. Drummond (1980, pp. 27–29) classifies inputs to health care, particularly, as

1. health service resources, including land, buildings, personnel, equipment, and consumable supplies
2. other support services (outside the health services)
3. patients' (and their families') resources, including personal time, drugs and dressing provided by the family, transportation, home adaptation, special diets, and other expenditures

In establishing the relevant inputs for assessing the cost of any specific program, it will almost certainly be necessary to draw up a list of program costs from the beginning, rather than assuming that it will be possible to rely on some predetermined list of inputs. In particular, it will be necessary to determine which inputs are actually going to be considered as important. Certainly in the overall societal assessment of costs of a given program, patient time may be considered as an important input. A program manager on the other hand, may be little concerned about patient time when considering whether a centrally directed immunization campaign is more cost effective than one in which vaccine is available through local health clinics. But in order to know what items should be valued and included as part of the costs of a program, it is reasonable to start with the broadest set of definitions possible.

Illustration

To examine in somewhat more detail the issue of program costs, consider the assessment of the cost of a campaign-based approach to immunization. The Ministry of Health (MOH) projects that it will use four teams of five persons each. An initial assessment of the input categories for such an immunization effort might be as listed in Table 17-3. Table 17-3 also shows those items that will be explicitly valued because they are direct costs to the Ministry of Health, and those items that will, in essence, be ignored because they are costs either to external donors or to patients themselves.

In any cost-benefit or cost-effectiveness analysis, there are two levels of costs: those that accrue directly to the person or organization that is the decision maker with regard to the conduct of the program, and those that accrue to the larger society. Frequently, as in the valuation shown in Table 17-3, the decision maker, in this case the Ministry of Health, is disinterested in costs to the larger society because these do not effect the decision that the campaign approach is more or less costly than some alternative program, for example, locally available immunization. If the Ministry of Health decided to launch an immunization campaign lasting eight and one-half days (the estimated time required to immunize 33.15 percent of eligible children), the Ministry assessment of costs based on Table 17-3 would be $3,060.

But $3,060 is clearly an understatement of the total cost of the campaign. It is an understatement for two reasons: first, because it ignores costs not accrued to the ministry, and second, because it ignores some costs accrued to the ministry but for which the ministry does not have to make a cash payment at the time of the immunization campaign. Both of these costs deserve some discussion.

Cost as payment or resource use

Before continuing with a discussion of the two sources of cost that are not valued in Table 17-3, it will be useful to spend a little time discussing the nature of valuation of cost in general. Costs can be considered

Table 17-3 Program Inputs for a Centrally Directed Immunization Campaign

	Valued by MOH	Not Valued by MOH
Project Staff		
Salaries		
Team leaders	4 at $5.50/day	
Team members	12 at $5.25/day	
Drivers	4 at $5.25/day	
Expenses (daily)		
Meals	40 at $1.65/day	
Lodging	20 at $1.40/day	
Transportation		
Vehicle costs		Use MOH vehicles
Gasoline, oil	$30.00/day	
Supplies (tires)	$340.00	
Space for Immunizations		Use local clinics
Supplies and Equipment		
Syringes		USAID
Vaccine		USAID
Sterlizing equipment		USAID
Clerical supplies		Use existing MOH
Technical Assistance		UNICEF/WHO
Patient Time		
Travel time		Not valued
Waiting time		Not valued

in two ways, as payments made for a particular input or as resources used in supplying the input. The Ministry of Health, as shown in Table 17-3, has placed a dollar value on the time of its personnel that in all likelihood refers to the actual amount of money that the ministry must pay for that personnel time on a daily basis. In essence, this is the payment method of valuing inputs. The alternative approach to valuing personnel as an input would be to consider it as a resource that can be used in many alternative ways. The cost of using the personnel for immunization is essentially equivalent to the best alternative use of the same resources. In economic terms, this is the concept of *opportunity cost*. The opportunity cost of using a person as part of an immunization team for a day is equal to the next best alternative use of that person's time that will be forgone during the same day because the person is part of the immunization team.

In 1983, a colleague, while working with an international technical assistance organization, was part of a survey assessment of primary health care services in Sri Lanka, organized in part by the assistance organization. The assessment lasted three weeks and involved about 40 people, mostly Sri Lankans. At the end of the assessment, our colleague submitted a report to the organization that included an estimate of the cost of the activity. As part of the estimate, he included the cost of his time, which was significantly higher than costs for other persons who were involved in the assessment and which greatly inflated the overall cost of the assessment, because he was working at a generally accepted Western wage. The deputy director at the assistance organization recommended that he remove the estimate of his time from the estimate of assessment costs because, as the deputy pointed out, if he had not been involved in the assessment he would simply have been sitting in his office.

There was without doubt an element of politics in the recommendation of the deputy director. The assessment appeared very costly with the inclusion of the technical assistant's time, and that time was clearly valued at a much higher level than the time of host country personnel. But at the same time, there was a very clear element of logic. In many cases the alternative uses of a particular resource at a particular point in time—the opportunities forgone because of the use of that resource in a particular way—may be zero. If not for the program, the resource would not be used at all. If not for the immunization program, the Ministry of Health personnel might simply sit in their offices for the eight and one-half days. In this sense, the cost of using these persons in the immunization program is, in fact and in practice, zero because no alternatives are forgone.

On the other hand, it may well be true that the use of a particular resource in a particular way means that other opportunities are indeed forgone. If the Ministry of Health personnel are not engaged in the immunization program, they may be providing much needed well-baby care or prenatal care, care that will be unavailable while they are participating in the immunization program. If so, the cost of their time in the immunization program is the value of the medical care forgone.

While the idea of opportunities forgone, or alternative use of resources, is intuitively appealing as a measure of cost, in practical terms, the value of an alternative use of a particular resource may be very difficult to establish. Further, most people would intuitively agree that the value of a resource in any alternative use is exactly what one would have to pay for it to use it in that way. Finally, the idea of a payment for a resource is relatively easy for program managers to grasp when compared to the concept of alternative resource uses. In consequence, the cash or payment basis for valuing inputs is more likely to be seen than the resource use basis.

The value of all inputs

As indicated above, the actual cost of the program as laid out in Table 17-3 is not the $3,060 recognized by the Ministry of Health, but some other amount that may be substantially more. It may even be more for the ministry itself. To see this, it is useful to consider costs incurred by the ministry that are not valued and costs incurred by other than the ministry.

Costs to the ministry not valued by the ministry

There are two clear sources of costs, that is, inputs, that accrue directly to the ministry but are not valued by the ministry in their calculation of $3,060. Probably the larger and more important of these will be the four vehicles needed to take the immunization teams to the immunization sites each day. The ministry will use vehicles already owned by the government, and so have assigned no cost to their use. But these vehicles indeed represent a cost to the ministry. That cost may be viewed as large or small (or as is the case in Table 17-3, as zero) depending on how the value of the vehicles is assessed. There are at least three alternative ways in which the vehicles could be valued:

1. as a resource that may be used in some alternative way
2. as equivalent to the cost of alternative rented transportation
3. as a capital expenditure depreciated over an expected operational life

We have already discussed the possibility that the alternative may be no use at all. In this case, the value of the alternative is zero and the use of the vehicles is free. If this were not the case, then it is likely that any valuation of the use of the vehicles would have to fall back on one of the two other methods.

Taking the second alternative, the Ministry of Health could rent transportation, along with a driver. It would not be unreasonable to expect that the cost of a vehicle and driver for one day in a typical developing country would be as high as $100. In this case, the value of the vehicles would be $100 per day minus the cost of the driver, which at about $10 per day would make the cost of the vehicles $90 per day, or $3,060 ($90 · 4 teams · 8.5 days), an amount equivalent to all other program costs!

Finally, if we take the third alternative, it might be estimated that a Ministry of Health vehicle may last five years under the conditions that prevail on the roads of the country under discussion. The ministry may assume a straight-line depreciation of the value of the vehicles from purchase at $17,500 each for the five-year period, thus making the use of the vehicles equivalent to $3,500 per year. If a working year was considered to be 260 days, this would make the use of the vehicles equal to $13.64 per day, for a total cost of about $458, substantially less than the $3,060 when valued as rental vehicles, but still a significant program cost. However, it is not unlikely that the Ministry of Health originally received the vehicles as donations from an international assistance agency, and thinking in these terms, that the vehicles were free to begin with, rather than in terms of the replacement value of the vehicles, may still be justified in valuing them at zero.

The second clear area of cost to the ministry not valued by the ministry is the category of clerical supplies. This may be a small item but would probably be best represented not as a no-cost item, but at the replacement cost value of the supplies that will be used.

Costs to others not valued by the ministry

The second realm of costs that will accrue as part of this program that are not explicitly valued by the ministry are all inputs provided to the program from other sources. These include the use of local clinics as immunization sites; the syringes, vaccine, and sterilizing equipment being donated through USAID; the technical assistance being provided through UNICEF/WHO; and finally, the time being provided by the people who will bring children for immunizations, and even the time of the children themselves.

It will not be necessary to belabor these costs in detail. We have discussed above the concept of alternative uses of the resources as well as cash value of the resources. But clearly, if local clinic space was not being used for the immunization campaign, it is possible, even likely, that it would be serving a useful alternative. The value of this might be assigned on the basis of some reasonable local rental price for space. If the immunization supplies and equipment were not being used in this campaign, it might be used in a different immunization program in a different country entirely. In that case it clearly represents a resource forgone by the other country and a cost that might be best estimated by the price of the equipment and supplies on the international market. If, however, the supplies and equipment are clearly earmarked as the property of the country and the question is simply whether they be used in the campaign approach or through locally available immunization, then the cost of the supplies and equipment is zero.

Technical assistance from UNICEF/WHO is a potentially valuable commodity, which when valued at the salary level of a person providing such assistance, plus travel and housing for the time of the program, may easily be at the level of $650 to $750 per day. Such a level would clearly make this the most costly component of the campaign. But as the deputy director might point out, if the technical expert was not involved in the campaign, he would probably just be sitting in his office anyway.

Finally, the costs to the people who come for the service might be valued. This is in no way a cost of the campaign either to the Ministry of Health, to the local clinics, or to the other sponsoring agencies. But it clearly represents a cost to the society in terms of lost production and resources that must be used in this way as opposed to some alternative way. Just as an estimate, suppose that each person who brings children for immunization must travel two hours round trip and wait one hour for the immunization. In a developing country context, such travel and waiting times are not an unreasonable expectation. Suppose further that travel costs are equivalent to $.25. Finally, suppose that each person brings two children, on average, for immunization. The total cost to the society for this activity might reasonably be estimated as $4,000 to $4,500, based on an average annual income of about $250 and assuming a working year of 230 to 250 days. This may seem like little for the time of all these people, but it still represents the single largest program cost after the technical advisors.

Valuing benefits

The section above has concentrated on the valuation of inputs, or costs. Now we will consider the valuation of outputs, or benefits. The title of this chapter is "Cost-Benefit and Cost-Effectiveness Analysis." We have already noted that the difference between these two forms of analysis is that in the former, dollar values are actually assigned to the outputs, or at least to those outputs that are the primary interest of program decision makers, while in the latter, no dollar values are assigned and assessments are made on the basis of the relative output levels (immunizations performed, hospital discharges, neonatal deaths, etc.) per se. With this in mind, it is clear that the valuation of outputs in dollar terms is applicable only to the case of cost-benefit analysis.

The conscious dollar-based valuation of health care or social welfare programs is an extremely difficult task. What, for example, is the dollar value of an immunization? Is it the positive value of the cost of treating a disease that if not immunized against, may occur? Or is it the amount of money that the average person will be willing to pay for immunization, or willing to pay to be treated for the disease that the immunization is aimed at preventing? Or, from another perspective, is it the value of a productive life that may be terminated by disease in the absence of the immunization? And is it useful or not useful to try to assess the dollar value of pain and suffering? Depending on how benefits are valued, the results of the same program may be quite different in benefit terms. Moreover, the dollar level assigned to benefits under differing valuation strategies will also differ substantially from one culture to another. The average person, for example, may be willing to pay little for immunizations in one culture, but may be willing to pay a significant amount in others. The value of each additional year of productive life in a Western culture may be several thousands of dollars, while in a less developed society may be only a few hundred dollars.

These problem issues in valuing benefits of health programs have plagued those who have sought to carry out cost-benefit analyses of health programs. It should be clear that the problems associated with valuing the outputs of an immunization program are equally problem issues in attempting to value, for example, an early cancer screening program, a renal dialysis or a kidney transplant program, an infant-feeding program, or any other type of program that has improved health states as the primary outcome. It is probable that the best thing that can be said in regard to such valuation efforts is that they will always be subject to some level of controversy over whether a valid dollar figure has been applied. Where two different types of programs producing similar results are being valued, the specific valuation strategy may not be too important because both programs may be assessed under specified and similar conditions. But when programs may produce different types of results (for example one program produces additional years of life for middle-aged adults, while another improves nutritional status for children) or when programs may take place in substantially different settings (for example, one program may be directed toward hypertension screening among urban poor populations, while another may be concerned with breast self exams by middle-class women), then dollar valuation becomes extremely difficult. This is particularly problematic, too, because these are precisely the types of situations where cost-benefit analysis should be able to provide the most useful information. Because valuation of health outcomes in ways that enjoy widespread acceptance and agreement remains an unattained goal, cost-benefit analysis applied to health programs is less useful than it might otherwise be.

Discussion Questions

1. Distinguish between cost-benefit and cost-effectiveness analysis? What type of program decisions are appropriate to each type of analysis?
2. Discuss the advantages and disadvantages of the market value and willingness-to-pay approach to assigning values to program outputs. Under what conditions might each be the preferred approach?
3. What is discounting? Why is it so important to decision making regarding health service programs—and particularly health promotion and disease prevention programs?

Glossary

Accuracy. The extent to which the estimate of the population is close to the true population value, regardless of whether the estimating was done on a biased or unbiased sample.

Analysis of covariance. A mechanism for comparing two groups or two areas, or sets of groups or areas, when the effects of differences in other characteristics of the groups or areas are held constant.

Analysis of variance. A test or an assessment of whether two distributions in total can be considered different from one another.

Analytic surveys. Surveys concerned chiefly with describing relationships between real-world phenomena. *See also* Descriptive surveys.

Association. The notion that as one measure, phenomenon, or attribute changes, another measure, phenomenon, or attribute will change.

Autocorrelation. Correlation of error terms across individual observations, usually associated with time series data.

Bias. The extent to which the expected value of an estimator being used is not the same as the true value being estimated.

Case study. The selection and observation of a single unique activity, organization, or entity (or of one example from a number of activities, organizations, or entities), and the formation of conclusions based on the observations.

Cause-and-effect diagram. A graphic tool used to display all the factors that may produce a given effect; often referred to as an Ishikawa diagram.

Checklist. A form providing an exhaustive list of items for recording data.

Chi-Square statistic. A statistical test that measures variation from expectation. The larger the chi-square value, the less likely that a particular distribution is a chance occurrence.

Cluster sampling. A sampling technique whereby the sample is drawn in two or more stages: in the first stage the total population to be sampled is divided into several clusters (mutually exclusive and all inclusive) on the basis of some meaningful variable; in the second and subsequent stages, smaller units within clusters are drawn. Sampling is random or systematic at each stage. *See also* Simple random sampling; Stratified sampling.

Cohort changes. Systematic changes associated with one particular age group of the population.

Communality. The portion of the variance in each of the variables in a data set that is shared with one or more other variables.

Community clinical oncology program (CCOP). A community-based research network involving hospitals, physicians, and support staff funded by the National Cancer Institute.

Content analysis. A technique for making inferences by objectively and systematically identifying specific characteristics of written and oral communications.

Content validity. An assessment of whether the measure being used to describe some real-world phenomenon seems to be, prima facie, describing that phenomenon.

Contingency table. The tabular joint array of two or more frequency distributions showing the number of cases falling simultaneously into a category of each distribution.

Control chart. An extension of the run chart that includes a statistically determined upper and lower limit for the normally expected variation.

Correlation. The joint relationship of two variables; the extent of correlation is generally assessed by a correlation coefficient such as Pearson's *R*.

Cost-benefit analysis. A comparison of the costs of a program to the benefits to be derived that converts all benefits (outputs) to dollar terms. *See also* Cost-effectiveness analysis.

Cost-effectiveness analysis. A comparison of costs of a program to benefits derived that does not convert the benefits of the program to dollar terms. *See also* Cost-benefit analysis.

Criterion validity. An assessment of whether the current measure of a phenomenon produces results that are closely related to other reasonable or accepted independent measures of the same phenomenon.

Critical path. In PERT and CPM, the sequence of activities and events that defines or determines the longest time from the start of a project to its end.

Critical path method (CPM). A method for scheduling the component parts of a complex project, similar to PERT, but with the addition of information about a critical path. *See also* Critical path; Program evaluation and review technique.

Cybernetic decision making. Decision making where information about the state of a program is used to make decisions that bring the program closer to the verifiable ends desired (no accepted process; ends verifiable).

Cybernetics. The science of program control based on program information.

Decision mode drift. A tendency for decision making to drift to the random walk model or the traditional model.

Degrees of freedom. The number of observations in a set of observations that remain free to vary when some subset is fixed. For example, the sequence: $2 + ? + ? = 11$ has one degree of freedom because when either question mark is determined, the other is fixed.

Delphi technique. A data collection technique involving an iterative series of questionnaires and feedback reports to a designated panel of respondents; usually associated with forecasting and large surveys, but of use also in providing structure to case studies.

Dependent variable. A variable whose particular value is assumed to be determined by, is dependent on, the values of some set of other *independent* variables.

Descriptive surveys. Surveys concerned with producing as accurate a picture as possible of a real-world situation. *See also* Analytic surveys.

Double-blind experiment. An experiment conducted so that neither the subjects, those conducting the experiment, nor the evaluators know which subjects are members of the experimental group and which subjects are members of the control group.

Dummy variable. A dependent or independent variable that takes on only two (or occasionally three) values (i.e., 1, 0).

Durbin-Watson test. A common test for autocorrelation.

Economic ordering quantity. A technique for determining the size of an order that results in the lowest inventory cost given some specific assumptions about storage and use.

Effectiveness. The degree to which program results meet predetermined objectives, with an emphasis on program outputs or the immediate results of program efforts and whether these outputs are as expected.

Efficiency. The degree to which program results are obtained as inexpensively as possible.

Efficiency tests. Determination of whether the specific means employed is the most efficient means for producing the ends desired; critical to the mechanistic model.

Evaluability assessment. The determination of whether program objectives are well-defined and plausible and whether the intended uses of evaluation information are well-defined.

Evaluation. The collection and analysis of information by various methodological strategies to determine the relevance, progress, efficiency, effectiveness, and impact of program activities.

Evaluation research. As typically defined, results based not on the evaluator's judgments, but on the scientific method.

Expert bias. Predetermined notions that many experts may have about what the actual problem or solutions to the problem may be.

External validity. The issue of whether what is observed from the sample is true of the whole population. *See also* Internal validity.

Face validity. *See* Content validity.

Factor analysis. A technique for finding composite weights involving a certain empirical logic for determining the weights and at the same time ensuring that the resulting weighted scores will not be such that midpoint values are ambiguous.

Factor loadings. In factor analysis, the values of the vector or vectors that best reproduce the original correlation matrix.

Flow diagram. A graphic representation of the flow of all actions involved in a given process, providing a detailed picture of specific activities involved in the process under study.

Formative evaluation. Evaluation of activities associated with the ongoing operations of a program, with an emphasis on decisions to improve the program and its management. *See also* Summative evaluation.

Frequency distribution. The one-dimensional array of the categories of a variable, showing the number of cases falling into each category.

***F*-test.** A statistical test associated primarily with regression or analysis of variance that shows whether results could be expected by chance or not.

Gantt chart. A visual means of indicating the sequence of events or activities that make up a project as it proceeds through time.

Guttman scaling technique. A technique based on the assumption that dichotomous attributes can be ordered in such a way that, for the least common attribute to exist or have a positive value for a given respondent or organization, all other attributes will also exist or be positive responses for the same respondent or organization; for the next least common attribute to exist, all attributes except the least common are assumed to exist, and so forth.

Hawthorne effect. The tendency for people to act differently when they know that they are part of an experiment, thus obscuring the expected effects of interventions.

Impact. The long-term outcomes of a program.

Incidence. The number of persons (scaled to an appropriate base, such as percentage or per 100,000) who succumb to a disease within a given time range. *See also* Prevalence.

Independent variable. A variable that serves to determine the value of some *dependent* variable, but is not itself determined by some other variable.

Inputs. The resources and guidelines necessary to carry out a program.

Instrumental tests. Determination of whether in the broad sense it is possible to demonstrate empirically that the means employed produces the ends desired; primarily appropriate within the cybernetic model.

Interactive problem solving. The resolution of problems by actions rather than by thought.

Internal rate of return. The discount rate at which the net present value of a given project is equal to zero.

Internal validity. The issue of whether the evaluator's observations or conclusions about relationships within the sample drawn actually exist for that sample. *See also* External validity.

Interval scale. A scale where the points are ordered and spaced at equidistant intervals.

Interview. An instrument or schedule that an interviewer administers.

Ishikawa diagram. *See* Cause-and-effect diagram.

Likert scale. A statement or series of statements made in either a positive or negative manner, concerning which respondents are asked to check one category—from among several categories of answers—that best represents their feeling about or belief in the statement.

Linear programming. A quantitative technique for maximizing some program output subject to program constraints.

Management by objectives (MBO). A management technique that focuses on objectives rather than process.

Mean. Average value of the variable of interest found by summing all values and dividing by the number of values.

Mean square. The total sums of squares divided by the degrees of freedom for the sums of squares.

Measurement. The assignment of one set of entities—generally numerical values—to another set of entities—generally some empirical fact or phenomenon.

Mechanistic decision making. Decision making where the ends are verifiable and the appropriate decision process is known and accepted.

Model specification. The description or elucidation of a causal model of how program inputs and process produce program outputs and outcomes.

Monitoring. The continuing comparison between a program process or results and expectations, with the aim to improve the quality of the program.

Multiple regression. A technique for regressing a single dependent variable simultaneously on two or more independent variables.

Needs assessment. The process of determining the nature and extent of the problems that a program is designed to address—the first stage in program implementation.

Net present value. The value today of an amount of money to be received or expended at some time in the future.

Nominal group technique. A technique used to generate data systematically within a case study format, involving a structured group meeting in which individuals are given a specific task.

Nominal scale. A scale where only a distinction between similar or dissimilar items is made.

Nonresponse. The unwillingness or the inability of persons selected for the sample to cooperate in answering either the questionnaires or interviews.

Operations research. The study and application of a variety of quantitative methods for management and decision making.

Opportunity cost. A term used to denote the loss of opportunities to use resources in ways alternative to a specific use strategy.

Ordinal scale. A scale in which the categories are ordered by magnitude.

Ordinary knowledge. Knowledge that does not owe its origin, testing, degree of verification, truth status, or currency to distinctive professional social inquiry techniques but rather to common sense, causal empiricism, or thoughtful speculation and analysis.

Ordinary least square. A mathematical technique for solving regression problems.

Outputs. The products of the program, which consist of direct outputs, intermediate effects, and long-run or ultimate effects or outcomes.

Pareto chart. A bar graph used to arrange information in such a way that priorities for managerial action can be established.

Pattern matching. A process in which empirically based patterns are compared with predictor patterns, and data from each case are assessed to determine if they support a set of theoretical propositions that are formulated as questions.

Poisson distribution. A statistical distribution that provides the likelihood of outcomes for rare events.

Precision. A measure of the degree of variation in the estimates that might be made on the basis of all possible samples drawn in a particular manner.

Prevalence. The number of persons at any time (scaled to an appropriate base, such as percentage or per 100,000) who actually show evidence of a disease. *See also* Incidence.

Probability sample. *See* Random sample.

Process. The specific set of activities, their sequencing, and timing for the sequencing, which actually represents program operation.

Program evaluation and review technique (PERT). An evaluation technique that (1) divides a project into self-contained activities, (2) develops a precedence table for them, and (3) produces a network of circles representing discrete events and arrows representing activities, and (4) determines a critical path of activities and events.

Progress. The degree to which program implementation complies with the plan for it.

Questionnaire. An instrument or schedule for collecting data that the respondent self-administers.

Queuing theory. A body of knowledge useful for examining the nature of waiting lines.

Random sample. A sample drawn on a random basis.

Random walk decision making. Making decisions through a random process (no accepted process; ends nonverifiable).

Ratio scale. A scale where the points are ordered by magnitude and spaced at equidistant intervals and which has a true zero point.

Reactiveness. The effect of knowledge of a situation on subsequent measures of the situation. *See also* Self-fulfilling prophecy.

Regression. A technique for describing the relationship between two continuous variables, one considered as dependent and the other as independent, associated with one another in a linear fashion.

Regression coefficients. A number, found by regression, that describes the amount of change in a dependent variable associated with a one unit change in the independent variable.

Regression discontinuity. A point of change in a regression line or the slope of the line associated with a change in a program variable.

Regression to the mean. The tendency for any time-related data to "regress," or come back, to the long-term trend line.

Relevance. The necessity of a program or service.

Reliability. The extent to which a measurement device will produce the same result when used more than once to measure precisely the same item.

Representative sample. A nonrandom sample where units are selected because they seem to be representative of the population as a whole.

Reproducibility. The extent to which a given researcher or evaluator can reproduce measures used in one setting to apply to the same phenomenon in other settings.

Run chart. A simple display of the average time of the occurrence of the event of interest displayed over time.

Sample of convenience. Sample chosen by selecting units that are conveniently available.

Scale. *See* Interval scale; Nominal scale; Ordinal scale; Ratio scale.

Self-fulfilling prophecy. An initial preconception concerning the way a program may work or its relative success that becomes one of the findings of an evaluation, even though it might not be true. *See also* Reactiveness.

Sensitivity. The ability of a measure to reflect changes in the state of the real-world phenomenon under evaluation.

Sensitization. *See* Hawthorne effect.

Sentinel events. Medical conditions and stages of conditions that indicate a lack of access to acceptable quality primary care.

Simple random sampling. A sampling technique where every sample of a given size from a population has an equal probability of being selected. *See also* Cluster sampling; Stratified sampling.

Simplex method. A technique for solving a variety of linear maximization problems. *See also* Linear programming.

Social learning. The actual participation in ongoing social phenomena through which individuals learn new behavior.

Social tests. Determination of whether the means employed meets relevant social criteria; appropriate to the random walk and traditional decision-making models.

Split halves. A reliability test, where the results of half of the measurements are correlated or compared with the results of the other half.

Spurious relationship. An apparent relationship between two variables that can be shown to be a result of their relationship to a third variable.

Standard deviation. The square root of the variance.

Standard deviation of the sample mean. *See* Standard error of the mean.

Standard error of the mean. The average squared difference between the mean for each sample and the true population value.

Stratified sampling. A sampling technique where the population is first divided into two or more strata that are assumed to be closely associated with the characteristic of the population to be estimated, and then sample members are drawn from every strata. *See also* Cluster sampling; Simple random sampling.

Structured observations. The development of categorical schemes during and after observation.

Summative evaluation. Evaluation of activities associated with outputs and outcomes of a program. *See also* Formative evaluation.

Sums of squares. The summation of the squared difference between each observation and the mean of all observations.

Survey research. An approach to knowledge that uses information collected through questionnaires or interviews directed to a sample of persons drawn from some population of interest.

Time series analysis. *See* Trend analysis.

Tracer condition. A particular disease entity around which observations in data collection efforts are structured that is used to characterize a range of diseases or treatment of these diseases.

Traditional decision making. Decision making where a decision process has become accepted in the absence of confirmation that the accepted process will produce a verified desired end.

Transferability. The extent to which other researchers or evaluators can use a measurement tool in similar settings or in other settings.

Trend analysis. A general evaluation strategy that depends on data analyzed over a series of discrete points in time.

***t*-Test.** A statistical test that two values are different from one another, usually applied to results of experiments.

Type one error. The finding of a program result when none actually exists.

Type two error. The finding of no program result when one actually exists.

Type three error. The assumption that a program was implemented, when in fact it was not.

Validity. The extent to which a measurement device actually represents reality. *See also* Content validity; Criterion validity; External validity; Internal validity.

Variance. A measure of the extent to which a number of observations differ from one another for some variable of interest.

Von Morganstern Standard Gamble. Technique for assigning a numerical value to individual choices or preferences among hypothetical states of health.

Bibliography

Arkin, H., and R. R. Colton. 1963. *Tables for Statisticians*. New York: Barnes and Noble.

Arnold, J., A. Zuvekas, J. Needleman, and P. Hochberg. 1987. "Incorporating Health Status Indicators into the Measurement of Medical Underservice." Prepared for the Department of Health and Human Services, Health Resources and Services Administration, Lewin and Associates, Inc.

Aulin, A. 1982. *The Cybernetic Laws of Social Progress*. Elmsford, NY: Pergamon.

Bainbridge, J., and S. Sapirie. 1974. *Health Project Management: A Manual of Procedures for Formulating and Implementing Health Projects*. Geneva: World Health Organization.

Berelson, B. 1952. *Content Analysis in Communications*. Glencoe, IL: The Free Press.

Berman, P. 1978. "The Study of Macro- and Micro-Implementation." *Public Policy* 26(2): 157–84.

Berwick, D., A. Godfrey, and J. Roessner. 1990. *Curing Health Care: New Strategies for Quality Improvement*. San Francisco: Jossey-Bass.

Blau, P. M., and W. R. Scott. 1962. *Formal Organizations: A Comparative Approach*. San Francisco: Chandler.

Boadway, R. W., and D. E. Wildasin. 1984. *Public Sector Economics*, 2d ed. Boston: Little, Brown & Co.

Bohannan, H. M., R. C. Graves, J. A. Disney, J. W. Stamm, J. B. Abernathy, and J. D. Bader. 1985. "Effect of Secular Decline in Caries on the Evaluation of Preventive Dentistry Demonstrations." *Journal of Public Health Dentistry* 45(2): 83–89.

Bosk, C. L. 1979. *Forgive and Remember: Managing Medical Failure*. Chicago: University of Chicago Press.

Boyle, C. 1989. "The Challenge to Operationalize Research Methods from a Management Perspective." *Journal of Health Administration Education* 17(3): 557–66.

Brassard, M. 1989. *The Memory Jogger Plus*. Methuen, MA: GOAL/QPC.

Browne, A., and A. Wildavsky. 1987. "What Should Evaluation Mean to

Implementation." In D. Palumbo (Ed.), *The Politics of Program Evaluation*. Beverly Hills: Sage Publications.

Bryen, S. D. 1971. *The Application of Cybernetic Analysis to the Study of International Politics*. The Hague: Martinus Nijhoff.

Campbell, D. T. 1969. "Reforms as Experiments." *American Psychologist* 24(4): 409–29.

Campbell, D. T., and J. C. Stanley. 1963. *Experimental and Quasi-Experimental Designs for Research*. Chicago, IL: Rand McNally.

Cochrane, A. 1972. *Effectiveness and Efficiency*. London: The Nuffield Provincial Hospitals Trust.

Cohen, D., B. Littenberg, C. Wetzel, and D. Neuhauser. 1982. "Improving Physician Compliance with Preventive Guidelines." *Medical Care* 20(10): 1040–45.

Cohen, D. I., and D. Neuhauser. 1985. "The Metro Firm Trials: An Innovative Approach to Ongoing Randomized Clinical Trials." In *Institute of Medicine, Assessing Medical Technologies*. Washington, DC: National Academy Press.

Delbecq, A. L., A. E. Van de Ven, and D. H. Gustafson. 1975. *Group Techniques for Program Planning: A Guide to Nominal Group and Delphi Processes*. Glenview, IL: Scott, Foresman.

Deming, W. E. 1986. *Out of the Crisis*. Cambridge, MA: Massachusetts Institute of Technology.

Denzin, N. K. 1978. *The Research Act: A Theoretical Introduction to Sociological Methods*. New York: McGraw-Hill.

Deuschle, J. M., B. Alvarez, D. N. Logsdon, W. M. Stahl, and H. Smith. 1982. "Physician Performance in a Prepaid Health Plan: Results of the Peer Review Program of the Health Insurance Plan of Greater New York." *Medical Care* 20(2): 127–42.

Deutsch, K. W. 1968. "Toward a Cybernetic Model of Man and Society." In W. Buckley (Ed.), *Modern Systems Research for the Behavioral Scientist*. Chicago: Aldine Publishing Company.

Dornbusch, S. M., and W. R. Scott. 1975. *Evaluation and the Exercise of Authority*. San Francisco: Jossey-Bass.

Drummond, M. F. 1980. *Principles of Economic Appraisal in Health Care*. Oxford: Oxford University Press.

Drummond, M. F., G. L. Stoddart, and G. W. Torrance. 1987. *Methods for the Economic Evaluation of Health Care Programmes*. Oxford: Oxford University Press.

Federal Register. 1987. "Medicare Program: Selected Performance Information in Hospitals Providing Care to Medicare Beneficiaries." 52(158): 30741–45 (August 17).

Freeman, H., and P. Rossi. 1981. "Social Experiments." *Health and Society: Milbank Memorial Fund Quarterly* 59(3): 340–73.

Friedman, B., and S. Shortell. 1988. "The Financial Performance of Selected Investor-Owned and Not-for-Profit System Hospitals before and after Medicare Prospective Payment." *Health Services Research* 23(2): 237–67.

Gillings, D., D. Makuc, and E. Siegel. 1981. "Analysis of Interrupted Line

Series Mortality Trends: An Example to Evaluate Regionalized Perinatal Care." *American Journal of Public Health* 71(1): 38–46.

Gujarati, D. 1988. *Basic Economics*, 2d ed. New York: McGraw-Hill.

Gurel, L. 1975. "The Human Side of Evaluating Human Services Programs: Problems and Prospects." In E. L. Struening and M. Guttentag (Eds.), *Handbook of Evaluation Research, Vol. II.* Beverly Hills: Sage Publications.

Hage, G. 1974. *Communication and Organizational Control: Cybernetics in Health and Welfare Settings.* New York: Wiley.

Hauver, J. H., and J. A. Goodman. 1980. "The Evaluation of Performance and Cost in a Hypertension Control Program." *Medical Care* 18(5): 485–502.

Holsti, O. R. 1968. "Content Analysis." In G. Lindzey and E. Aronson (Eds.), *The Handbook of Social Psychology, Vol. 2*, 2d ed. Reading, MA: Addison-Wesley, pp. 596–692.

Horn, S., and J. Williamson. 1977. "Statistical Methods for Reliability and Validity Tests: An Application to Nominal Group Judgments in Health Care." *Medical Care* 15(11): 922–28.

Hsiao, W. C., and D. L. Dunn. 1987. "The Impact of DRG Payment on New Jersey Hospitals." *Inquiry* 24: 216.

Hyman, H. H. 1955. *Survey Design and Analysis: Principles, Cases, and Procedures.* Glencoe, IL: The Free Press.

JCAHO. 1990. *Primer on Clinical Indicator Development and Application.* Chicago: JCAHO.

Jain, A. K. 1989. "Fertility Reduction and the Quality of Family Planning Services." *Studies in Family Planning* 20(1): 1–16.

Kahan, J., D. Kanouse, and J. Winkler. 1984. "Variations in the Content Style of NIH Consensus Statements: 1979–83." RAND note (November).

Kaluzny, A. D., and Associates. 1987. *Cancer Control in the Rubber Industry.* NCI Final Report.

Kaluzny, A. D., R. Harris, and V. Strecher. 1990. "North Carolina Cancer Early Detection Program." NCI/DCPC-funded research. University of North Carolina at Chapel Hill.

Kaluzny, A., T. Ricketts III, R. Warnecke, L. Ford, J. Morrissey, D. Gillings, E. Sondik, H. Ozer, and J. Goldman. 1989. "Evaluating Organizational Design to Assure Technology Transfer: The Case of the Community Clinical Oncology Program." *Journal of the National Cancer Institute* 81(22): 1717–25 (November 15).

Kaluzny, A. D., and J. E. Veney. 1980. *Health Services Organizations: A Guide to Research and Assessment.* Berkeley: McCutchan.

Kanouse, D. E., J. D. Winkler, J. Kosecoff, S. H. Berry, G. M. Carter, J. P. Kahan, L. McCloskey, W. H. Rogers, C. M. Winslow, G. M. Anderson, L. Brodsley, A. Fink, L. Meredith, and R. H. Brook. 1990. *Changing Medical Practice through Technology Assessment: An Evaluation of the NIH Consensus Development Program.* Ann Arbor, MI: Health Administration Press.

Katz, D., and R. L. Kahn. 1978. *The Social Psychology of Organization.* New York: Wiley.

Kendall, M. G., and B. B. Smith. 1939. *Tables of Random Sampling Numbers* (Tracts for Computers XXIV). London: Cambridge University Press.

Kerlinger, F. N. 1973. *Foundations of Behavioral Research*, 2d ed. New York: Holt, Rinehart & Winston.

Kerlinger, F. N., and E. J. Pedhazur. 1973. *Multiple Regression in Behavioral Research*. New York: Holt, Rinehart & Winston.

Kessner, D. M., C. K. Snow, and J. Singer. 1974. *Assessment of Medical Care for Children*. Washington, DC: Institute of Medicine.

Kleinbaum, D. G., and L. L. Kupper. 1978. *Applied Regression Analysis and Other Multivariable Methods*. North Scituate, MA: Duxbury Press.

Kmenta, J. 1971. *Elements of Econometrics*. New York: Macmillan.

Knaus, W. A., E. A. Draper, D. P. Wagner, and J. E. Zimmerman. 1986. "An Evaluation of Outcome from Intensive Care in Major Medical Centers." *Annals of Internal Medicine* 104: 410–18.

Kosecoff, J., and A. Fink. 1982. *Evaluation Basics: A Practitioner's Manual*. Beverly Hills: Sage Publications.

Kotch, J., A. Kaluzny, and J. Veney. 1991. "The Performance-Based Management System to Reduce Prematurity and Low Birthweight in Local Health Departments: Final Report." Submitted to the Association of Schools of Public Health and the Centers for Disease Control.

Kralewski, J., B. Dowd, L. Pitt, and E. Briggs. 1984. "Effects of Contract Management on Hospital Performance." *Health Services Research* 19(4): 479–98.

Lawler, E. E., III. 1985. "Challenging Traditional Research Assumptions." In E. E. Lawler III, A. M. Mohrman, Jr., S. A. Ledford, Jr., and G. E. Cummings and Associates (Eds.), *Doing Research That Is Useful for Theory and Practice*. San Francisco: Jossey-Bass.

Lazarsfeld, P. F. 1958. "Evidence and Inference in Social Research." *Daedalus* 87: 99–130.

Lazarsfeld, P. F., and M. Rosenberg. 1955. *The Language of Social Research*. Glencoe, IL: The Free Press.

Leape, L. 1990. "Practice Guidelines and Standards: An Overview." *Quality Review Bulletin* 16(2): 42–49.

Leverett, D. H., O. B. Sveen, and O. E. Jensen. 1985. "Weekly Rinsing with a Fluoride Mouth Rinse in an Unfluoridated Community: Results after Seven Years." *Journal of Public Health Dentistry* 45(2): 95–100.

Levesque, B., E. DeWailly, R. Lavoie, D. Prud'Homme, and S. Allaire. 1990. "Carbon Monoxide in Indoor Ice Skating Rinks: Evaluation of Absorption by Adult Hockey Players." *American Journal of Public Health* 80(5): 594–97.

Lieu, Ben-Chiek. 1976. *Quality of Life Indicators in U.S. Metropolitan Areas*. New York: Praeger.

Lindblom, C. E., and D. K. Cohen. 1979. *Usable Knowledge: Social Science and Social Problem Solving*. New Haven, CT: Yale University Press.

Lohr, K. N. 1988. "Outcome Measurement: Concepts and Questions." *Inquiry* 25: 37–50.

Manfredi, C., R. Czaja, and G. Nyden. 1989. "Adoption of PDQ by Community Physicians." NCI Final Report. Survey Research Laboratories. University of Illinois.

March, J. G., and H. A. Simon. 1958. *Organizations.* New York: Wiley.

Marshall, C., and G. Rossman. 1989. *Designing Qualitative Research.* Beverly Hills: Sage Publications.

McKinney, M. M. 1989. "CCOP Site Visits: Findings and Recommendations." Unpublished report. Health Services Research Center, University of North Carolina at Chapel Hill.

Mick, S. S. 1989. "Research Methods and Management Control for Master's Students in Health Management." *Journal of Health Administration Education* 7(3): 507–23.

Miles, M. B., and A. M. Huberman. 1984. *Qualitative Data Analysis: A Source Book of New Methods.* Beverly Hills: Sage Publications.

Miller, D. C. 1977. *Handbook of Research Design and Social Measurement,* 3d ed. New York: David McKay.

Mintzberg, H. 1987. "Crafting Strategy." *Harvard Business Review* 87(4): 66–75.

Mintzberg, H. 1989. *Mintzberg on Management.* New York: The Free Press.

Mishan, E. J. 1988. *Cost-Benefit Analysis,* 4th ed. London: Unwin Hyman.

Moser, C. A., and G. Kalton. 1972. *Survey Methods in Social Investigation,* 2d ed. New York: Basic Books.

National Planning Association. 1974. "Community Hospital-Medical Staff Sponsored Primary Care Group Practice Program of the Robert Wood Johnson Foundation." Mimeographed.

Neter, J., and W. Wasserman. 1974. *Applied Linear Statistical Models.* Homewood, IL: Richard D. Irwin.

New York Times. 1990. "Study Says Nutrition Report Mislead Congress." January 19.

Norusis, M. J. 1988. *SPSS-X: Advanced Statistics Guide.* Chicago: SPPS, Inc.

Palumbo, D. (Ed.). 1987. *The Politics of Program Evaluation.* Beverly Hills: Sage Publications.

Park, R. E., A. Fink, R. Brook, M. Chassin, K. Kahn, N. Merrick, J. Kosecoff, and D. Solomon. 1986. "Physician Ratings of Appropriate Indications for Six Medical and Surgical Procedures." *American Journal of Public Health* 76: 766–72.

Patton, M. Q. 1990. *Qualitative Evaluation and Research Methods,* 2d ed. Beverly Hills: Sage Publications.

Petasnick, W. 1989. "Expectations of What an Entry-Level Manager Should Know about the Application of Health Service Research Methods: Perspectives of an Administrator of a University Teaching Hospital." *Journal of Health Administration Education* 17(3): 567–72.

RAND Corporation. 1988. "Health Insurance and the Demand for Medical Care: Evidence from a Randomized Experiment." Santa Monica, CA.

Rockett, I. R. H., E. S. Lieberman, W. H. Hollinshead, S. L. Putnam, and H. C. Thode. 1990. "Age, Sex and Road-Use Patterns of Motor Vehicular Trauma in Rhode Island: A Population-Based Hospital Emergency Department Study." *American Journal of Public Health* 80(12): 1516–18.

Roethlisberger, F. J., and W. J. Diskson. 1939. *Management and the Worker.* Cambridge, MA: Harvard University Press.

Rooks, J. P., N. L. Weatherby, E. Ernst, S. Stapleton, D. Rosen, and A. Rosenfield. 1989. "Outcome of Care in Birth Centers." *New England Journal of Medicine* 321(26): 1804–11.

Rosenberg, M. 1968. *The Logic of Survey Analysis.* New York: Basic Books.

Rosenthal, R., and L. Jacobson. 1968. *Pygmalion in the Classroom.* New York: Holt, Rinehart & Winston.

Rossi, P. H., and H. E. Freeman. 1989. *Evaluation: A Systematic Approach,* 4th ed. Beverly Hills: Sage Publications.

SAS Institute. 1988. *SAS/STAT User's Guide.* Cary, NC: SAS Institute, Inc.

Schaefer, M. 1973. *Evaluation/Decision Making in Health Planning and Administration.* HADM Monograph Series, Number 3, Department of Health Administration, School of Public Health, University of North Carolina at Chapel Hill.

Scheirer, M. A. 1989. "Implementation and Process Analysis in Worksite Health Promotion Research." In *Methodological Issues in Worksite Research.* Bethesda, MD: National Heart, Lung and Blood Institute.

Scheirer, M. A., and F. L. Rezmovic. 1983. "Measuring the Degree of Progressive Implementation: A Methodological Review." *Evaluation Review* 7: 599–633.

Scriven, M. 1967. "The Methodology of Evaluation." In R. W. Tyler, R. M. Gagne, and M. Scriven (Eds.), *Perspective of Curriculum Evaluation.* Chicago, IL; Rand McNally.

Schroeder, S. 1989. "Organization and Management Indicators." Memorandum to the JCAHO Organization and Management Task Force." JCAHO, Chicago.

Shortell, S. M., and W. C. Richardson. 1978. *Health Program Evaluation.* St. Louis: C. V. Mosby.

Shortell, S. M., T. M. Wickizer, and J. R. C. Wheeler. 1984. *Hospital-Physician Joint Ventures.* Ann Arbor, MI: Health Administration Press.

Steckler, A. 1989. "The Use of Qualitative Evaluation Methods to Test Internal Validity." *Evaluation and the Health Professions* 12(2): 115–33.

Steckler, A., and R. Goodman. 1989. "How to Institutionalize Health Promotion Programs." *American Journal of Health Promotion* 3(4): 34–44.

Suchman, E. A. 1967. *Evaluative Research.* New York: Russell Sage Foundation.

Swain, R. L., and E. D. Nichols. 1965. *Understanding Arithmetic.* New York: Holt, Rinehart & Winston.

Swartz, K., and T. D. McBride. 1990. "Spells without Health Insurance: Distributions of Durations and Their Link to Point-in-Time Estimates of the Uninsured." *Inquiry* 27: 281–88.

Theil, H. 1971. *Principles of Econometrics.* New York: Wiley.

Thompson, J. D. 1967. *Organizations in Action.* New York: McGraw-Hill.

Torrance, G. W., and D. Feeny. 1989. "Utilities and Quality-Adjusted Life Years." *International Journal of Technology Assessment in Health Care* 5(4): 559–75.

Torrance, G. W., W. H. Thomas, and D. L. Sackett. 1972. "A Utility Max-imization Model for Evaluation of Health Care Programs." *Health Services Research* 7(2): 118–33.

Veney, J. E., and J. W. Luckey. 1983. "A Comparison of Regression and ARIMA Models for Assessing Program Effects: An Application to the Mandated Highway Speed Limit Reduction of 1974." *Social Indicators Research* 12: 83–105.

Warner, D. M., D. C. Holloway, and K. L. Grazier. 1984. *Decision Making and Control for Health Administration*, 2d ed. Ann Arbor, MI: Health Admin-istration Press.

Weiner, N. 1948. *Cybernetics, or Control and Communications in the Animal and Machine*. New York: Wiley.

Weiss, C. H. 1975. "Evaluation Research in the Political Context." In E. L. Struening and M. Guttenag (Eds.), *Handbook of Evaluation Research, Vol. I*. Beverly Hills: Sage Publications.

Weiss, C. H. 1983. "Ideology, Interests and Information." In D. Callahan and B. Jennings (Eds.), *Ethics, the Social Sciences, and Policy Analysis*. New York: Plenum Press.

Weiss, C. H. 1989. "Congressional Committees as Users of Analysis." *Journal of Policy Analysis and Management* 8(3): 411–31.

Weiss, C. H., and M. J. Buculavas. 1977. "The Challenge of Social Research to Decision Making." In C. H. Weiss (Ed.), *Using Social Research in Public Policy Making*. Lexington, MA: Lexington Books.

Wennberg, J. E. 1984. "Dealing with Medical Practice Variations: A Proposal for Action." *Health Affairs* 3: 6–32.

Wennberg, J. E. 1990. "Outcomes Research, Cost Containment, and Fear of Health Care Rationing." *New England Journal of Medicine* 323(17): 1202–3.

Wholey, J. S. 1979. *Evaluation: Promise and Performance*. Washington, DC: Urban Institute.

Williamson, J. W. 1978a. *Assessing and Improving Health Care Outcomes: The Health Accounting Approach to Quality Assurance*. Cambridge, MA: Ballinger.

Williamson, J. W. 1978b. "Formulating Priorities for Quality Assurance Ac-tivity." *Journal of the American Medical Association* 239(7): 631–37.

Williamson, J. W., H. R. Braswell, and S. D. Horn. 1979. "Validity of Medical Staff Judgments in Establishing Quality Assurance Priorities." *Medical Care* 17(14): 331–46.

Williamson, J. W., H. R. Braswell, S. D. Horn, and S. Lohmeyer. 1978. "Priority Setting in Quality Assurance: Reliability of Staff Judgments in Medical Institutions." *Medical Care* 16(11): 931–40.

Winer, B. J. 1962. *Statistical Principles in Experimental Design*. New York: McGraw-Hill.

Wonnacott, R. J., and T. H. Wonnacott. 1979. *Econometrics*, 2d ed. New York: Wiley.

Workman, S., A. Zili, A. Balshem, and P. Engstrom. 1988. "Cancer Control in a Defined Population: Results of the 'Beat the Odds' Education Campaign." In P. F. Engstrom, P. Anderson, and L. Mortenson (Eds.), *Advances in Cancer Control: Cancer Control Research and the Emergence of the Oncology Production Line.* New York: Alan R. Liss, Inc.

World Health Organization. 1980. "Measurement of Coverage, Effectiveness and Efficiency of Different Patterns of Health Care." SHS/78/1. Geneva: World Health Organization.

World Health Organization. 1981. "Health Programme Evaluation: Guiding Principles, Health for All, Series No. 6." Geneva: World Health Organization.

Wortman, P., A. Vinokur, and L. Sechrest. 1982. "Evaluation of NIH Consensus Development Process, Phase I: Final Report." Center for Research on Utilization of Scientific Knowledge. Institute for Social Research, University of Michigan, Ann Arbor, MI.

Wortman, P., A. Vinokur, and L. Sechrest. 1988. "Do Consensus Conferences Work? A Process Evaluation of the NIH Consensus Development Program." *Journal of Health Politics, Policy and Law* 13(3): 469–98.

Index

About the Authors

The authors, both of whom are professors of Health Policy and Administration at the School of Public Health of the University of North Carolina at Chapel Hill, have extensive experience in research and evaluation in the domestic and international arenas. Dr. Veney has been the director of research for the National Blue Cross Association, has taught courses in research and evaluation for a number of years, and has directed a program to train postdoctoral fellows in program evaluation techniques in mental health programs. Dr. Veney has also spent time as a technical specialist with the World Health Organization Southeast Asia Regional Office in New Delhi, where he worked specifically in helping country health planning units to improve their program evaluation efforts. During that time he worked with health planning personnel in India, Burma, Nepal, Sri Lanka, and Thailand. From 1984 to 1989 he was the evaluation officer for the program for International Training in Health at the University of North Carolina, a United States Agency for International Development project for training of family planning personnel in Africa and Asia, that involved him in field-based evaluation efforts in several countries of sub-Saharan Africa and south Asia. Most recently, Dr. Veney is the principal investigator of a project funded by the National Institute of Allergy and Infectious Diseases (NIAID) to develop an evaluation design to assess the NIAID Community Program for Clinical Research on AIDS. He is presently director of the Doctoral Program in the Department of Health Policy and Administration.

Dr. Kaluzny has been involved with various domestic and international evaluation research activities. He is a consultant to various federal and state governmental agencies, as well as a number of private research corporations. His evaluation and research efforts include work with the National Cancer Institute (NCI), National Heart,

449

Lung and Blood Institute, the Agency for Health Care Policy and Research (AHCPR), and the Institute of Medicine as well as with the United States Agency for International Development, the Ford Foundation, Project HOPE, and the United Nations. Dr. Kaluzny has been the principal investigator of the NCI-funded contract to evaluate the Community Clinical Oncology Program (CCOP), and most recently is the principal investigator of an NCI grant to evaluate methods to increase the use of cancer detection regimens among primary care physicians.

Drs. Veney and Kaluzny have collaborated on a number of research and evaluation efforts. They have been coprincipal investigators of a major study of innovation in hospitals and health departments funded by the National Center for Health Services Research and an evaluation of drug treatment centers in North Carolina funded by the National Institute for Mental Health. They have recently collaborated on research in local health departments, where they have carried out evaluations of state-imposed standards and primary care programs and the implementation and evaluation of performance evaluation systems to prevent low birth weight and prematurity. Most recently Drs. Veney and Kaluzny, and other colleagues from the University of North Carolina at Chapel Hill, have collaborated on an AHCPR-funded project assessing the attributes of clinical protocols as part of the larger NCI-funded CCOP evaluation.